V&R Academic

Jaap Grave / Rick Honings / Bettina Noak (eds.)

Illness and Literature in the Low Countries

From the Middle Ages until the 21st Century

With 10 figures

V&R unipress

MIX
Papier aus verantwortungsvollen Quellen
FSC www.fsc.org FSC® C083411

Bibliografische Information der Deutschen Nationalbibliothek

Die Deutsche Nationalbibliothek verzeichnet diese Publikation in der Deutschen Nationalbibliografie; detaillierte bibliografische Daten sind im Internet über http://dnb.d-nb.de abrufbar.

ISBN 978-3-8471-0520-6
ISBN 978-3-8470-0520-9 (E-Book)
ISBN 978-3-7370-0520-3 (V&R eLibrary)

Weitere Ausgaben und Online-Angebote sind erhältlich unter: www.v-r.de

Gedruckt mit freundlicher Unterstützung der Deutschen Forschungsgemeinschaft.

Printed in Germany.
Titelbild: Ary Scheffer, La mort de Géricault 1824, Musée du Louvre
Druck und Bindung: CPI buchbuecher.de GmbH, Zum Alten Berg 24, 96158 Birkach

Gedruckt auf alterungsbeständigem Papier.

Contents

Acknowledgements

The editors wish to thank all contributors for their patient and committed work on the book. Furthermore we would like to express our gratitude to the DFG (German Research Foundation), the NWO (Netherlands Organisation for Scientific Research) and the Niels Stensen Foundation for the sponsoring of the projects from which this book resulted. Many thanks to prof. dr. Jaap Goedegebuure for his useful peer review and to Eli ten Lohuis for the translation of the introduction. Finally we are grateful for the help of Tatjana Schoenaich for finishing the manuscript.

Rick Honings and Bettina Noak

Introduction

In 1807 Willem Bilderdijk published *De Ziekte der Geleerden (The Illness of the Scholars)*. Amounting to over three thousand lines, the work is to be considered a milestone in the history of the Dutch didactic poem that need not shun comparison with international melancholy literature.[1] The subject suited the poet to a tee. In a colourful manner all his own, he depicted the 'Iliad of plagues' that could assail men of learning together with its origins, accompanying symptoms and any remedies developed to cure it. He discussed, for example, melancholy, sleeplessness and the 'weakening' of the brain.

Yet the fascination with being ill was hardly a new phenomenon in the nineteenth century. From as early as classical antiquity there has been an interplay between literature and medicine. The first book of Homer's *Iliad* recounts the plague that swept the camp of the Achaeans, supposedly sent by Apollo out of revenge. While this instance concerns a full-length book, it is the aphorism that is of greater importance as a literary technique for the dissemination of medical knowledge, from the *Corpus Hippocraticum* of antiquity until the *Aphorismi de cognoscendis et curandis morbis* (1715) by Herman Boerhaave. In addition, the subject of illness and its impact on mankind was explored by great numbers of poetic scholars and scholarly poets.

A number of topoi keep recurring in the relationship between literature and medicine. Magic has a place in both domains as magical words, sayings and songs were believed to have a healing effect. Since classical antiquity, physicians have been viewed as priests with access to secrets that remain hidden from patients. This is where the distrust of physicians stems from. On the one hand, they are suspected of charlatanism, as if their knowledge were mere bluff; on the other hand, medicine has to the present day been an 'arcane' science, riddled with – at least to the uninitiated – incomprehensible notions and concepts. Further, arrogance and greed on the part of physicians already constitute an

1 Cf. Joris van Eijnatten, 'Bilderdijk's Head. Meta-medical Reflections of an Afflicted Poet', in: *Social History of Medicine* 18 (2005), pp. 337–356.

important motif in *De Medicina*, the history of medicine by classical physician Celsus. Another topos concerns the concept of injury (trauma). Again, the *Iliad* sets the tone: the first surgeon is Machaon. He may have been able to dress incurable wounds but he could not heal the trauma of Iphigenia's sacrifice, which was thus left to spread through the doomed history of the Atrides.

Three research domains

The relationship between literature and medicine has received a relatively great deal of attention in the research conducted over the past decades.[2] Here, only those aspects that are relevant to the present collection are discussed. Despite the fact that since the nineteenth century literature and medicine have come to be seen as separate entities, and the natural sciences are increasingly placed in a positivistic light, the communication between the two areas as sketched above remains.[3] In all likelihood, the two cultures of the *humanities* and the *sciences* have never even functioned as separate worlds. The research on literature and medicine generally distinguishes three lines of approach:

2 For a short overview of the research on medicine and literature cf. Carsten Zelle, 'Medizin', in: Roland Borgards [e.a.] (eds.), *Literatur und Wissen. Ein interdisziplinäres Handbuch*, Stuttgart 2013, pp. 85–95; Harald Neumeyer, 'Medizin und Literatur', in: Ansgar Nünning (ed.), *Metzler Lexikon Literatur- und Kulturtheorie. Ansätze – Personen – Grundbegriffe*, 5th edition, Stuttgart 2013, pp. 504–505. For subjects and authors cf. Dietrich von Engelhardt, *Medizin in der Literatur der Neuzeit. Bd. I: Darstellung und Deutung*. Hürtgenwald 1991; Dietrich von Engelhardt, *Medizin in der Literatur der Neuzeit. Bd. II: Bibliographie der wissenschaftlichen Literatur 1800–1995*, Hürtgenwald 2000; Bettina von Jagow and Florian Steger, *Literatur und Medizin. Ein Lexikon*, Göttingen 2005. Some recent publications on this topic are: Sarah Anderson, *Readings of Trauma, Madness, and the Body*, New York 2012; Jan Frans van Dijkhuizen and Karl Enenkel (eds.), *The Sense of Suffering. Constructions of Physical Pain in Early Modern Culture*, Leiden 2009; Marc Priewe, *Textualizing Illness. Medicine and Culture in New England 1620–1730*, Heidelberg 2014; Allan Ingram [e.a.], *Melancholy Experience in Literature of the Long Eighteenth Century. Before Depression, 1660–1800*, Basingstoke [etc.], 2011; Stephanie Siewert and Antonia Mehnert (eds.), *The Morbidity of Culture. Melancholy, Trauma, Illness and Dying in Literature and Film*, Frankfurt/M. etc. 2012. On art and medicine cf. Renée van de Vall and Robert P. Zwijnenberg, *The Body Within. Art, Medicine and Visualization*, Leiden 2009.

3 C.P. Snow, *The Two Cultures and a Second Look. An Expanded Version of The Two Cultures and the Scientific Revolution*, Cambridge 1979. On the communication between literature and medicine cf. Bettina Jagow and Florian Steger, *Was treibt die Literatur zur Medizin? Ein kulturwissenschaftlicher Dialog*, Göttingen 2009.

1.

The functionalist angle is strongly represented in the research. What is studied here is the *literary function* of medical knowledge and the reception of this knowledge in literature. The fact that a great number of authors were themselves physicians or at least possessed medical expertise plays an important role. Well-known German examples are Friedrich Schiller or Gottfried Benn. For Dutch literature, such authors as J.J. Slauerhoff or Simon Vestdijk come to mind. From classical antiquity, medical knowledge was held to be a necessary asset for the moneyed, well-educated (male) elite, and this affected the uses of this knowledge in literature. Conversely, however, literature also fulfils a function in the history of medicine. After all, literary works can be used as a source of information on the state of affairs of the medical sciences in the past; they serve as representations. Indeed, disease and good health are frequently reflected upon in literary texts. Ethical matters, such as the reputation of physicians, their social duty and the balance of power between physician and patient are also often thematised in functionalist research.[4]

2.

A second angle is provided by *cultural studies.* In the background stand the various 'turns' in the cultural studies of the past decades, such as the *linguistic turn* or the *affective turn.* Culture is perceived as a fabric of linguistic expressions that has come about according to discursive rules. In this manner, the functionalist separation of literary and medical texts is removed; medical texts too are texts that go back to a certain cultural discourse. Hence, methods of discourse analysis – building on the theoretical principles of Michel Foucault – play an important role. This also comprises the idea of disease as cultural construct, as, for instance, in the research by Ludwik Fleck. Studies on the functions of corporality, research into traumata or the development of particular metaphors for the discussion of disease are also considered part of this domain. Since text and culture are closely interwoven, medical concepts define social and political observation, and vice versa.[5]

4 Cf. F. Meulenberg, J. van der Meer and A.K. Oderwald (eds.), *Ziektebeelden. Essays over literatuur en geneeskunde,* Utrecht 2002; Sofie Vandamme, *Koele minnaars. Medische verwoording en literaire verbeelding van ziekte in verhalen*, Leuven 2007.

5 Cf. Michel Foucault, *Naissance de la clinique – une archéologie du regard médical,* Paris 1963 and *Les mots et les choses – une archéologie des sciences humaines*, Paris 1966; Ludwik Fleck, *Denkstile und Tatsachen. Gesammelte Schriften und Zeugnisse*, Berlin 2011.

3.

Connected with the second angle is the idea that the linguistic articulation of medical knowledge has *a poetics of its own.* The methodological merits of literary analysis, particularly in the field of narratology, are brought to bear on medical texts: historical, ancient or Biblical exemplum literature, casuistry, *medical case histories* or medical *observationes.* Although these genres ranging from classical antiquity to the (post-)modern period define the observation of medical phenomena, historical differences in writing about disease are indeed perceived. Moreover, a direct interaction with literary texts takes place here as well. The influence of the Freudian *case histories* on the literature of the fin de siècle is a case in point.[6]

Content of this collection

In this collection, all these angles recur in the approaches adopted by authors as they discuss texts roughly ranging from the Middle Ages up to the twenty-first century. A central place is especially allotted to texts from the Low Countries: from mediaeval non-medical literature, early-modern works by learned poets and physicians, texts from the Enlightenment (when literature and knowledge entered into a fruitful symbiosis in the learned societies) and from the nineteenth-century Romantic period, to subjects from the twentieth and twenty-first century. The various perspectives and subjects of the various contributions are sketched against the backdrop of the angles mentioned above. Thereby the collection covers a wide range of different sorts of texts and genres. It might be needful to remember that the concept of an autonomous literature (although always under discussion) is the product of cultural processes in the 19th and 20th century. In the research about the topic the mentioned broad choice of texts proved to be very useful. As could be seen in the following delineation of the articles it challenges chronological and thematic boundaries and opens up a differentiated view on the relationship between illness and literature.

6 Cf. Nicolas Pethes and Sandra Richter (eds.), *Medizinische Schreibweisen. Ausdifferenzierung und Transfer zwischen Medizin und Literatur (1600–1900)*, Tübingen 2008; Yvonne Wübben and Carsten Zelle (eds.), *Krankheit schreiben. Aufzeichnungsverfahren in Medizin und Literatur*, Göttingen 2013.

1.

The articles by Gerard Bouwmeester and Mark van Vledder, Arnold Lubbers and Wouter Schrover address the socio-cultural position of medicine and of physicians, and the role of literature and the literary field in the dissemination of medical knowledge. They thus follow the functionalist paradigm. In their corpus-based study 'Medical Actors and Actions in Non-Medical Middle-Dutch Literature', Bouwmeester and Van Vledder examine the social position of physicians and the status of medical knowledge in mediaeval texts. Their conclusion is that even in the Middle Ages, the physician's position was a controversial one. While the physician held a high social position as adviser to the king and, even, as a political agent, there were, on the other hand, warnings against fraud, together with pleas in favour of medical knowledge on the part of laymen. Knowledge of medical sciences was considered a competence that was of great importance to civilized persons from the upper classes.

Wouter Schrover's article 'Reading Literature through Medical Sociology: The Doctor-Patient Relationship in Thomas Rosenboom's *Publieke werken* (*Public Works*) and a Poem by Neeltje Maria Min' highlights similar questions. Here, the main starting point is the subject of 'power', a far from unimportant one in the history of medicine. In his analysis of the power of physicians Schrover uses the concepts *Aesculapian, charismatic* and *social power.* Dependence on physicians increased, as did the helplessness of the sick. Especially in the nineteenth century, which is also the setting for Thomas Rosenboom's *Public Works*, progress in medical knowledge is achieved at the expense of lower-class patients. An important tool with which to break the power of the medical sciences and the medical elite is irony. In the sonnet 'My body is crawling with streptococci' by Neeltje Maria Min, the irony of the already deceased 'I' constitutes a last resort to protect some personal dignity from the clutches of the doctor (and 'healthy' fellow beings!).

Up-to-date medical knowledge, of the connection between macrocosmos and microcosmos, for instance, already plays a role in the mediaeval texts, revealing a social interest in natural sciences that at an early stage becomes part of popular culture. In other words, scientific interest is not a phenomenon exclusive to the Enlightenment or the nineteenth century. How this interest takes shape in the nineteenth century in book clubs in the United Kingdom of the Netherlands between 1815 and 1830, is the subject of Arnold Lubbers's contribution 'Oddities, or Illness and Health as Topics in the Early 19th-Century Dutch readers' digest'. Apart from books on general knowledge and reference books on health, it is especially two major discussions, hotly debated in early-nineteenth-century Europe, which resonate in the book clubs: those on *animal magnetism* and on *cowpox vaccine.* With respect to the first debate, the influence is notable of authors translated from the German, such as the influential publication by C.A.F. Kluge, *Proeve eener voorstelling van het dierlijk Magnetismus* (*An attempt to present animal Magnetism,*1812) or C.W. Hufelands *Belangrijke waarnemingen omtrent het slaapwandelen, of het droomleven, zonder den invloed van het magnetismus* (*Important observations concerning somnabulism, or the dream life, without the influence of Magnetism, 1817*). In the Dutch discourse there is admiration to be found for the reputed treatment successes of mesmerism, besides criticism (on religious grounds) of these methods. A similar discussion takes place with regard to the *cowpox vaccine.* While inoculation was promoted by the government, Abraham Capadose expressed his fierce opposition to the scheme.

2.

The subsequent articles in the collection have been influenced by the said cultural studies approach. The contribution by Helmer Helmers, 'Illness as Metaphor: The Sick Body Politic and Its Cures', shows how medical concepts helped shape the political metaphors of the early-modern period. Here, too, classical tradition plays a decisive role. The Galenistic paradigm of the harmony of the body fluids is brought to bear on the state. Disturbances in this order result in the *body politic in crisis* as analysed by Helmers. The influence of Paracelsian medicine can be detected in political concepts purporting to remove such 'foreign social phenomena' as deviant convictions or political opponents (i.e. *the xenobiotic other*) from the body politic by means of iron and fire, thereby echoing the surgical practices of the day. In curing the body politic, the healing powers of the royal charisma may perform an important role. Medical metaphors may, in this manner, contribute to the development of a national ideology.

Attention is also given, in this collection, to mental disorders and delusions, from the early-modern period to the present day. Even more so than purely physical illnesses, failings of the human brain seem to appeal to many an author's imagination. Again, precursors can be found in classical antiquity. As the contribution by Ronny Spaans, 'Diagnosing the Poetic Inspiration: Medical Criticism of Enthusiasm in the Poetry of Jan Six van Chandelier (1620–1695)', shows, poets and Humanist theologians and physicians from the early-modern period reflect upon the Platonic inheritance of the *furor poeticus*, both at the literary, ethical and medical level. Around 1648, the learned Humanist, writer and pharmacist Jan Six van Chandelier sketches in his poem *Verrukkinge der Sinnen* (*Rapture of the Senses*) a satiric and self-critical image of inspired poethood. To him, poetic ecstacy is a form of frenzy that may impair the health of poets and readers alike. Yet the idea of literature as remedy is here as well. Against wordly passion stands Christian enthusiasm; early-modern man had to learn the difference between the Christian rapture that could only benefit mental health, and delusions and melancholy that were thought to be prompted by the devil.

Four of the collection's contributions analyse the melancholy concept in the early-modern period and the nineteenth century. In his article 'Melancholy and Fantasy: Johan Wier's Use of a Medical Concept in his Plea for Tolerance', Hans de Waardt examines how the concepts *imagination, brain* and *demonic possession* are handled in the famous work *De praestigiis daemonum* (1563) (*Delusions of Demons*) by Johan Wier. Although Humanist circles did not rule out the possibility of demons seizing the human body, it is not so much the direct action of anthropomorphic satanic powers that is involved here as medical concepts of evil powers. Demons were deemed capable of disturbing the human brain by effecting a disturbance of the *humores* in the body. This led to illnesses which could then be diagnosed and treated by physicians. In imitation of such (neo-)Platonic theoreticians as Marsilio Ficino, Johan Wier views the devil as an abstract idea that may cause disease in the human mind but cannot be present as a living person capable of entering into a pact with people. He instrumentalizes this idea in order to argue against the persecution of witches, which was advocated by the church in this period.

The possibility that demons may act on the human body and thus cause mental illness was also acknowledged by the British scholar Robert Burton in his book *Anatomy of Melancholy* (1621), a work that was also influential in the Netherlands. Here, it provides the theoretical underpinning of the subsequent articles. In her article 'Pictures of Melancholia in Four Tragedies by Joost van den Vondel', Bettina Noak shows that the concept of *demonic possession* is still active in the seventeenth-century author Vondel, although ultimately it is the Humanist-medical approach that prevails with him. His predilection for dichotomies not only emerges in the structure of his plays but also in the way in which he deals with the 'melancholy' syndrome: on the one hand, he examines the melancholy of unbelievers and tyrants and, on the other, that of martyrs. The contribution uses four analytical concepts: the sickly imagination of the *conscience* in the downfall of the tyrants, the cannibalistic *incorporation* that connects the poet with, especially, religious delusion, the martyr's *ego impoverishment* and, lastly, chances of a *breakthrough* in the melancholy disposition through faith in the *Christus medicus.*

With lovesickness the subject of her contribution, Olga van Marion examines in 'Lovesickness on Stage: Besotted Patients in 17th-century Medical Handbooks and Plays' one specifc aspect of melancholy that was also discussed extensively in the medical literature of the early-modern period. A dichotomic structure is also discernible in the Humanist concepts on love and its medical effects: Burton distinguishes between *nuptial love* and *tyrant love* or *heroical melancholy*, in other words, honourable love versus deluded love. Sufferers from tyrannical love present particular symptoms, in his view: a quickened pulse (*pulsus amatorius*), blushing, sweating or paling in the presence of the beloved and panting. These topoi are deployed in both G.A. Bredero's tragi-comedy *Lucelle* (1616) and Theodoor Rodenburgh's *Vrou Iacoba* (1638). While love-struck male characters present all the symptoms described here, the female protagonists display what is, according to Van Marion, a specific form of love melancholy: noxious vapours in the female brain cause a flood of tears.

Melancholy was also a *hot item* during the Romantic period. In their 'The Poet as Patient. The Curious Case of Willem Bilderdijk: A Retrospective Approach', Rick Honings and Steven Honings analyse how Bilderdijk the patient can be diagnosed with the use of modern-day psychiatric insights. Time and again he complained about all kinds of physical and mental ailments, expressing a wish to die soon. Just like authors from the early-modern period, he adduced religious reasons to account for illnesses; in his view, they could be traced to the Fall of Man. Exercising all due methodological caution (it is dangerous to diagnose someone from the nineteenth century) Rick and Steven Honings lay Bilderdijk on the exam table. They sketch a picture of a patient who as early as childhood developed a personality disorder (*pervasive developmental disorder*) because of his limited social contacts, and ever since suffered from persistent depression and a longing for death. Later in life Bilderdijk may have suffered from bipolar disorder, with manic and productive periods alternating with periods of depression.

3.

Historical exempla and medical case histories constitute important genres in which literary techniques and medical knowledge are bound up. A different type of text is the *confession*, which goes back to Saint Augustine. In her contribution "'Am I Not Punished Enough?' Confessions of Homosexuals in Medical Studies Around 1900" Mary Kemperink discusses the genre of the *confession* in medical studies on homosexuality. She is critical of Foucault's opinion that the evolution of the concept of 'homosexuality' was a mere tale of power and suppression. In contrast, Kemperink argues that the evolution of a clearer image of homosexuality was brought about by cooperation between patients and physicians, with literary techniques being of overriding importance. She examines this discourse by means of confessions in three influential publications: Richard von Krafft-Ebing's *Psychopathia sexualis* (1903), Dr. Laupts' *Tares et poisons* (1896) and Magnus Hirschfeld's *Ursachen und Wesen des Uranismus* (1903). The confessions are to illustrate the worked-out concepts of homosexuality but in the texts, they assume a literary life of their own. They are rendered by first-person narrators through interior monologue, rhetorical questions, metaphors, symbols and rhetorical topoi. These narratives are further connected with then prevailing genres, such as the adventure story, the love story, the naturalistic or the decadent novel. Patient narratives are thus literalized besides being infused with medical knowledge, which makes the question whether we are dealing here with medical case histories or, rather, literary stories with a medical purport almost unanswerable.

The development of a new concept of disease is also the subject of the article by Joost Haan and Liesbeth Minnaard: 'The Shaking Palsy in the Low Countries: Representations of Parkinson's Disease in Dutch and Flemish Prose'. They demonstrate that the representation of the 'shaking palsy' stands in a long tradition that goes back to Shakespeare. In their contribution, they analyse six Dutch texts. Parkinson's disease proves to be an interesting subject since a complex of physical and mental problems are observed in the clinical picture. The novel *Duivelskermis* (*Devil's Carnival*) by Gerrit Krol imparts a meaning all its own to the subject of *demonic possession:* the hallucinations that go with the syndrome bring about changes in the characters. Their perception of reality, of time and space, is no longer reliable and they are haunted by visions and distortions. Their 'healthy' environment is consequently suspicious of the patients. The enlightening work that the medical sciences ought to carry out to promote the rights of these sick people does not achieve the desired effect so that the patients are completely at the mercy of the physicians. Their distress sometimes stems from inner and physical injuries sustained in the past and may be transmitted to the next generation, as the unprocessed traumatic experiences in Jeroen Brouwers' *Bezonken Rood* (*Sunken Red*) show.

The last three articles in this collection focus attention on trauma and how to combat trauma. In his article 'Poet-Judge-Physician. Literature as Cicatrix: The Case of Maria Dermoût', Frans-Willem Korsten examines the role of the author against the background of the concept of the 'cultural physician', as developed by Nietzsche and Deleuze. According to Korsten, Dermoût not only writes *case histories* but these have a simultaneous healing effect as well: as they are being narrated, they can heal wounds. The decisive figure of thought in the article is the *cicatrix*, which not only denotes a scar marking an injury that will disappear over time but 'material in its own right': newly grown tissue to cover an old wound. Literature becomes a tool for justice: normally silent distress is finally given a voice.

The question whether it is possible to put into words the unutterable and unpresentable of war experiences is the main subject of the article by Sander Bax: 'The Legacy of Incomprehensibility: Trauma, Experience and Historiography in Harry Mulisch's Historical Novel *The Stone Bridal Bed*'. Taking the concept of *traumatic memory* for his starting point, he shows how Mulisch uses the modern myth in order to still express the unutterable in his novel *Het Stenen Bruidsbed* (*The Stone Bridal Bed*). In autobiographical texts Mulisch himself underlines literature's ability to 'keep open' events from the past, to make them present for readers, while the literary work as such proves to be a complete whole. Against the background of *memory studies* and *trauma theory* Bax demonstrates the ability of the medical but also, in particular, narrative trauma concepts to offer a framework for the expression of traumatic experiences. In recounting the traumata from the past, myth plays a crucial role. It may represent a 'liminal experience' and be the narrative of an extreme crossing of borders that can only be clad in the a-historical form of the myth. In *The Stone Bridal Bed* Mulisch deploys Homer's *Iliad* and *Odyssey* in order to still give expression to the unutterable war experiences of main character Norman Corinth.

A new form of *memory culture* is what Stephan Besser proposes in his article 'Mixing Repertoires: Cerebral Subjects in Contemporary Dutch Neurological Fiction', which ends this collection. The fascination with the workings of the human brain also comes to the fore in contemporary novels. Besser studies three: Robbert Welagen's *Porta Romana*, Jeroen van Rooij's *De eerste hond in de ruimte (The First Dog in Space)* and Yves Petry's *De maagd Marino (The Virgin Marino)* – including their use of the concept of *brainhood* against the background of some influential theoretical concepts from the *neurocultures.*

Thus, this collection offers fourteen articles that showcase a multitude of subjects and approaches yet have in common that they all highlight the relation between disease and literature. This entails a first-ever overview of Dutch-language research in this field, whereby in some cases actual cooperation was entered into with experts from the medical sciences. Of course, we do not pretend to sketch an exhaustive picture of this research area. We merely wish to demonstrate that this is a fascinating subject that merits more attention – and we sincerely hope that this collection will boost further research into the subject.

Gerard Bouwmeester and Mark G. van Vledder

Medical Actors and Actions in Non-Medical Middle Dutch Literature*

People have certain opinions about their doctors. Watching popular television series such as ER, Grey's Anatomy, House or the Dutch classic Medisch Centrum West, one is tempted to perceive medical practitioners as mostly young, handsome, smart, emphatic, well educated. Moreover, they have high moral and ethical standards. And are we not lucky? These people will take care of us when we are ill or injured!

In an era in which the advancements in public health are huge (e.g. the discovery of antibiotics, the evolution of surgical techniques and powerful diagnostics), doctors are heroes. At the same time, opening a newspaper or digging into any internet forum regarding health care professionals, the chances are significant that a whole different picture will arise. Recent examples of malpractice, scientific fraud and financial scandals committed by medical personae gain increasingly broad media attention and have taken as much away from the doctors' good reputation as centuries of science and ER's George Clooney have added to it. The criticism did not go by unnoticed by the medical world, resulting in a multitude of measures to avoid and prevent future incidents, such as the design, development and implementation of new, stricter guidelines, safety measures and moral codes.[1]

We are fascinated by these ambiguities: firstly, the extremely positive image of often fictional doctors *versus* the hypercritical social attitude, and secondly, that critical, sometimes even negative popular attitude towards doctors *versus* the (by now: long-term) medical-professional reflex to improve and be transparent. Starting from that fascination, we have set out to investigate public opinion on medical acting and actors in literature from the medieval Low

* We would like to thank the editors of this volume, and especially Dr. Bettina Noak, for their comments on an earlier draft of this contribution. Likewise, the colleagues at the University of Utrecht and the Erasmus MC in Rotterdam for sharing their thoughts.

1 Literature on medical reputation and medical reputation management is vast. An interesting (recent) historical perspective is given by Dana Ploeger, 'Van het voetstuk gevallen', in: *Medisch contact* 64 (2009)-15, pp. 660–663.

Countries. We have chosen the (late) Middle Ages for two reasons: it is a period in which the medical profession underwent major changes (think of the foundation of medical schools and/at universities, translation of innovative Arabic medical treatises into Latin, but also the Black Death) and secondly, Middle Dutch medical texts recently received much scholarly attention, especially by Erwin Huizenga.[2]

This attention creates an interesting parallel to our contribution, as we have chosen to study the opinion on medical acting and actors through non-medical texts. We will write about the late medieval image of doctors not by sketching how doctors wrote about themselves (a matter already addressed in the recent *hausse*), but by analysing how they (and their actions) were represented in texts that did not strive for medical instruction or audience. We will hypothesize that this approach will offer a whole new vision on the public opinion on the medical profession in the late Middle Ages.

Methodology

The method applied in this contribution contains three steps. First, a 'medical word field' was made: a list of Middle Dutch words associated to medical acts and actors.[3] This list was inspired by the terminology encountered in Erwin Huizenga's recent ground breaking work on surgery texts in the late medieval Low Countries.[4] The words chosen to employ for further study were: aersater, visiker, surgien, medicyn, fisisciene, meester – (including variant spellings and forms, like aersatrie). Secondly, the transcendent *Geïntegreerde Taalbank* (GTB) was used.[5] The GTB is an online collection of historical Dutch dictionaries, such as the *Oud-Nederlands Woordenboek*, *Vroegmiddelnederlands Woordenboek* and the *Middelnederlands Woordenboek*.[6] The GTB makes it possible not only to

2 Most notably Erwin Huizenga, *Tussen autoriteit en empirie. De Middelnederlandse chirurgiën in de veertiende en vijftiende eeuw en hun maatschappelijke context*, Hilversum 2003, but also, earlier: Erwin Huizenga, *Een nuttelike practijke van cirurgien. Geneeskunde en astrologie in het Middelnederlandse handschrift Wenen*, Österreichische Nationalbibliothek, 2818, Hilversum 1997. Also internationally, there are plenty of recent studies of historical medical acting, for example by Nancy Siraisi and Michael McVaugh.

3 The idea of composing and using a word field was inspired by Laura van der Wijden, *Scheve ogen in de Lage Landen. De functie en betekenis van afgunst en jaloezie in Middelnederlandse teksten*, Santpoort Zuid, 2011. Discussion on methodology on pp. 15–20.

4 See note above. A. Dewitte, *De geneeskunde te Brugge in de Middeleeuwen*, Brugge 1973 was also conducted; the glossary (pp. 65–69) is extremely extensive, but because it is not very specific (it lists words, but does not cite them) it turned out to be not very useful for a contribution like this.

5 http://gtb.inl.nl [last retrieved on March 12, 2015].

6 The pros and cons of using the GTB for philological research (and beyond just looking for the

look up the meaning of the words, but also cites them in an enormous corpus of (among others) Middle Dutch texts. This feature helped to create a list of Middle Dutch texts in which one of the words from the word field is presented. The last step – in order to let the corpus match the research interest explained above – was to exclude all the medical texts.

Results

The list of Middle Dutch texts containing one or more items from the medical word field was significantly more extensive than expected; the assumption, based on (the lack of) earlier literature on the topic, that the results would be scarce, soon proved to be incorrect. As it is impossible to discuss all the material in a limited contribution like this, focus has been given to several texts (table 1).[7] Together, these texts cover the broadness of the material found; dating from the early to the late Middle Dutch period, a remarkable geographic dispersion, and different genres. In the next section, the results will be discussed into more detail. This will be done along the lines of explicitness: the first text has the most explicit opinion on medical act(or)s, the last text the least explicit one. This is a rather pragmatic order; other options (like genre) would be just as justifiable. The advantage of this choice is that it allows the presentation of a gradual description, starting with texts that have very explicit opinions on medicine towards texts that contain more concealed opinions.[8]

Text	Date	Genre
Moriaen	1200 (c.)	Chivalric romance
Ferguut	1250 (c.)	Chivalric romance
Leven van Lutgart	Shortly after 1264	Saint's life
Boec van Catoene	1290 (c.)	School text
Natuurkunde van het Geheelal	Late 13th century	Artes ('scientific') literature

meaning of a word) are shown and (critically) discussed in Jack Hoeksema, 'Het WNT: een Waarlijk Nuttige Tool?', in: *Nederlandse Taalkunde* 16 (2011)-2, pp. 152–159, and Marijke Mooijaart, 'Discussie: de historische woordenboeken online. Van 'acht' (507) tot 'zwangerschap' (1851): historische lexicografie van boek tot internet', in: *Nederlandse Taalkunde* 16 (2011)-2, pp. 141–151.

7 One willing to test and/or extend our corpus could start by searching through GTB on our world field. The hypothesis, based on the broadness of the corpus, is that the findings will be representative of what could be found elsewhere, but obviously this view is open to change upon further research.

8 It should be stressed that this 'development' is the result of the ordering principle of this contribution; the reader should not be tempted to interpret it as if such a change was a contemporary, thus: medieval, chronological process.

(Continued)

Text	Date	Genre
Die Rose	1300 (c.)	Allegory
Der Leken Spieghel	1325–1328	Moral instructions
Melibeus	1342	Dialogue cf. *Liber de consolatione*
Reinaerts Historie	1373/1417–1470	Animal epic

Table 1: Texts used in this contribution in chronological order[9]

Discussion

1 Medicine and astrology

The first passage discussed comes from a text called the *Natuurkunde van het geheelal* ('Physics of the Universe').[10] It is a short (just under 1800 lines), rhymed treatise that claims to discuss 'astronomy, nature and the seven planets.'[11] The text is divided into chapters, and the first relevant passage is found in the closing part of the chapter on the zodiac and the influence of celestial bodies on people and human behavior. There, the text stresses the importance of (what can be called) astrology for those engaged in medicine, headed: 'Waer bi dat een recht fisiker emmer astronomie connen moet'.[12] The text reads: 'Wilde hi wesen goet phisicijn, hi en soude van astronomien leren. So mocht hi vrouwen ende heren seker cureren, ende ghenesen.'[13] A little further, a more general paragraph title is used ('Welc dat een goed fisiker es').[14] The desired astrological knowledge allows medical practitioners to know 'als hem ziecheyt comet an, wat planete regneert

9 Refrain was taken from discussing the complete contents of these texts as this would be beyond the scope of this contribution; all of the cited editions of these texts, however, have extensive introductions. In addition, the most recent literary histories could be consulted, resp.: Frits van Oostrom, *Stemmen op schrift. Geschiedenis van de Nederlandse literatuur vanaf het begin tot 1300*, Amsterdam 2006, pp. 274–281, p. 269 et sqq., pp. 395–397, p. 345, and Frits van Oostrom, *Wereld in woorden. Geschiedenis van de Nederlandse literatuur 1300–1400*, Amsterdam 2013, pp. 79–85–89, pp. 347–358, pp. 151–158, pp. 142/143–164–174–477, pp. 322–331.

10 The text has been edited in [anonymous], *De natuurkunde van het geheelal. Een 13de-eeuws Middelnederlands leerdicht*, edited by Ria Jansen-Sieben, Brussel 1968 (2 volumes). The introduction discusses the combination of medicine and astrology/astronomy: vol. I, pp. 36–37.

11 Natuurkunde (see n. 10), vol. 1, p. 275.

12 Natuurkunde (see n. 10), vol. 1, p. 361. Why a proper physician should always know astronomy.

13 Natuurkunde (see n. 10), vol. 1, p. 362, ll. 1248–1251. If he wants to be a good physician, he should learn about astronomy. Then he may certainly cure and heal people.

14 Natuurkunde (see n. 10), vol. 1, p. 363. What a good physician is.

dan, daer bi so mach hi weten al of hi ghenesen of steruen sal.'[15] Too often, so the text says, a doctor prescribes the wrong potion, with sometimes disastrous consequences: 'Nochtan en batet niet een caf. Maer den zieken hi verseerde ende sijn ziecheyt hi oec meerde.'[16] The *Natuurkunde* contains what could be called very normative remarks on physicians. Although not primarily concerned with medical education (and most would agree nowadays that the stars have little to do with good medical practice), it is explicit in its opinion that knowledge of celestial bodies should be a part of the curriculum; good doctors know of planets and stars. Even less explicit, it could be concluded that the author regards knowledge as an essential condition for good medical practice. At the very least this suggests that doctors were regarded as good scholars and wise man, capable of reading, studying and interpreting scientific works.

2 Find yourself a proper doctor

The second passage presented is very short: 'Bestu siec, kies enen man, die wel van ersatrien can.'[17] This rhyme couple is one of the lessons from the *Boec van Catone*, a Middle Dutch translation of the medieval *Disticha Catonis*, a medieval Latin school book.[18] This passage is interesting, because it contrasts with many other findings in two ways. Firstly, it is directed not at medical practitioners, but at patients; the text does not prescribe anything to doctors, but teaches the reader to find a good doctor when she or he is ill. That leads to the second point: by stressing the importance of finding the best doctor, the text implies the existence of bad doctors. Obvious as it may seem, a message such as this is rarely encountered.

15 Natuurkunde (see n. 10), vol. 1, p. 363, ll. 1261–1264. When illness overtakes him, what planet reigns? – thus he will know whether he will be cured or die.

16 Natuurkunde (see n. 10), vol. 1, p. 365, ll. 1278–1280. Yet, it [the medical interference] doesn't help anything. Instead, the patient and his illness deteriorate.

17 Quoted from the so-called Oudenaarde Book of Rhymed Texts, Oudenaarde, Stadsarchief, hs. 5576, through [anonymous], *Den duytschen Cathoen. Naar de Antwerpse druk van Henrick Eckert van Homberch, met als bijlage de andere redacties van de vroegst bekende Middelnederlandse vertaling der Dicta Catonis*, A. M. J. van Buuren, O. S. H. Lie and A. P. Orbán (eds.), Hilversum 1998, p. 128, ll. 19–20. When you are ill, pick a man who knows his medicine.

18 *Den duytschen Cathoen* discusses the tradition, before editing a Middle Dutch translation.

3 Medicine as labour

Not prescribing anything to doctors, nor patients, is Jan van Boendale's *Der Leken Spieghel* ('The Lay Mirror'). Nevertheless it is included it in this contribution, because it gives an insight in the position of medicine in medieval society.[19] Nowadays, medicine is everything a field or profession needs to be regarded a science: it is – for example – taught and studied at universities, it has scholarly journals and conferences, and much of its research is funded by institutions with names like Nederlandse Organisatie voor Wetenschappelijk Onderzoek (Netherlands Organisation for Scientific Research). According to Van Boendale's Mirror, the medieval situation was different. In chapter 14 of the third part of this text, the author writes about the origins and nature of poetry and science.[20] After listing and explaining the seven 'aerten liberale' of the clergy (grammar, logic, geometry, arithmetic, rhetoric, astronomy, theology), the text turns to the seven arts 'inder leekere hant'.[21] These 'lay arts' are what perhaps are called 'crafts':

> Nu hoort, ic salse u wisen: smeden ende lantwinninghe, wolle werc ende scepinghe, nayen ende arsatrie dan, conste van ghietene volghet hier an, gout, metael, zilver ofte loot, ofte ander mine, clein of groot.[22]

These are the 'bastard' or 'hybrid' arts ('bastaerde', l. 121), because they are applied by hand ('mitter hant', l. 122). Without necessarily suggesting a normative hierarchy (the text positions rather than judges), Van Boendale's text shows us a perception in which medicine is a craft rather than a science; it is placed among loot casting and spinning instead of geometry and astronomy. Therewith, this passage can easily be contrasted with the one from the *Natuurkunde*, where medicine is associated with knowledge of the cosmos.

---

19 The simplification of such a statement is self-evident; there is no such thing as 'medieval society'.

20 The most recent (!) edition of *Leken spieghel* is Jan van Boendale, *Der leken spieghel. Leerdicht van den jare 1350 door Jan Boendale, gezegd Jan de Clerc*, Matthias de Vries (ed.), Leiden 1844–1848 (3 volumes). There is a more recent, strongly abbreviated translation: Jan van Boendale, *Lekenspiegel. Een leerdicht uit Antwerpen, samengesteld en vertaald door Ludo Jongen en Miriam Piters*, Amsterdam 2003.

21 Van Boendale, Der leken spieghel (see n. 20), vol. III, p. 151, l. 101, l. 111. Liberal Arts; in the hands of the laity. (Note that the list of liberal arts in *Der leken spieghel* is different than the 'normal' seven arts: grammar, rhetoric, logic (=dialectics), arithmetic, geometry, music, astronomy. Why theology replaces music is not clear.)

22 Van Boendale, Der leken spieghel (see n. 20), p. 152, ll. 114–120. Listen, I will enumerate them: forgery, farming, spinning and weaving, shipping, sewing, healing and the casting of various metals, like gold, silver or lead.

4 Doctors as moneygrubbers

What *Die Rose* has in common with Van Boendale's text, is that it also puts a medical aspect in context. Whereas *Der Leken Spieghel* positions medicine among the crafts, a passage in Hein van Aken's translation of the Old French classic *Roman de la Rose* contains a different, more opinioned attitude towards medical practitioners: 'Avocate ende fisiciene, dese gaen alle die straten gemene, ende sijn blide ende sere in hogen alsi den penninc winnen moegen ende hare const vercopen wale: Hoe sere die sieke si gepijnt, si wouden datter sestich ware.'[23] This passage is part of a lengthy speech by Redene ('Reason'). In this monologue, this allegorical character states that 'Goet en maect den man niet rike, no scat, no have des gelike, mare wient genoget dat hi hevet, hi es rike vor al dat levet.'[24] The merchant, for example (l. 4907), and likewise lawyers and doctors, are people attaching too much importance to (earthly) possession. This shows two things. Firstly, it suggests that doctors ought to not attach too much to earthly possessions but should aim at something higher (although not specified, this might be god, or the task of healing, or high ethical standards) according to the author. Secondly, the opinion on doctors is not very explicit, but as Van Aken uses them as an example of people with a wrong attitude towards 'earthly possessions', it is clear that he does not hold them in very high esteem. Whatever the reason might be, it suggests that either the author or his environment has been a victim of high medical costs.

5 The doctor and non-medical ethics

This contribution makes use of a word field in which various words for 'doctors' are sought in Middle Dutch texts. Often, these words seem to be applied randomly, as it does not seem to have interpretational consequences what words is used exactly. One case, however, shows that there is at least some awareness of the differences between the various words for 'doctor'. That case is the *Melibeus*, a Middle Dutch translation of Albertanus of Brescia's *Liber de consolation*. In this corpus (and thereby in Middle Dutch literature), the *Melibeus* is the only

23 Hein van Aken, *Die Rose [van Heinric van Aken]*, Eelco Verwijs (ed.), Utrecht 1976, p. 81, ll. 4925–4929; 4932–4933. Lawyers and physicians, they go through the streets together and are happy and proud when they gain the money and sell their art. [...] It doesn't matter how much the ill are in pain; they wanted there to be sixty of them.

24 Van Aken, Die Rose (see n. 23), p. 79, ll. 4823–4826. Goods do not make a man rich, and neither do treasure or property, but he who settles for what he has, has a rich life.

text that distinguishes different kinds of doctors: both 'medicinen', 'surginen' and 'visikers' are used.[25]

The first 'medical encounter' is in the introductory part of the text. Melibeus' daughter is abused and he and his wife Prudentia discuss whether (and if, how) he should take revenge. He seeks council and among many, there is 'een meester, een surgien' present.[26] The surgeon speaks:

> Dambacht van Surgyen heeft inne sulke goedertierenheit van binnen, dat het niemen wille deren, maar hulpen hen allen dies begheren. Het valt dicke dat liede die striden ghequetst werden in beyde siden en een meester te hen beyden en helpt hen met sire wijsheyden even ghelijc spade ende vroe. Daer om en hoert ons niet toe dat wi raden in eneghe sake ten orloghe of ter wrake. Al es u dochter ghequetst swaer wi willen daer toe nemen waer en ghenesense na onse macht metter hulpen vanden Gods cracht. Anders en raden wi niet daer toe.'[27]

After the words of the surgeon, another man stands up:

> Een medicyn stont op doe en sprac met rade twaren der visikers die daer waren ghelijc dat dandere hadden ghesproken; maer hine woude raden no stoken ten orloghe wien lief of leet: maer sine consten waren ghereet sijnre dochter te staen bi. Een woert sprac hi: in onsen boeken men leest dat contrarie contrarie gheneest. Also machmen orloghe en wrake ghenesen met sulker sake.[28]

The surgeon stresses the goodness of his profession: surgeons help everyone in need, on both rival sides, including Melibeus' daughter. The 'medicus' does not claim similar goodness; instead, the basis of his knowledge is foregrounded, namely what he read in books. Therewith, both medical professions are present at Melibeus' council, but the text presents them quite differently: the practical and the intrinsically good surgeon *versus* the bookish and not necessarily good 'medicus'.

When Melibeus has received all the advice, Prudentia suggests: 'Nu laet ons

25 See for example F. A. Snellaert, *Nederlandsche gedichten uit de veertiende eeuw van Jan van Boendale, Hein van Aken e.a.*, Brussel 1869, pp. 11–12, ll. 247, 248, 284.

26 Snellaert, Nederlandsche gedichten (see n. 25), p. 11, l. 262; 'a master, a surgeon'.

27 Snellaert, Nederlandsche gedichten (see n. 25), pp. 11–12, ll. 265–281. The craft of surgery has such internal goodness, that is does not strive to hurt anyone, but helps everyone desiring help. It often happens that in battle, people at both sides are wounded and that a master [surgeon] assists them equally with his wisdom, just as late and early [anytime]. That is why it does not fit us to advise in matter of war and revenge. If your daughter is badly wounded, we will notice that and cure her as best as we can, with God's help. We do not advise anything else.

28 Snellaert, Nederlandsche gedichten (see n. 25), p. 12, ll. 282–294. Then, a *medicus* stood up and he took council with the physicians who were there, just like the other did that. He did not want to advise or spur anyone to war, but his arts were ready to support his daughter. He spoke a word: 'In our books we read that contraries cure contraries. Thus, war and revenge are cured with similar matter.'

dan examineren te wat orbore dat mach keren den raet die ghi hebt ghenomen.'[29] She starts:

> Der meester raet van surgyen selen wi der waerheyt lyen; dien was gherecht ende goet, want te haren ambacht, des sijt vroet, behoert wel dat si nieman en haten, maer dat si allen lieden baten.[30]

But she goes even further: 'Leent hen oec mildelijc van uwen goede, ghi sijt rijc, so dat si met willen claer tuwer dochter nemen waer, so dat si mach in corter stont mids Gods hulpe werden gesont.'[31] The surgeon's words have the desired impact: the audience accepts his claims. The 'medicus' however gets less understanding: 'Hets dicke geseyt en noch doet dat medicine in haren sin vore vrienscap setten hare ghewin.'[32] When Prudentia asks Melibeus how he interpreted the medicus' words, her word choice is very far from neutral: 'Nu willic van u weten saen, hoe ghi dat woert hebt verstaen dat u die dwase spraken toe.'[33] It should be noted that Prudentia has an agenda: throughout the whole story, she does not want Melibeus to take revenge. Therefore, the statement 'contrarie gheneest contrarie' is to her detriment, because it stresses that war can only be met with war.[34] Prudentia 'neutralizes' this statement by mocking the *medicus* even before Melibeus gets to give his opinion. Due to this agenda, we would not go as far as to conclude that the *Melibeus* considers surgeons as 'good' doctors and the *medicus* as a bad one. However, even when one does not want to draw such conclusions, it is interesting to see that the two groups are opposed: none of them speaks on behalf of all (what we would call) medical practitioners, their words are weighed differently and whereas the surgeon's profession is called a craft (l. 2165), the *medicus* is presented as quoting from his books (l. 291). The *Melibeus* is the only text discussed in this contribution that distinguishes the medical professions in this degree of explicitness.

---

29 Snellaert, Nederlandsche gedichten (see n. 25), p. 78, ll. 2156–2158. Now let us examine to what profit the council you took can be brought.

30 Snellaert, Nederlandsche gedichten (see n. 25), p. 79, ll. 2162–2167. We will esteem the master surgeon's advice correct; it was just and right, because that craft, as you know, has the quality that it hates no one, but helps everyone.

31 Snellaert, Nederlandsche gedichten (see n. 25), ll. 2168–2173. Also, generously share your property with them, as you are rich, so that they observe your daughter with a clear mind, in order that she will be healthy as soon as possible, with God's help.

32 Snellaert, Nederlandsche gedichten (see n. 25), ll. 2178–2182. It is often said that *medici* put their profit before friendship.

33 Snellaert, Nederlandsche gedichten (see n. 25), ll. 2186–2188. Now I quickly want to know how you have understood the words these fools said to you.

34 Another interpretation of this passage was also considered: 'contraries cure contraries' can also be interpreted as if war should be 'cured' by its opposite, peace. This interpretation however does not seem to make sense in the context of this *Melibeus* passage: if indeed the *medicus* suggests a peaceful attitude, why would the peace-seeking Prudentia mock him?

6 Playing doctor

Manuscript The Hague, Royal Library, 129 A 10 contains a compilation of ten Middle Dutch chivalric, more precisely Arthurian, romances: the Lancelot Compilation.[35] One of those romances is the *Moriaen.* In the *Moriaen*, Walewein is one of the main characters. Being one of Arthur's most important knights, this information is not very significant, but what is fascinating is that in the *Moriaen*, Walewein has a talent unknown in other stories: a doctor.[36] This talent already pops up in the opening phase of the text. A wounded knight appears at Arthur's court and immediately, Walewein performs first aid; not surprisingly, the narrator adds, because 'men hadde niet te dien stonden arsatere vonden also goed alse verre als god de sonne scinen doet. Van dat hi hem wilde onderwinden ende daer hi dlijf an conste vinden dat en mochte niet bederuen noch van genen wonde steruen.'[37] Walewein confidently addresses the wounded: 'Her riddere, nv sijt al sonder hoede vander doet op desen tijt [...] want ic sal v hulpen scieren.'[38] He treats him with a herb 'behandelt dat was also goet dattet stelpte mans bloet ende verlichte al ongesonde';[39] 'doe verlichte therte sijn.'[40] When set out on a quest, Walewein gets into trouble in a distant castle. He is so badly beaten that 'en leefde ertsce man ne geen die also ware nv beraden dat hem man mochte staen in staden noch artsatere oec genesen. Nv wouts god, hi sal gewesen van sire smerte van sire scande.'[41] And so it happened: God intervenes and Walewein is liberated by Moriaen. The latter also expresses his fear that Walewein is too injured to be treated (ll. 2600–2603), but it is Walewein himself who convinces his colleague

35 An extensive study of this compilation is available in English: A. A.M. Besamusca, *The book of Lancelot. The Middle Dutch Lancelot compilation and the medieval tradition of narrative cycles,* Cambridge 2003.

36 Even in the *Roman van Walewein*, a romance completely devoted to this knight, this competence is not mentioned once. The only medical acting is done by other, unnamed doctors ('arsaters'); Penninc and Pieter Vostaert, *De jeeste van Walewein en het schaakbord,* G.A. van Es (ed.), Zwolle 1952, p. 215, ll. 7502. In the *Roman van Walewein* are, however, magical elements, including for example the healing bed. See for a discussion of magic in this book John Verbeek, "Hare herte stont te storme van groten wondere!' Wonderen in pluskwadraat in de "Roman van Walewein"', in: *Queeste. Tijdschrift over middeleeuwse letterkunde in de Nederlanden* 14 (2007), pp. 33–44.

37 [anonymous], *Moriaen,* Hanneke van Buuren and Maurits Gysseling (eds.), Zutphen 1971, p. 55, ll. 84–89. In those days, there was no better doctor in the World then Walewein. The knights he cured, never died of their wounds, if they were alive when brought to him.

38 Moriaen (see n. 37), p. 56, ll. 108–111. Sir knight, refrain now from being afraid of death, because I will help you quickly.

39 Moriaen (see n. 37), p. 56, ll. 113–115. [...] which was so good that it stopped the bleeding and eased all insalubrities.

40 Moriaen (see n. 37), p. 56, l. 118. Then his heart eased.

41 Moriaen (see n. 37), p. 132, ll. 2278–2283. In the whole world, there was no doctor who could heal his wounds; only God could save him from this misery.

that he knows enough about medical forces to cure himself – with some rest and God's help (ll. 2611–2617). Walewein turns out not to be overestimating his own abilities, because even though initially Moriaen and a hermit wash his wounds, he indeed treats himself:

> Hi begaetde sine wonden. Men hadde so goede meester vonden daer nie moder aue genas, alse her walewein selue was. Soe wat wonden Walewein plach, si heilden daermen toe gesach.[42]

The day thereafter, Walewein is sad because he cannot ride out. Nevertheless, he is fit enough to hurry himself to the window when a third knight approaches the hermit's house (l. 2863). At dinner, Walewein explains that he is too weak to continue his quest, but: 'Margen salic vromer sijn! Dan selewi porren sonder fijn rechte alst begint dagen.'[43] And so it happens: two days after being more dead than alive, only one night after not being fit enough to mount his horse, and receiving no medical treatment apart from his own, Walewein declares himself cured and continues his quest.

This text is different from the other discussed so far, because it does not explicitly say anything about doctors: no attitudes, no opinions, no remarks even are made about actual medical practitioners. Instead, medical talents are attributed to another character, a knight, Walewein. It is beyond doubt that Walewein can be interpreted as a good, honorable character. The author of the *Moriaen* adds another endowment to Walewein, already known for (for example) his sword abilities and his skills with women, therewith enlarging the his authority of the character.

7 (Ab)use of the doctor's reputation

A similar matter of authority seems to be at stake in *Reinaerts Historie*, the fifteenth century reworking and expansion of the more famous *Van den vos Reynaerde*. King Nobel is – in the added part – close to expelling Reinaert from the court, but the fox tries to convince the lion of his value. Reinaert reminds the king of an incident in the past, when his father provided medical assistance to the king's father:

> [My father] quam hier in van der scolen tot Mompelier, dair hi studeerde der jaren vier in recepten van medecinen ende alle die teyken van urynen kende hi so wel als sijn hant,

42 Moriaen (see n. 37), p. 150, ll. 2795–2800. But he treated his own wounds, as nowhere in the world, there was a doctor as good as he: whatever the nature of the wounds treated by Walewein, they healed while watching.

43 Moriaen (see n. 37), p. 166, ll. 3237–3239. I will have to be totally cured [before I can come along]. Tomorrow I will be better. We will leave at dawn.

> ende alle die crude die men vant treckende, viscose ende laxitive, die kende hi bet dan sulke vive die grote meisters nu willen wesen. Hy was van consten sou ut gelesen, dat hi syden ende bont mocht dragen.[44]

Reinaert aims to establish his position at court, by not just emphasizing his ties with his father, but by a detailed description of his father's credentials as a doctor. Reinaert disguises his own wickedness by pointing at the best quality of a family member: his father was a doctor. These ascriptions are debatable; earlier on in the story, Reinaert described his father as a conspirator against the king, hiding a treasure. This treasure does not exist, and probably neither did the conspiracy Reinaert's father ought to be a member of – Reinaert just used his father and the king's fear to set himself free. The same process could be at hand here; the fox emphasizes that Nobel was too young to remember the incident, so there are no witnesses, and he should just be trusted. But what is true or not in and outside the story does not really matter in our contribution; what is significant, is that the author makes Reinaert plea for his credibility by referring to his father who was a *doctor* – not a lawyer or nobleman or merchant or priest, but a doctor. Even if Reinaert is lying again about his father, this passage only works if the status of a doctor is undisputable; the audience might have thought that Reinaert was lying again, but must have understood that the king accepted Reinaert's claim as an argument to keep him at court.

8 There is nothing more we can do

This paragraph is not devoted to a single text, but to a topos that is present in multiple texts. Three examples have been selected in which a text refers to medical acting by stating things like 'there is nothing more to do'. Remarks like this do not say a lot about medicine or about what medical practitioners actually can or cannot do, but they nevertheless reflect a certain awareness of doctors; after all, one cannot say 'don't call the doctor, it has no use' if one does not have at least some perception of doctors and what they can do.

The first example is from a chivalric, Arthurian romance which was translated from Old French into Middle Dutch towards the end of the thirteenth century: *Ferguut.* In this story, the protagonist is sent on a quest by King Arthur and at some stage, he spends the night at Castle Idel. There, the lord's niece falls in love

44 *Reynaert in tweevoud. Vol. II: Reinaerts Historie*, Paul Wackers (ed.), Amsterdam 2002, p. 254–255, ll. 5933–5944. [My father] came here after graduating in Montpellier, where he studied four years in medicine and he knew all the signs of urine as good as his own hand, and all the stimulating, viscous and relaxing herbs one found, he knew them all better than the great masters nowadays claim to do. He was so educated in the arts, that he was allowed to wear silk and fur.

with him. That very moment is described as such: '[Die Minne] sette een scicht in haren boge ende scoet der joncfrouwen dore doge in therte so diep, hen conste verdriven noit meester; het moeste met haer bliven.'[45] The arrow of love was shot into her heart so deeply, that no doctor would ever be able to remove it.

The other examples in this paragraph are taken from William of Affligem's Middle Dutch translation of the saint's life of St. Lutgart. This text contains multiple passages in which the limitations of medical acting are mentioned. The first one is when the state of a certain Ysabel is described. She was so ill, 'so dat met rade noch met talen, noch fisicien, noch ander man [...] en conste nit en twint gehelpen der siker nonnen.'[46] Another example is encountered in the chapter on the illness of duchess Mary of France, the second wife of duke Henry I of Brabant.[47] The illness was developing so badly, that 'fisicien negheen' could help by any means.[48] A third interesting mentioning of the word 'fisicine' is also found in this chapter; a messenger is sent from the court of the abbey where Lutgart lives, in order to ask Lutgart to pray for Mary. The messenger emphasizes how ill Mary is by referring to the powerlessness of the doctors.[49]

9 Conclusions and General Discussion

Modern doctors can rest assured; strong opinions have been around for many years, for the best and for the worst. In this essay, we have studied the presentation of medical actors and actions in Middle Dutch, non-medical literature. By creating a word field and searching through an extensive corpus of non-medical texts, we found a significant amount of texts using words regarding medicine. We selected several remarkable cases, which were discussed above.

When reviewing the texts used in this contribution, one can safely conclude that medical personae are seldom presented in a neutral way: their appearance never goes unnoticed. For instance, in *Melibeus* the surgeon and doctor repre-

45 [Anonymous], *Ferguut*, E. Rombauts, N. de Paepe and M.J.M. de Haan (eds.), Hilversum 1982, p. 86, ll. 1233–1236. [Love] putted an arrow in her bow and shot the damsel through her eyes into the heart so deeply, that no doctor would ever be able to remove it; it was there to stay with her.

46 [Anonymous], *Leven van Sinte Lutgart. Tweede en derde boek*, François van Veerdeghem (ed.), Leiden 1899, p. 65, ll. 6486–6490. That with advise nor language a doctor, nor any other man, could help the sick nun. (The identification of William of Affligem as author/translator of this text is firmly established in Erwin Mantingh, *Een monnik met een rol. Willem van Affligem, het Kopenhaagse Leven van Lutgart en de fictie van een meerdaagse voorlezing*, Hilversum 2000, but (logically) unknown to Van Veerdeghem, who considered several author options.)

47 Sinte Lutgart (see n. 46), p. 123, n. 1.

48 Sinte Lutgart (see n. 46), p. 124, l. 12576. No doctor.

49 Sinte Lutgart (see n. 46), p. 124, ll. 12620–12624.

sent are among the top advisors of the king and their words weigh heavy on his decision. Especially the surgeon seems to carry an intrinsic goodness and literacy. The medical skills attributed to Walewein and abuse of the title by Reynard the fox are other examples of the idea that mentioning medical actors or attributing medical talents to a person adds status. That 'status' should not be automatically read as a positive thing is shown by *Die Rose*, where it is suggested that not everyone was impressed with the medical profession and the financial compensation that sometimes came with treatment.

This contribution aimed to give an overview of attitudes towards medicine in medieval, vernacular Dutch literature. By choosing this aim, we have refrained from explaining the different attitudes actually encountered. This lacuna is an interesting starting point for further research, which could question – for example – whether there is a chronological or geographic explanation for the similarities and differences we have encountered. Another matter is the world field; in our attempt to catch as many finding places as possible, we have thrown out our net and treated all cites equally. This method surely works for our aims, but a more exhaustive study might benefit from an etymological or multilingual study of words such as visiker, arsatrie and surgine. These are often applied without any additional information, but what was the perception of such words by the medieval audiences of a text? Are they as synonymous as most texts from our corpus seem to indicate? Other directions for follow-up research include a study of differences between genres (are 'Arthurian' doctors different from 'epic' doctors?) or a study of translations (did Middle Dutch translators add or omit information when translating from – for example – Old French?). In addition, the amount of text found using our search strategy resulted in an enormous number of texts. Describing all of these separately would have been too extensive for the scope of this chapter. Instead we have selected several texts of interest of which we thought would represent the whole body as best as possible, although there might valuable information regarding our topic in the excluded texts.

The main goal of this contribution was to answer the question regarding what opinions on medical actors and acting can be derived from medieval non-medical literature. We have shown that the medieval public opinion on these topics is diverse. Thereby, this essay does not only prove that the medical profession has been a subject of equal praise and criticism since at least the middle ages, it also shows us that something volatile as a long gone public opinion can be 'caught' in written texts.

Hans de Waardt

Melancholy and Fantasy: Johan Wier's Use of a Medical Concept in his Plea for Tolerance

1 Introduction

> As a result of sootiness of their black bile, the victims of this disease believe that they have changed into wolves or even dogs. They therefore go out of their houses, especially by night, imitating wolves or dogs in their every action.
> They are pale, and their eyes are sunken and dry. They see but dimly and have a dry tongue and a great thirst, while their mouth lacks salvia. Their legs are so covered with sores that they cannot be healed – because of frequent injuries and dog bites.[1]

This description of symptoms is from Johan Wier's *De praestigiis daemonum* (*Delusions of Demons*) which was first published in 1563.[2] The book brought its author instantaneous fame as a major opponent of the witchcraft trials; but also brought disrepute as an ultra-sceptic who undermined the very basis of religion.[3] Johan Wier (1515–1588), or Weyer as he is also called, was born in Grave in Brabant.[4] In 1529, he moved to Antwerp where he joined the household of the very erudite champion of natural magic Agrippa of Nettesheim (1486–1535).[5] He

1 Johann Weyer, *De Praestigiis Daemonum*, ed. George Mora a.o., Binghamton/New York 1991, p. 343. Johan Wier, *Opera Omnia*, IV, xxiii, Amsterdam 1660, p. 336, § 3–4.

2 Johan Wier, *De Praestigiis Daemonum*, Basel 1563. In 1564, 1566, 1568, 1577, and 1583 new, each time revised, editions appeared. Apart from these Latin editions a number of German and French translations appeared of which Wier only accepted his own German version *De Praestigiis, Von Ihrer Ursprung, Underscheid, Vermögenheit, und Rechtmessiger Straaff*, [S.l.] 1578. Wier introduced this story in the second edition of his book, Johan Wier, *De Praestigiis Daemonum*, Basel 1564, p. 357.

3 A good example of a negative qualification is the one given by King James VI/I in his *Daemonlogie, in Forme of a Dialogue*, Edinburgh 1597, p. 2v.

4 Literature on Wier is vast. For an overview of relevant literature see Hans de Waardt, 'Witchcraft, Spiritualism and Medicine: the Religious Convictions of Johan Wier', in: *Sixteenth Century Journal* 42 (2011), pp. 369–91.

5 The standard biographical study on Agrippa still is Charles G. Nauert, *Agrippa and the Crisis of Renaissance Thought*, Urbana, Ill 1965. But see also Marc van der Poel, *Cornelius Agrippa: The Humanist Theologian and His Declamations*, Leiden 1997; Christopher I. Lehrich, *The Language of Demons and Angels: Cornelius Agrippa's Occult Philosophy*, Leiden 2003.

then studied medicine in Paris and in 1550 he was appointed first physician to Duke William of Cleves and Jülich.

His description of a werewolf fantasy contains most of the central elements of the argument Wier develops in this book. Under the influence of an excess of black bile, a person's fantasy may run wild, resulting in a loss of the sense of reality and even in a – fully imagined – physical transformation. In this case as in many others in his book, it is the patient himself who concocts a story he perceives as totally true but is in reality completely delusional. What is really vexing these hapless people is a humoural unbalance. Their cold and dry condition is a symptom of melancholy.

Here, the patient is male, but in most of Wier's case histories, it is women who suffer such a loss of control over their imagination. He, for instance, discusses in great detail the case of a twenty-year old girl who in 1562 was convinced that a knife was hidden in her left side. Initially, it was assumed that the girl 'was distressed by melancholia or that she was somewhat delirious'. However, when a real knife was discovered under her skin, it was concluded that she was bewitched. Wier, on the other hand reasoned that if a real knife had been enclosed within her body, it would have been completely impossible for her to move, to sit, or stand. It should be noted, he adds, that she had previously been vexed by a quartan fever caused by 'an excess of heavy, bitter, melancholic humor putrefied within the body'. The girl's brain was therefore saturated with black bile, the humour that the devil often used to induce phantasms in his victims. People thus possessed were open to all sorts of demonic delusions and could even be driven into a suicidal frenzy.[6]

2 Fantasy and the brain

The medical concept on which Wier constructed his argument was in itself not innovative. Most if not all physicians shared his view that demons could invade the body of a melancholic human. In 1549, for instance, Jason Pratensis (1486–1558) from the Dutch province of Zeeland wrote in his *De cerebri morbis* (*Brain diseases*):

> It happens truly that demons, inasmuch as they are thin and incomprehensible spirits, insinuate themselves into the bodies of men, hidden in the guts they weaken him secretly, causing diseases. They frighten souls with dreams, and shake minds with

6 Erik Midelfort, *A History of Madness in Sixteenth-century Germany*, Stanford, Cal 1999, p. 77; see also Michael MacDonald and Terence R. Murphy, *Sleepless Souls. Suicide in Early Modern England*, Oxford 1990, pp. 50–51.

> furies, so that on the whole it may be wondered whether the madman was attacked by mania of whether he was not rather beaten by the spirit.[7]

Wier does not refer explicitly to this passage, but he was certainly familiar with Pratensis's book. He for instance borrowed from it a story about a priest who believed that each night a woman pressed him down in his bed with such force that he could hardly breath. According to Pratensis this was all 'pure imagination, simple illusion' a viewpoint Wier of course fully endorsed.

Wier's claim that an excess of black bile could easily lead to a corrupted perception of reality and thus to an acceptance of fantasies as impressions of the real world was also rather traditional. In the view of many scholars, this causal relationship had a sort of vice versa character in the sense that fantasy in its turn could lead to a humoural imbalance. In 1538, for instance, Juan Luis Vives (1493–1540), who was born in Spanish Valencia to a *converso* family but spent most of his active live in Flemish Bruges, wrote:

> A mere commotion of our fantasy bearing some resemblances to an opinion or judgment that a given object is good or bad, is enough to disturb our soul with all emotions: we fear, rejoice, cry, feel sad. This is also why our emotions seem to converge toward that part of the body where the fantasy prevails, and also why we will actually attribute bodily qualities to emotions and call them warm, cold, dry, or a mixture of those. Internal and external causes can exacerbate and repress the influence of our bodily temperament. Among the internal causes we find the emotions themselves: sadness makes us cold and dry, joy makes us warm and wet. Emotions both reflect and contribute to the temperament of the body.[8]

Already in 1557, the famous Italian physician Girolamo Cardano (1501–1576), whose work Wier repeatedly quotes, had emphasized that melancholy caused witches to imagine that they did many wondrous and horrible things.[9]

However, Wier based his plea not only on medical theories but also on what he had found in the works of theologians, lawyers, philosophers, and philologists. His fellow courtier Andreas Masius (1514–1573), a recognised philologist and expert on Hebrew, supplied him for example with neutral translations of Bible

7 Jason Pratensis, *De Cerebri Morbis*, Basel 1549, p. 224. The translation is from Midelfort, A History of Madness (see n. 6), p. 153. Sidney Anglo was the first to point to this influence by Pratensis on Wier, see his 'Melancholia and Witchcraft: The Debate between Wier, Bodin and Scot', in: *Folie et Déraison à la Renaissance*, Brussels 1976, pp. 209–22.

8 Juan Luis Vives, *The Passions of the Soul: The Third Book of De anima et vita*, ed. Carlos G. Norena, Lewisson, NY 1990, p. 2, as quoted in Noga Arikha, *Passion and Tempers. A History of the Humours*, New York 2007, p. 218.

9 On Cardano's influence on Wier see Stuart Clark, *Thinking with Demons. The Idea of Witchcraft in Early Modern Europe*, Oxford 1995, p. 238. Wier may have met Cardano in person when the latter in the course of an extended trip through France, England, and the Empire also visited Cleves in 1557, cf. Girolamo Cardano, *The Book of my Live (De Vita Propria Liber)*, transl. Jean Stoner, intr. Anthony Grafton, New York 2002, p. 89.

verses that were traditionally used to vindicate the witch trials. From legal experts Wier borrowed, as Erik Midelfort shows in his *History of Madness in Sixteenth-Century Germany*, two fundamental juridical ideas that helped him to dismantle the binding quality of the diabolic pact: Contracts are not binding if one of the parties has kept the other party uninformed about facts that are essential for the impact of the agreement. The demonic pact was therefore not valid because the Devil always kept his human accomplices in the dark about the consequences of the pact. The second one was the insanity plea that was already acknowledged in the sixth century in the *Corpus Iuris* of Emperor Justinian. By the mid sixteenth century, German lawyers were completely familiar with Roman law and Wier invited them to accept these arguments.

3 Demonic possession

In Book Four of his *De praestigiis* (281–358), Wier discusses the problems of 'those who are thought to be afflicted by the witchcraft of *lamiae*'.[10] In Wier's time, there was no clear view on the exact nature of demonic possession, of the symptoms by which it could be recognized, or the ways in which it could be treated.[11] In her *La folie au Moyen Age*, Muriel Lahaire sums up a large number of, often contradictory, actions that in medieval times could be perceived as symptoms of demonic possession.[12] Even in the sixteenth century, this fogginess had certainly not been cleared. The Reformation had not been very helpful in this matter. Stuart Clark's contention that 'in France and England alike, both the theoretical debates about possession and exorcism [...] were heavily factionalized in terms of the complex religious and political controversies of the time.' That it 'was not just that possession and exorcism were contentious subjects dividing Protestants from Catholics; they divided the faiths internally as well', may have applied to other parts of Europe as well.[13] As Walter Stephens convincingly shows in his *Demon Lovers*, the concept of demonic possession was

10 'Lamiae' is a Latin term for witches. Originally *De praestigiis* counted five books, but starting with the fourth edition (1568) it was subdivided in six books. This later arrangement is followed here. Quotations in this section are from the edition by MORA (see n. 1). For the sake of brevity the references are given in the main text between brackets.

11 On this see HANS DE WAARDT, 'Demonic Possession. An Introductory Note', in: *Dämonische Besessenheit. Zur Interpretation eines Kulturhistorischen Phänomens / Demonic Possession. Interpretation of a Historico-Cultural Phenomenon*, HANS DE WAARDT a.o. (ed.), Bielefeld 2005, pp. 20–35.

12 MURIEL LAHAIRE, *La Folie au Moyen Age XIe-XIIIe Siècle*, Paris 1991, pp. 29–32.

13 STUART CLARK, 'Witchcraft and Magic in Early Modern Culture', in: BENGT ANKARLOO, STUART CLARK and WILLIAM MONTER, *Witchcraft and Magic In Europe*, Vol. 4, *The Period of the Witch Trials*, London 2002, p. 138.

initially even quite vague for the Dominican friar Heinrich Kramer, who wrote *Malleus Maleficarum,* the handbook for the prosecution of witchcraft, first published in 1487.[14]

Another aspect that blurred the view was the indistinct conception of the essence of demonic possession as it belonged both to the domain of the priests and to that of the physicians. Clergymen emphasized the preternatural element of the demonic activity, whereas physicians saw it on the first place as a disturbance of the brain as a result of a humoural imbalance. Both, however, admitted that the other party could also play a significant role. The *Rituale Romanum*, the compendium of church rites proclaimed by the pope in 1614, prescribed that Catholic clergymen, before agreeing to start an exorcism, should establish wether the afflicted person was not suffering from black bile or another natural illness.[15] If individuals commanded 'unknown languages', knew about things that were hidden or put away out of their sight, and showed physical strength that did not match their age or bodily complexion, then it could be assumed that they were possessed.

The *Rituale* also stressed that there were many other signs, without giving any details about their nature, that could indicate that a person was the victim of this affliction. It furthermore stressed that a demon could seem to have departed from a human body, but in reality was still present. Demons could also trick observers by having their victim imitate the symptoms of a natural disease. So the official Catholic handbook left much room for the priests or physicians to attach a diagnosis of their liking to the behaviour of a patient. After the Reformation, Catholic clergymen, especially in France, used public exorcism sessions as a, at times very effective, propaganda tool. However, doubt about the reliability of both the people who claimed to be possessed and the individuals who presented themselves as expert exorcists always remained strong, also among Catholic protagonists.[16]

The takeover by demons of human minds and bodies was the central element of Wier's argument, but his description of the causes and maturation of demonic possession was also rather dim. The first sentences of Book four of his *De Praestigiis* discuss the circumstances that cause a demonic possession:

> When with God's permission the Devil assails bodies in various ways, often strange and preternatural ways, the victims – be they men or cattle – are said to be afflicted by witchcraft. At some point the Devil enters into these bodies, or does not even enter in

14 Walter Stephens, *Demon Lovers. Witchcraft, Sex, and the Crisis of Belief*, Chicago, Ill. 2002, pp. 343–51.

15 *Rituale Romanum Pauli V. Pont. Max. Jussu Editum*, Rome 1826, p. 342.

16 Sarah Ferber, *Demonic Possession and Exorcism in Early Modern France*, London 2004, pp. 17–22.

> but agitates and infects the useful humors of the body, or carries the harmful humors into the principal bodily parts, or blocks the veins and natural ducts of these parts, or dislocates the structure of the organs, or disturbs the brain's spirits and imbues them with multifarious forms, and sometimes excites them so that the vital force in these people comes forth more powerfully than in sane people. Or else he fouls and defiles the bodies with poisonous matter or with vapors within or without and does other things of this sort, so that countless strange and serious diseases are produced.[17]

So, demons affected corporeal functions both from within and without the body. They could corrupt the humours, but were also able to import them or poisonous matter into a human body. They, therefore, induced a wide variety of strange and serious illnesses. Wier does not give any description of the nature or symptoms of these diseases apart from the observation that they are 'strange'. In other words, it is up to the beholder to decide whether the behaviour of a human being is deviant enough to identify it as the result of a demonic possession. In itself, this point of view was not very original. It was, for instance, not fundamentally different from that which the pope, as we saw above, presented a few decades later. What matters here, however, is that Wier, more than other contemporary authorities, put such great emphasis on the autonomy of the demons. Being the opening paragraph of one of the books in which the whole work was subdivided, these lines have a crucial position. It is therefore important to note that he did not refer to any other factor that could cause a patient to fall prey to a demonic attack. The victims had no other option than to undergo it and could only hope for able healers like Wier to assist them. It is contended here that Wier actually made the most of the indistinct character of the whole concept to build up his argument that the mind of women who voluntarily confessed that they had concluded a pact with the devil, had actually been taken over by demons. In his *De praestigiis*, but not in any of his other publications, when discussing women in general, he repeatedly states that members of the female sex simply miss any real understanding. This claim of course helped him to make his point. However, when he, in other places, discusses his contacts with individual women, he often presents them as worthy interlocutors. Of his second wife Henrietta, he even said that her 'lively faith' made her 'a fierce opponent of diabolical trickery'.[18] This suggests that in reality he appreciated the intellectual abilities of women much more than he seemed to do in his general pronouncements. It was indeed a matter of rhetoric.

17 Wier, Opera omnia (see n. 1), V, i, p. 278; Mora (ed.), *De Praestigiis* (see n.1), p. 284.
18 De Waardt, Witchcraft, Spiritualism and Medicine (see n. 4), p. 390.

4 Natural magic and fantasy

Another example of this approach in which a derogatory tone prevailed in general assessments, but a more sympathetic one in regard of individual cases, is notable when Wier discusses natural magic. Remarkably enough, he borrowed arguments from heroes of natural magic whose trustworthiness he emphatically disavowed elsewhere. His chapter 'Concerning Fantasy and how it is impaired' starts with a long quotation from the 1497 translation by the Florentine Marsilio Ficino (1433–1499) of *De mysteriis* (*Mysteries*), a work of the third century AD Neo-Platonist Iamblichus:

> The imagination is naturally joined to all the powers of the soul, and it shapes and fashions likeness and apparitions of all external forms, and it carries over the sights or impressions of one set of powers to another, forming a notion or opinion from the impressions which flicker forth from the senses. Secondarily, it presents to the notion or opinion information which proceeds from the intellect, but in itself it embraces images from every source. In fact, it fashions and expresses all the activities of the *anima*, accommodating the external to the internal.[19]

This passage is followed by an even longer quote from Ficino's *Theologia Platonica* were it is stated that the human imagination is so powerful that it can change or at least influence a person's physical condition.[20] In the mid-sixteenth century, the reliability and integrity of advocates of natural magic like Ficino or Wier's mentor Agrippa were called into question by people who felt more inspired by Aristotle and they still formed the majority. The fact that Wier chose to refer to Ficino while there were other less conspicuous texts available like that, for instance, of Vives, suggests that he still considered the Tuscan advocate of magic an authoritative source.[21]

Several references to less questionable authors follow these two long quotations. With the exception of Aristotle, none of these, however, receive so much

19 Mora (ed.), De Praestigiis (see n. 1), pp. 186–87.

20 On Ficino's views concerning the power of imagination see Guido Giglioni, 'Coping with Inner and Outer Demons: Diseases of the Imagination and Imaginary Diseases in Marsilio Ficino', in: *Diseases of the Imagination and Imaginary Disease in the Early Modern Period*, Yasmin Haskell (ed.), Turnhout 2011, pp. 19–50.

21 There was at least one such idea that was quite common in this period, namely that a fetus could turn into a monster if, during the pregnancy, the mother was terrified by some sort of fearful impression or fantasy. In his study of monstrous birth the famous surgeon Ambroise Paré devoted a separate chapter to this subject, see chapter 9, 'An Example of Monsters that Are Created through Imagination', in: Ambroise Paré, *On Monsters and Marvels*, trans. and ed. Janice L. Pallister, Chicago 1982, pp. 38–42. The first edition of this work appeared in 1573. It is not inconceivable that Wier, who studied medicine in Paris in the mid-1530s, has met Paré in person who at that time was living as house-surgeon in the Hôtel-Dieu, the chief public hospital of Renaissance Paris.

attention as the Neo-Platonist Ficino. Wier even finishes this chapter with a quote from yet another, though spurious (but Wier was unaware of that), Neo-Platonist namely the pseudo-Dionysius, whose *De divinis nominibus* (*The Divine Names*) is also mentioned as a valid authority.

There is another contradiction that deserves to be mentioned. In his *De praestigiis*, the role of the Devil and his demons is overpowering. However, in the medical casebook Wier published in 1567, the devil is completely ignored.[22] Neither does Wier ever refer to any diabolical influence as the source of illnesses or other mishaps in his studies of pathological anger and prolonged fasting, nor does he mention it in his correspondence.[23] This suggests that in his view the capacities of the demons were not so all-pervasive a power as he presented them in his *De Praestigiis*. We may, as it seems, conclude from this that he used the spectre of the power of Hell, an image many people were evidently familiar with in the sixteenth century, as a rhetorical device to exculpate witches.

This approach is actually in full accord with how spiritualists perceived the power of demons. For them, the devil really was the abstract principle of evil that could dominate the mind-set of human beings, but he certainly was not an anthropomorphous horror that could establish direct contacts with humans, conclude pacts with them, let alone have sexual relations with them.[24]

5 Medicine, rhetoric, and history writing

It was Wier's aim to exonerate the usual suspects of witchcraft, or as he referred to them, 'these demented old women' (*vetulas illas dementitas*) decried as witches. His *De praestigiis* was meant to convince his readers and especially the judges and other magistrates that it was pointless to prosecute and sentence such defendants. However, in order to exonerate them, he had to furnish the judges with other possible culprits. To that end, he stated that crimes that were attributed to witches were in reality committed by demons who infested these females with the conviction that they had brought all sorts of evil to their fellow

22 Johan Wier, *Medicarum observationum rararum*, Basel 1567. Wier also issued a German translation Johan Wier, *Artzney Buch*, Frankfurt/M. 1580. An enlarged edition of his translation appeared in 1588.

23 Johan Wier, *De Ira Morbo, eiusdem Curatione Philosophica, Medica & Theologica*, Basel 1577. This book was also translated Johan Wier, *Vom Zorn Iracundiae antidotum*, Wittenberg 1585. *De commentitiis jejuniis*, his case study of a young girl who pretended not to have eaten for an extended period appeared for the first time in the fifth edition of the Latin version of his *De praestigiis*, Basel 1577.

24 Gary Waite, "'Man is a Devil to Himself': David Joris and the Rise of a Sceptical Tradition towards the Devil in the Early Modern Netherlands, 1540–1600", in: *Nederlandsch archief voor kerkgeschiedenis* 75 (1995), pp. 1–30, here 9–11.

human beings. In other words, he used his medical knowledge and expertise as arguments in a debate of a judicial nature. Here, the rules of rhetoric, a discipline which was rapidly gaining in importance in the sixteenth century, could be very useful.

With the renascence of the liberal arts, oratory had re-claimed in the intellectual life of Western Europe the central position it had had in classical times.[25] Sixteenth century humanists fully agreed with Cicero that there was a direct connection between '*eloquentia*' and '*sapientia*', between eloquence and 'wordly wisdom'. A growing number of universities explicitly wished to install in their students a 'wise and eloquent piety'.[26] This was the intellectual atmosphere in which Wier had done his studies, first with Agrippa and then in Paris.

By training, Wier was a physician and in his time physicians not only attached a high status to oratory qualities, but also to the historical profession.[27] In the classic age, physicians and historians had been aware of the many similarities between their professions in the ways in which they selected and interpreted disparate data.[28] Early modern humanist physicians believed that the study of the past would sharpen their observatory qualities.[29]

Wier's use of history fitted in with a dominant characteristic of contemporaneous history writing. Most early modern historians were convinced that their work should not just describe what had happened but should also buttress a didactical aim.[30] They realized that they should serve their message in a form that their listeners could digest. From classic authors like Cicero, humanists understood that to get their message over to the intended public, they had to adapt it to their capacities. How an orator expressed himself was about as important as the actual content of his speech.[31] As a true advocate of toleration, Wier indeed tried to present his arguments as convincingly as possible.

From other sources, he had also learned that a message was more effective if one did not overfeed the audience with data too complex for them to understand. His mentor Agrippa, who was one of the main protagonists of natural magic,

25 On this see Heinrich F. Plett, *Rhetoric and Renaissance Culture*, Berlin 2004.
26 Walter Ruegg, 'Introduction', in: *A History of the University in Europe*, vol. 2, *Universities in Early Modern Europe, 1500–1800*, Hilde de Ridder-Symoens (ed.), Cambridge 1996, pp. 28–29.
27 Cf. Nancy G. Siraisi, 'Oratory and Rhetoric in Renaissance Medicine', in: *Journal of the History of Ideas* 65 (2004), pp. 191–211.
28 Arnaldo Momigliano, 'History between Medicine and Rhetoric', in: *Ottavo contributo alla storia degli studi classici e del mondo antico*, Arnaldo Momigliano (ed.), Rome 1987, pp. 13–25.
29 On this see Nancy Siraisi, 'Anatomizing the Past: Physicians and History in Renaissance Culture', Renaissance Quarterly 53 (2000), pp. 1–30.
30 Anthony Grafton, *What Was History? The Art of History in Early Modern Europe*, Cambridge 2007, pp. 34–49.
31 Gary Remer, *Humanism and the Rhetoric of Toleration*, University Park, PA 1996, p. 14.

held that most mortals never managed to free themselves of the limitations of the material world as a result of which their perceptions and understandings were mere products of misconceptions. A similar principle was part of the lessons of Hendrick Niclaes and David Joris, spiritualist prophets in whose teaching Wier took great interest during the 1550s.[32] His brother Matthias, who was a sort of small-scale spiritualist prophet in his own right, held that: 'To them who are rude as yet, nothing of the Sublime Mysteries may be talked of.'[33]

For Wier, it was evident that he should take his readers by the hand, confront them with arguments they could handle, and introduce them step-by-step into what he considered the ultimate truth. Most people in his time were convinced that preter-natural forces could indeed bring about changes in the domain of nature. He therefore made this principle the basis of his argumentation, but he did so in a very pragmatic way.

6 Demonic possession and other diabolically provoked afflictions

He begins this part of his book with two stories from the Bible; of course the most reliable source in the eyes of all or at least most of his readers. It is related in the Old Testament how, with God's permission, Satan vexed both Job and Nebuchadnezzar, killing the children and destroying all the property of the first, and causing the second one to lose his mind. Job ended in misery, covered with ulcers and with a dung-heap as his only abode. The King of Babylon was brought to believe that he had turned into a cow which made him roaming about and grazing the fields. Wier subsequently shifts to stories from the New Testament in which Jesus expels demons from possessed individuals like the Gadarene who was infested with a whole legion of evil spirits. Nowhere in these Bible texts, Wier emphasizes, is it stated that Satan or any of his devils needs the assistance of human beings. Even the *Malleus*, the witchhunters' manual that had been published a century earlier by the Dominican Inquisitor Institoris viz. Kramer,

---

32 On Wier's religious convictions see DE WAARDT, Witchcraft, Spiritualism and Medicine (see n. 4). There were actually quite a few similarities between the teachings of Agrippa and some of the views held by spiritualist prophets, cf. PAOLA ZAMBELLI, 'Magic and Radical Reformation in Agrippa of Nettesheim', in: PAOLA ZAMBELLI (ed.), *White Magic, Black Magic in the European Renaissance: From Ficino, Pico, Della Porta to Trithemius, Agrippa, Bruno*, Leiden 2007, pp. 138–182.

33 MATTHIAS WIER, *The Narrow Path of Divine Truth Described from Living Practice and Experience of its Three Great Steps*, London 1683, p. 52. This is an English translation of his *Dat Boeck der Sproecken*, Rotterdam [ca. 1560].

admits, Wier stresses, 'that the Devil works evil by himself and does not need the consent of a malicious woman' (285).

On this firm Biblical basis, he then constructs the rest of his argument, first discussing the symptoms that were often perceived as indications that a witch was at work. In the second and the following chapters he then presents a large number of case histories, several of which came from his own medical practice. Victims of witchcraft may throw up all sorts of strange things:

> The objects are often strips of coarse woollen cloth, iron nails (sometimes of fairly large size) and fragments thereof, iron and brass clasps, needles, pins (sometimes fastened together or inserted into a piece of cloth), and balls of thread. I have seen these things for myself. Sometimes, too, bones are vomited forth, and undergarments, and other still more ridiculous oddities. (286)

Wier fails to see how all this is possible. Where did all these objects come from? Certainly not from the stomach! The human oesophagus simply was too narrow for objects of that size to pass from the stomach to the mouth. People who for the fun of it had swallowed things like an egg or a stone ran a serious risk of suffocating or dying in another very unpleasant way. Wier's colleague Solenander (1524–1601) had in his possession a stone that he had found in the lungs of a young man who in 1553 had died after years of terrible coughing (287). Wier himself had, when he was living in Arnhem, examined a girl of sixteen who was thought to be bewitched by her female neighbours (291).[34] When the girl was about to vomit, Wier opened her mouth and found a piece of cloth in it. This was, however, completely clean and it was therefore unlikely that it had been in her stomach. To explain why it was possible that this piece of cloth was hidden in the girl's mouth, Wier suggested that a demon had put it there who had acted so swiftly that none of the bystanders had noticed his action.

In the remainder of Book Four, Wier gives a really impressive number of other, similar examples of which the werewolf diagnosis and therapy, and the story about the hidden knife with which this contribution began, are only two. In many of these stories Wier himself appears as a close witness. However, he had only hearsay as evidence regarding many other incidents, or he had found them in existing literature. Sometimes Wier's version can be compared with other sources and in most of these cases his account is pretty much in line with these other data. For obvious reasons his rendering of cases he had not witnessed

34 In 1550 the case was brought before the Court of Gelderland. Four women who had been accused of witchcraft were acquitted, the cunning man who had accused them, was banished. See on this case Hans de Waardt, 'At Bottom a Family Affair: Feuds and Witchcraft in Nijkerk in 1550', in: *Witchcraft in the Netherlands from the Fourteenth to the Twentieth Century*, Marijke Gijswijt-Hofstra and Willem Frijhoff (ed.), Rotterdam 1991, pp. 132–48.

himself, is often less reliable. His account of the demonic possessions by which the orphanage of Amsterdam was overtaken in 1566 is, for instance, not really very accurate.[35] His information in this case was really third-hand as he had received it from his old friend, the chancellor of Gelderland, who had not been personally involved in this case either.

Wier also used material from sources like the work of the classic poet Virgil. 'Credulous and superstitious people of Antiquity would have it that many men are changed into beasts by the evil doing of witches', he writes (337). He then quotes some ancient myths like that of Circe and Ulysses, only to undercut these immediately with the help of the Christian authority St. Augustine and the pagan encyclopaedist Pliny who had argued that such stories were either false or fiction (341). Demons could not alter the essential basics of nature, they could for instance not remove a man's testicles, but they could induce sexual impotence by natural means (332–35). Wier did, however, believe that the gender of human beings could change and to prove that he discussed a few case stories about women who had suddenly changed into men (344–6). But all these transformations, he emphasizes, had perfectly natural causes.

After thus defining what sort of accounts he found acceptable, and which stories he rejected, he states that individuals who claimed to be possessed were either impostors, or melancholic, or poisoned. Individuals from the first category deserved harsh punishment, people from the other two obviously needed treatment, and people who believed this nonsense should be educated. He also denounces the people who fed the superstition of the simple folk by offering magical treatment. Both cunning folk and exorcising clerics were nothing but fraudulent crooks in his eyes. Wier sincerely disliked such clergymen and then most of all the mendicant friars. In this he of course joined in with his mentor Agrippa, who had really hated the friars and of these especially the Dominicans, and of course Erasmus who has also repeatedly voiced his sincere aversion to these clergymen.[36] There is, however, perhaps also another reason why Wier felt the urge to bring down these healers, both the lay and the ordained exorcists. If demons were indeed so powerful as he claimed and if it was impossible for human beings to control these spirits, then it was also not feasible that some humans were able to force demons to depart from bodies or other natural objects. Be it as it may, Wier was perhaps not a very original thinker, there was, however, one element that was sincerely innovative. Essentially, he instrumentalized a medical concept in a debate that was not really about humoural

35 On this case see Hans de Waardt, *Toverij en samenleving. Holland 1500–1800*, Haarlem 1991, p. 70 and the literature mentioned there.

36 James D. Tracy, *Erasmus of the Low Countries*, Berkeley 1996, pp. 93–94, 207.

pathology but about tolerance.[37] He did not alter the basic contents of this concept, but he did emphasize the elements of it that served his purpose, while passing over less useful details. It was his goal to exonerate the usual suspects in witch trials and to achieve that he twisted the medical concept of demonic possession a bit, just enough to deploy it in the rhetoric of tolerance.

37 In his *De ira morbo* (see n. 23), he does something similar. Alarmed by the havoc of the religious wars in both France and his native Low Countries, he there discusses possibilities to mend the senseless anger that in his view was the basis of the unprecedented ferocity of these conflicts. Again he deployed his medical knowledge in the hope that it could further the case of tolerance. In this book, however, he says nothing about demonic influence. See on this Hans de Waardt, "'Lightning strikes, wherever ire dwells with power': Johan Wier on anger as an illness", in: *Diseases of the Imagination* (see n. 20), pp. 260–274.

Olga van Marion

Lovesickness on Stage: Besotted Patients in 17th-Century Medical Handbooks and Plays[1]

1 Introduction

Were we to follow the advice from Dutch physician and philosopher Johan van Beverwijck (1594–1647), we would live healthy lives in balance with our environment and love our partners wisely and in moderation. At least, this is what the Dordrecht town physician and councillor proffers in his medical handbooks *Schat der gesontheyt* (1636, *Treasury of Health*) and *Schat der ongesontheyt* (1642, *Treasury of Sickness*). However, upsets in the balance of our humours as the Galenic doctrine knows them, and between the dichotomies warm-cold and moist-dry that come with the four elements, will not only lead to such diseases of the head as melancholy and madness but also to 'lovesickness' or 'love melancholy'. Those whose love is unbridled lose weight, pine away, shrivel up and eventually meet their death. Truly a serious disease that requires firm action. Van Beverwijck is following in a tradition here that goes back, via mediaeval tractates, to the love lessons from classical antiquity. The phenomenon of lovesickness or *amor hereos* is of all time and has from time immemorial been illustrated with *exempla* from world literature, from Homer to the Bible. For his part, Van Beverwijck also trots out stories of such famous lovers as Paris and Helen, from whose lecherous lusts sprang the entire Trojan war, or King David, who even had a subject's murder on his conscience because of his passion for Bathsheba. Thus, the disease and its disastrous impact are always presented by means of literature. The disorder itself is impossible to evidence by removing a stone from someone's intestines or conducting a post-mortem on a dead body; its symptoms may cause death and their danger can only be shown with terrifying examples. In this paper I will put side by side insights from medicine about

1 This article was written as part of the NWO Veni-project *Indigenous roots of the Dutch Renaissance. The conceptions of the medieval in early modern Dutch literature.* Thanks to Eli ten Lohuis for translating this article and to research master student Tim Vergeer for his help with finding quotations.

lovesickness and plays featuring sufferers from the disease, written by the two Dutch poets and playwrights Gerbrand Adriaensz. Bredero (1585–1618) and Theodore Rodenburgh (1574–1644).

2 Love symptoms

Since people who are desperately in love do nothing but think of their beloved day and night, their brain abstracts necessary heat from their stomach, according to medical man Van Beverwijck. Restless, the afflicted are unable to digest food, and this causes great numbers of 'rauwe humeuren' ('crude humours') to be retained in their body. These humours clog their veins, giving their faces a bloated, pale and melancholy aspect.[2] People in love, then, look extremely unhealthy to start with, but they go from bad to worse when they lose all their confidence in ever being united with their beloved. They fall silent, become anxious, irritable and wrathful, and lapse into melancholy gloom. At first sight, being infatuated may seem pleasant, especially in the beginning, when the lovers look at each other and through their eyes beauty 'hits their heart more quickly than a flying arrow', but this condition always ends in violent emotions and a great anxiety with which the lovers torment themselves. Their bodies are undermined by melancholy 'moistures' that press heavily on the brain and that slowly consume their flesh and bones.[3]

Van Beverwijck cites numerous writers before him who likewise pointed out the dangers of passionate love, including Plato, Lucian, the Spanish poet Cristóbal del Castillo, Plautus, Plutarch, Petrarch and Ovid. Among them is also the English scholar and vicar Robert Burton, who in his exhaustive encyclopaedic study *The Anatomy of Melancholy* (1621) adopts a distinction between, on the one hand, 'nuptial love' and, on the other, 'tyrant love' or 'heroical melancholy'; he terms the latter a disease, frenzy, madness, hell: 'It subverts kingdoms, overthrows cities, towns, families, mars, corrupts, and makes a massacre of men; thunder and lightning, wars, fires, plagues, have not done that mischief to

2 Johan van Beverwijck, *Schat der gesontheyt. Met verssen verçiert door Jacob Cats*, Dordrecht 1637, pp. 136–137; cf. Johan van Beverwyck, *Schat der gesontheyt. Met veersen verçiert door de Heer Jacb Cats, Ridder &c*, Deel 1, Amsterdam, Jan Jacobsz Schipper, 1660, p. 42. On Van Beverwijk, see Lia van Gemert, 'Johan van Beverwijck als 'instituut'', in: *De zeventiende eeuw* 8 (1992), pp. 99–106, Lia van Gemert, 'The power of the weaker vessels: Simon Schama and Johan van Beverwijck on women', in: *Women of the Golden Age: An International Debate on Women in Seventeenth-century Holland, England and Italy*, E. Kloek, N. Teeuwen and M. Huisman (eds.), Hilversum 1994, pp. 39–50 and Lia van Gemert, *De schat der gezondheid. Ziekte en genezing in de Gouden Eeuw. Bloemlezing uit het werk van de Dordtse arts Johan van Beverwijck*, Amsterdam 1992.

3 Johan van Beverwijck, *Schat der ongesontheyt*, Dordrecht 1644, pp. 406–407.

mankind, as this burning lust, this brutish passion. Let Sodom and Gomorrah, Troy, and I know not how many cities bear record.'[4] Even though the patients know that these and many similar miseries, threats or torments will undoubtedly beset them – Burton continues – they still allow themselves to be led like an ox to the slaughter, either out of their own weakness, their depraved nature or because of love's tyranny, which rages so furiously. Symptoms or signs of melancholy love are similar in many writers. Burton, too observes paleness, leanness and dryness in the patients; they are hollow-eyed, 'they pine away, and look ill with waking, cares, sighs.'[5] In his opinion, the best *exemplum* is Queen Dido, immortalized by Vergil in *Aeneis* 4:

> Unhappy Dido could not sleep at all,
> But lies awake, and takes no rest:
> And up she gets again, whilst care and grief,
> And raging love torment her breast.[6]

There are many such bodily symptoms by which lovers can be distinguished, Burton continues. Two of the most notable signs lie in the *pulsus amatorius* and in the patients' countenance: love makes for an irregular pulse and makes lovers blush at one another's sight, it causes them to tremble, sweat or gasp for breath. But the symptoms of lovers' minds are almost infinite, and so diverse that no human skill or learning can grasp them; every poet is full of catalogues of love symptoms, but fear and sorrow may deservedly lay claim to being the most important features. What is their impact on the human body? It is said that Empedocles, the philosopher, was present at the cutting up of someone who had died for love; his heart was burnt up, his liver was the dark colour of smoke, his lungs dried up to such an extent that he truly believed his soul was either sodden or roasted through the vehemence of love's fire. Which probably induced a modern writer of amorous emblems to express love's fury through a pot hanging over a fire, with Cupid blowing on the coals. Just as its heat consumes the water, so love dries up the moisture that is naturally inherent in a person.

3 Patients on the Dutch stage

One of the seventeenth-century plays to centre around lovesickness is Bredero's tragi-comedy *Lucelle* (1616). The passionate longing the rich merchant's daughter Lucelle feels is for a different man than the baron who is besotted with

4 Robert Burton, *The Anatomy of Melancholy*. Part 3, Sect. II. Memb. I. Consulted on http://www.gutenberg.org/files/10800/10800-h/ampart3.html [last retrieved on February 27, 2015].
5 Robert Burton, The Anatomy of Melancholy (see n. 4), Part 3, Sect. II. Memb. III.
6 Robert Burton, The Anatomy of Melancholy (see n. 4), Part 3, Sect. II. Memb. III.

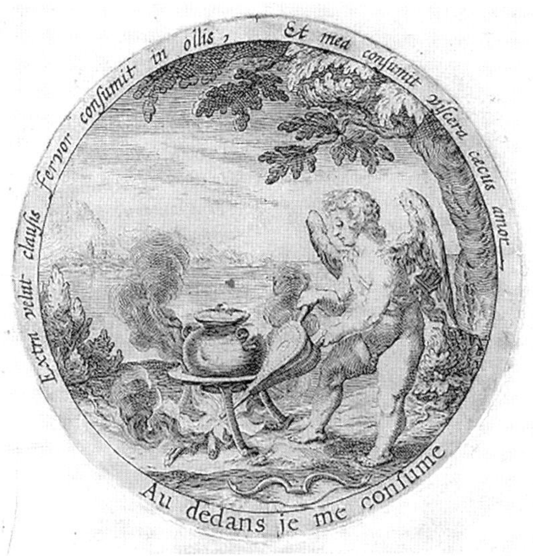

Fig. 1

her and to whom she is about to be married off. Voilà, the recipe for a box office hit that was performed for decades and whose printed version saw a great many reprints. The play opens on a dazzling dialogue between two men. Their conversation starts with how physical love traditionally begins: seeing the adored one. Baron has beheld Lucelle in person: 'This morning the fairest woman on earth showed herself 'oogenschijnlijck' (before my eyes).'[7] The glimpse has in an instant given the poor man more joy than he has experienced in his entire life.

This is immediately followed by a warning from a noble friend of the baron's, Adelaar, whose name, it is no coincidence, translates as 'eagle'. This clever man argues that love is blind, that Baron therefore cannot trust his own judgement:

> Love that is blind, and judges rashly
> Ugliness as a thing of beauty, just as it pleases her.[8]

His admonition falls on deaf ears. Baron plunges into misery and then there is no holding back: Lucelle's hair is as beautiful as the sun, as are her forehead, eyebrows, eyes, nose and chin; this enumeration of the beloved's beauties starts a Petrarchistic *catalogue-concetto* ending with Lucelle's virginity, which Baron eventually hopes to pluck.

As Adelaar makes another attempt to cure his friend of his mistaken views, his

7 G.A. Bredero, *Over-gesette Lucelle*, C.A. Zaalberg and M.J.M. de Haan (eds.), Culemborg 1972, p. 69.

8 G.A. Bredero, Over-gesette Lucelle (see n. 7), p. 69: 'De Minne die is blint, en oordeelt onvertsaacht / 'Tgoet voor quaat, 't lelijck schoon, na dattet haar behaacht.'

pleas turn out to be very similar to the precepts found in love tractates and medical handbooks. He argues that too strong a physical love is capable of conquering people as well as gods and of sending their passions in directions that are not good for them. Baron needs to understand that love damages our brain and that besides being blind, it is also completely unreliable:

The master of the gods, the ruler of mankind,
That governs our heart at his own discretion.
Love is blind, unpredictable, dissembling, deceitful,
Lawless, faithless, unchaste, untruthful.
Its arrows dipped in poison, blood, or grease,
He wounds whosoever he hits, whoever he hits he heals again.[9]

Once more, Adelaar is paid no heed. Rather than restrain himself, Baron continues to praise the divine power of love, the first thing to be created in prehistoric times by Chaos and the appointed ruler of the gods. Then Adelaar reproves his friend, reminding him of the famous literary *topos* of the two types of love or Eros: on the one hand, vulgar Eros, or earthly love, and, on the other hand, divine Eros, or divine love, well-known since Plato's *Symposium* and passed down in mediaeval tractates, as Mary Francis Wack demonstrates in her study of the Latin medical handbook *Viaticum* (where the particular type of love that is also called *eros* is considered a disease, *morbus*, of the brain involving desire and 'affliction of the thoughts')[10] and as Berhard Haage argues in his paper on *amor hereos* as a medical terminus technicus adopted in classical antiquity and the Middle Ages.[11] But it is not only via this route that playwright Bredero could have known about the by now widespread idea of two kinds of Venus – a chaste *Venus casta* and a shameless *Venus impudica:* he may also have come to the notion through the renewed attention that was directed to Plato's idea on the subject by the Neo-Platonist Marsilio Ficino in *De Amore* ('l'una Venere celeste, l'altra vulgare').[12] In any case, pal Adelaar wins the day with this point of view,

9 G.A. Bredero, Over-gesette Lucelle (see n. 7), p. 72: 'De meester van de Goon, de dwinger van de mensch, / Die onse sinlijckheyt bestuurt na wil en wensch. / De min is sichteloos, kindts, veynsend', logenachtich, / Wetteloos, trouweloos, onsuyver, onwaerachtich. / Sijn pijltjes zyn gedoopt in gift, in bloet, of smeer, / Het wondt al wie het raackt, wie't raackt die heeltet weer.'

10 The definition follows Galenic tradition in localizing sensation and passions in the brain rather than in the heart, where Aristotle puts them; Mary Frances Wack, *Lovesickness in the Middle Ages. The Viaticum and Its Commentaries*, Philadelphia 1990, p. 38.

11 Bernhard D. Haage, "'Amor hereos' als medizinischer Terminus technicus in der Antike und im Mittelalter", in: *Liebe als Krankheit. 3. Kolloquium der Forschungsstelle für europäische Lyrik des Mittelalters*, Theo Stemmler (ed.), Mannheim 1990, pp. 31–73.

12 Marsilio Ficino, *El libro dell'amore, a cura di Sandra Niccoli*, Olschki (ed.), Firenze 1987, cap. VII: 'l'una Venere celeste, l'altra vulgare; e la celeste esser nata da Celio sanza madre, la

emerging as the better debater. In his opinion, we should simply term the kind of love that his friend has in mind 'Cupid', or bestial lust or irrational will. This type weakens our body as well as our mind, is youth's enemy and may bring older people to the brink of disaster and – as Homer and Ovid showed through many an example – consume their intestines until death sets in:

> This Animal, or vermin, attractive and full of show,
> Seduces mankind with the flowers and the bees,
> But whoever tastes or swallows once this bitter sweet,
> He feels his insides shrivel up incurably,
> And he concludes his life with a miserable end.[13]

Again, the cautionary words are in vain. Baron is over the moon because of the glimpse he caught that morning of his beloved. That glimpse has sunk into his blood through his eyes and has gone straight into his stomach, where it now stirs his heart with sweet bitterness and pleasurable pain – Baron is fond of Petrarchistic imagery, while Adelaar again brings the classical examples to the fore: did not Biblical figures like Adam, David and Samson and mythological heroes such as Hercules, Paris and Jason suffer terribly at the hands of this intolerable brute, this 'love', this tyrant? With his next rejoinder, Baron unexpectedly gains the upper hand in the verbal duel with his friend. He gives him a dose of his own medicine. After all, isn't Adelaar himself deeply in love? Seeing as he behaves rather oddly when he is in the company of a certain beautiful Valerieke. As Baron describes Adelaar's amorous behaviour, we see some striking resemblances to medical observations as mentioned by Van Beverwijck: as soon as Adelaar is near his beloved, strong winds and thunderstorms blow up in his blood, upon which complete upheaval follows, with him no longer able to tense or move his muscles. Motionless, he stares ahead:

> How often I've seen you standing, removed from yourself,
> shattered and bereft of your senses;
> As soon as you saw that beauty, the woman of your soul,
> to whom your heart and brains are so devoted,
> then your limbs nor your muscles could tense anymore,
> and your brain can only run around in circles.[14]

---

volgare nata di Giove e di Dione.' Consulted on http://www.classicitaliani.it/ficino/ficino libro amore.htm [last retrieved on February 27, 2015].

13 G.A. Bredero, Over-gesette Lucelle (see n. 7), p. 75: 'Dit Dier, of ongediert, lieflockend' en schoonschijnich, / De menschen bloemtjes en de soete honich biet, / Maar wie dit bittre soet eens proeft of inne giet, / Die voelt zijn ingewant verscheuren en verschenden, / En hy besluyt zijn tijdt met een ellendich ende.'

14 G.A. Bredero, Over-gesette Lucelle (see n. 7), p. 78: 'Hoe dick sach ick u staan gelijck als uytgetogen, / Ontreddert en ontmant van menselijck vermogen, / Als ghy de schoone saacht,

That silences Adelaar and Baron leaves, his mind set on bringing about his conquest of the adored Lucelle.

4 Symptoms in female characters

How does Lucelle herself fare, the love-struck main character in Bredero's tragicomedy, who is an artistic and musical woman and, according to her father, composes verse in the style of the 'rederijkers' that sends her audiences into raptures? She does not appear on stage until the end of the first act, together with her lady companion. Rather surprisingly, she then does not say her lines but sings them as a stage song. At least, this much can be deduced from the fact that the lines are suddenly much shorter and are indented from the margin. The Meertens Instituut's Liederenbank (Song Bank) recognizes the lines as those of a stage song but has no melody to go with it, so we will have to make do with the text only.

Lucelle complains to Margrieta. She has no idea what has happened to her or what she might have swallowed to give her some inexplicable physical symptoms. She feels as if some kind of vapours has gone to her head: 'what kind of vapours has hit me in the head'. It is two months now, and her cheerfulness has changed to sorrow and her laughter turned into crying. She is seriously weakened and does nothing but complain and lament and weep all day. From her brain, a strange something seems to rush through her blood, tormenting her, a something that pervades her whole body and obtrudes itself into her heart:

> There's something in my brain,
> and something rushes through my blood,
> that gives me this torment,
> and goes through all my limbs,
> through all my senses and my mind.
> Yes, it spreads further
> until deep into my heart.
> There I often feel it obtrude itself
> making me terribly upset.[15]

Lucelle goes red and white by turns and feels all hot. Everything stinks, she thinks, and whatever she drinks tastes of bile. She has lost her appetite because

---

de vrouwe van u siel, / Daar hart en harsens bey soo heftich op an viel, / Dat ghy noch lijf noch le-en noch spieren niet en roerde, / En niet dan het gedacht zijn ambacht uyt en voerde.'

15 G.A. Bredero, Over-gesette Lucelle (see n. 7), p. 96: 'Daar leyt yet in mijn harsen, / En 'twemelt door mijn bloet / Dat my dees quelling doet, / En treckt door al mijn leden / Sinnen en sinlijckheden, / Ja 'twribbelt sich soo vart / Tot midden in mijn hart, / Daar voel ick't vaak opdringen / Met veel veranderingen.'

food tastes of nothing. What she does manage to get down, she retches, spits or vomits back out again. She is also plagued by sleeplessness. She is unable to lie quietly, keeps tossing and turning, and worries all night long:

I lie in bed, but cannot get to sleep,
I do nothing but lie awake,
I await with thousand worries
The so desired tomorrow.[16]

Once risen, she cannot concentrate and she will capriciously start on new activities without finishing any. It is, she says, a 'steady suffering', which eats her up as if 'consuming' her.

In the description Lucelle gives of her illness we recognize the traditional *topoi* of the pale, listless, emaciated and sleepless lover. Still, her account differs on two points from those the male lovers give of their symptoms. The first of these has already been mentioned: the strange vapours that have gone to her head. The other concerns an abundance of tears:

The best of my days
I waste (oh!) complaining,
Lamenting and in misery.
My eyes press hard from me
A sea of tears.[17]

These vapours and floods of tears are elements we did not encounter in the usually male examples of lovesickness given in the medical handbooks. Yet we do recognize something similar in a passage by Johan van Beverwijck where he writes about the moist nature of children and women. They are able to get rid of any surplus body fluids by crying.[18] We also find the vapours and tears in the seventeenth-century handbook on tears *De lacrymis* (1661) by the French philosopher and poet Pierre Petit. This handbook explains tears by means of the pneuma theory, according to which there is a connection between body and soul through various kinds of vapours: when someone feels sad, the vapours in the body are compressed, and this brings about crying.[19]

Tears are more suited to women than to men, according to Petit. This is very convenient when further on in the play all miseries reach a climax. Lucelle turns out to have secretly married her lover, who everybody believes to be of low birth.

16 G.A. Bredero, Over-gesette Lucelle (see n. 7), p. 97: 'Ick leg, en krijg geen vaack, / Ick doe niet dan ick waack: / Ick wacht met duysent sorgen / Na de gewenschte morgen.'
17 G.A. Bredero, Over-gesette Lucelle (see n. 7), p. 96: 'Het beste van mijn dagen / Verslijt ick (och!) in klagen, / In treuren en in wee: / Mijn oogen my een Zee / Van traantjes streng uytparsen.'
18 Lia van Gemert, Ziekte en genezing in de Gouden Eeuw (see n. 2), p. 25.
19 Pierre Petit, *De Lacrymis Libri tres*, Parijs 1661, passim.

When he is made to drain the poisoned cup as punishment, she despairs and decides to take poison as well to end her life. She does so theatrically besides her husband's dead body. The women and men who have gathered around the now deceased couple react in gender-specific ways. The besotted Baron lets loose a torrent of reproaches at the lifeless Lucelle on whom he has wasted so much time, while in the background Margrieta tearfully mourns the dead couple.

5 Lovesickness in a historical character

The second play to assign an important role to lovesickness takes us to the year 1638. When, in January of that year, the Amsterdam Theatre opens with a series of tragedies about mediaeval lords and counts (Vondel's *Gysbreght* and the plays by P.C. Hooft and Suffridus Sixtinus about the political murder of Floris V, Count of Holland), the end of the season has a play that features for its main protagonist a female ruler from the national past. It was to be the last play that prolific and controversial poet-diplomat Theodore Rodenburgh would write. His 'historial' play *Vrou Iacoba* is devoted to Countess Jacqueline of Bavaria (1401–1436). This combative Countess of Holland and Zeeland was especially known for having during her life suffered greatly with a series of failed love relationships. She had been married off as a child to John of Touraine, the French Dauphin, who died young, and as a girl, to her cousin, John IV, Duke of Brabant, who she divorced; as a young woman, she had chosen Humphrey, Duke of Gloucester, who did not keep his promises. Next, in 1428, at the Reconciliation of Delft, a political promise had been extracted from her that she would never again marry.

Poets and historiographers agreed that this young countess, widowed and fatherless at the age of sixteen, and then twice married unhappily, had plumbed the depths of misery when robbed of her counties and financially at rock bottom, she awaited the end of her life in loneliness, at a certain moment not even capable of properly rewarding a couple of envoys. The mediaeval chronicle *D'oude Chronijcke* that hides no secrets about Jacqueline's love life already makes a first move towards a sad play: 'Then she burst into bitter tears and went into her room, lamenting her shame and the fact that her friends had deserted her'.[20] Playwright Rodenburgh took up this sad story element, turning it into a scene for the stage. It must have made quite an impression. In the middle of the first act, the countess remains behind on stage, all by herself and it is at that moment that

20 Wouter van Gouthoeven, *D'oude Chronijcke ende Historien van Holland (met west-Vriesland) van Zeeland ende van Wtrecht. Van nieus oversien, vermeerdert, verbetert*, Dordrecht 1620, p. 457: 'Doe wert sy seer bitterlijc schreyende, ende ginc in haer kamer beclagende de ongetrouwigheyt van hare vrienden, ende hare confuselijcke schande.'

she starts a song about her misery. The tune to which this song can be sung is probably that of the Magnificat. Again, as in Bredero, a female protagonist is presented who suffers from lovesickness and expresses her sorrow in a sad stage song.

The song starts with the idea that most people who are ill or miserable seek distraction and a means to escape from their worries:

> Whoever has a heavily laden heart
> That is tormented by sorrow,
> Seeks distraction to cheer themselves up.
> Just like most people
> Who have exhausted their bodies
> Seek out a little spot to rest.[21]

From the second stanza onwards, Jacqueline identifies with the content. Others may find distraction, but that is not for her. In a triad that ends in a climax she explains to us that she cannot manage to forget her past. Her memories are too vivid, her memory too cruel and her experiences too harrowing:

> My joy I lost,
> as the sad choir of my senses
> showed me the past again,
> and as all my memories
> of the misery that fate has given me,
> appeared all too real before me.
> If only I could forget
> what fate has brought me,
> then I would feel so happy.
> But my memory is
> like an executioner unto my soul:
> nothing but sorrow and misery.[22]

We recognize in Jacqueline's description the restlessness that is characteristic of lovesickness as well as the phenomenon of the patient thinking of only one thing,

---

21 Theodore Rodenburgh, *Vrou Iacoba Erf-Gravinne van Hollandt, &c*, Amsterdam 1638, fol. B2r: 'Een overladen hert / Door droefheytsquel verwart, / Soeckt heugelijck vermaken: / Gelijck als int ghemeen / De af-ghesloofde leen / Nae rustingh plaetse haken.' For this play, also see: Olga van Marion and Tim Vergeer, 'Gezongen emoties. Toneelliederen in Rodenburghs *Vrou Iacoba* bij de opening van de nieuwe Schouwburg', in: *De zeventiende eeuw* 30–2 (2014), pp. 168–184 and Rick Honings and Olga van Marion (eds.), *Vrouw van het Vaderland. Jacoba van Beieren in literatuur en kunst*, Haarlem, 2011.

22 Theodore Rodenburgh, Vrou Iacoba Erf-Gravinne van Hollandt (see n. 21), fol. B2r: 'Mijn vreughde ick verloor, / Als 't droeve sinnens-koor / Verleden doent af-beelden, / Vermits dat het gedacht, / Van 't gun 't gheval my bracht, / Te werckelijck in speelden. / Dat ick vergeten mocht: 't Gun 't ongeluck my brocht, / Ick achten my gheluckigh, Maer het gheheugen wis / Mijn ziels beulinne is, / Te droevigh en te druckigh.'

running around in circles as if crazy and being seriously weakened. In Robert Burton's words: 'And when he is gone, he thinks every minute an hour, every hour as long as a day, ten days a whole year, till he see her again.'[23]

Also, the wish to die presents itself. The idea of ending her miserable life appears twice in Jacqueline's song. First, the countess raises the question in general whether she will renounce her God-given task (de 'Hemels-vooght versaken', forsake the Heavenly father) and 'like a cowardly woman' run from her duty as a ruler to act as a shepherd to her people. Obviously, her reaction is a resounding 'no'. By addressing herself in an exclamation with a double 'no' ('Jacqueline, no, oh, no!') she answers in the negative the desperate question whether she should run away from her duties. The next question is implicit: how could Jacqueline revenge herself or atone for everything that has gone wrong? The answer 'Revenge yourself through weeping' can be understood in the light of Christian ethics that especially women could wash away their sins by shedding tears. Crying had a cleansing effect and thus was a form of penance. Jacqueline's tears, sweeter than revenge, will be shed for the sake of her subjects:

> Jacqueline, no, oh no!
> Revenge yourself through weeping,
> and let your tears be a sacrifice.
> Be content with whatever falls to you,
> that will be a laurel wreath
> for all your subjects.[24]

The second time Countess Jacqueline contemplates suicide in her song surpasses the first. She has suffered so much that she cannot cope anymore:

> Of the world's sound and fury
> I have had, alas,
> so excessively much!
> Yes so that my soul is
> stirred most strongly
> to leave the world behind.[25]

At this point in the two plays, both female protagonists Lucelle and Jacqueline have, before the very eyes of their audiences, reached the point of suicide. Both women are driven by lovesickness, with the countess also bewailing her political

23 Robert Burton, The Anatomy of Melancholy (see n. 4), Part 3, Sect. II. Memb. III.

24 Theodore Rodenburgh, Vrou Iacoba Erf-Gravinne van Hollandt (see n. 21), fol. B2r: 'Jacoba, neen, ach neen! / Wreeckt u door u gheween, / En offert op u Tranen. / Ghenoeght u met u dans, / 't Sal zijn een Laure-krans / Voor al uw Onder-danen.'

25 Theodore Rodenburgh, Vrou Iacoba Erf-Gravinne van Hollandt (see n. 21), fol. B2v: 'Uyt Wereltsche geraes / Heb ick ghehadt, helaes! / Soo veel in over-maten, / Jae dat mijn ziele wort / Seer ernstigh gheport: / De Werelt te verlaten'.

defeats. Bredero's merchant daughter Lucelle throws herself on her husband's dead body, about to drink from the same poisoned cup, while Rodenburgh's Countess Jacqueline, in more abstract terms, adheres to her intended 'leave-taking from the world'. How will this end?

The two playwrights are not free to choose their endings. The author of the 'historial play', Rodenburgh has to abide by the facts in his historical source. This is the mediaeval chronicle mentioned earlier, which in his times was so widely read that in 1636, two years before *Vrou Iacoba* was staged, a new reprint appeared. It recounts extensively how Countess Jacqueline of Bavaria did not commit suicide but lived on for a few more years.[26] Poet Bredero too is bound to his source – the French play that he took for his starting point. His *Lucelle* is an adaptation of the *Lucelle* by Louis Le Jars (1576), which, for all that it was written in prose and contains no songs at all, yet as a tragi-comedy has a happy ending that audiences will have come to love.

Moreover, both poets will have felt bound to Christian ethics, within which suicide is unacceptable. Famous Dutch handbooks on love such as *Der minnen loep* (ca. 1411) by the Hague court poet Dirc Potter strongly denounce all cases of disastrous love relations ending in suicide. For instance, Dirc Potter adds a strong warning to the sorrowful story of the forbidden love of the mythological characters Hero and Leander, which ends with Hero's suicide. He urges his readers not to lose their head when loving and to always endure their suffering wisely if their partner has been unfaithful:

> And so I put my advice on paper for you:
> you should love wisely
> and suffer patiently
> when someone is unfaithful to you,
> since you must spare your soul at all times.[27]

If literary tradition and the renown of their protagonists made it impossible for the two playwrights to have the besotted patients Lucelle and Jacqueline commit suicide, what then did eventually happen with these characters?

26 Wouter van Gouthoeven, *D'oude Chronijcke ende historien van Holland (met West-Uriesland) van Zeeland ende van Utrecht. Beginnende vanden Jare onses Heeren 449. tot dit teghenwoordigh Jaer 1636*, 's-Gravenhage 1636, p. xxxxx.

27 Dirc Potter, *Der minnen loep* I, v. 454–458, P. Leendertz (ed.), Wz. Part 1. Leiden 1845, p. 19: 'Daer om scrivic u minen raet, / Dat ghi wiselic minnen sult, / Ende lyden een heymelic verdult / Wanneer u ontrouwe wedervaert / Die ziele moet ymmer sijn ghespaert.' Also see Olga van Marion, *Heldinnenbrieven. Ovidius' Heroides in Nederland*, Nijmegen 2005, p. 57.

6 Lovesickness and the means to be cured of it

To cure lovesickness, physician Johan van Beverwijck in his *Treasury of Sickness* recommends calling in a doctor to the sick person. He will quickly observe that the invalid's pulse has quickened and that his urine looks reddish and fiery because of the waking, fasting and the constant restlessness that has brought an infection to the blood and brain. The doctor cannot but judge that he has a 'binnen-koortsche' (internal fever) on his hands or that there is some other infection in the body. Should the doctor suspect a case of love pain, then he will need to look carefully for changes in the patient's exterior and pulse rate as soon as the object of love comes near the patient. Galen himself once exposed a secret love in this manner.[28] Still, Van Beverwijck has to admit that being cured of this disease is hardly possible. Even Apollo, the god of medicine who has power over medicinal herbs, once complained to the poet Ovid that he himself could not be cured of love. If one is quick, and fights the incipient love pain from its very start, one stands a chance of recovering but if the pain is already deep-seated and has the upper-hand in the body, the disease will turn into insanity. Those afflicted thus will slowly waste away, their bodies dehydrated. Some patients take their own lives.[29]

In his *Treasury of Health* Van Beverwijck is a fraction more optimistic. A sufferer of lovesickness may be cured by, as it were, throwing himself on his beloved to get rid of his complaint; however, care should always be taken that the relation is not incestuous in nature, or otherwise forbidden. In some cases blood-letting will help, as will a mixture of rue seed and, among other things, coriander.[30] A general remedy for all diseases is to seek recourse in God, whose grace constitutes a Christian medicine. And, we should always tell the truth to those who are tormented by lovesickness: make clear that they have taken leave of their senses and better judgement and that they will be ill until they meet their death, a therapy that, as the author states, goes back to Aristotle's *Ethics*. It is a great pity, though, that the disease is so persistent and that the patients ignore all advice and are impervious to reason.[31]

In the first play examined in this paper, Bredero's *Lucelle*, sound advice was of no avail. For a long time, the 'patient' Baron races like a madman after the woman he is besotted with and he does not regain his senses until at the end of the play when the rival he intends to murder turns out to be a relative. By that time, the rival himself has already ended his life. Beside the dead body of her

28 Johan van Beverwijck, *Schat der ongesontheyt, ofte genees-konste van de sieckten*, 2nd ed., Dordrecht 1644, pp. 410–411.

29 Van Beverwijck, Schat der ongesontheyt 1644 (see n. 28), p. 417.

30 Van Beverwijck, Schat der ongesontheyt 1644 (see n. 28), pp. 419–420.

31 Van Beverwijck, Schat der gesontheyt 1660 (see n. 2), p. 43.

beloved, Lucelle has drunk of the poison and she would surely have died if it had not been for an apothecary who rushes up to reveal that he has merely concocted a sleeping draught. Towards the end of the fifth act the couple has recovered, everyone's honour has been saved, and a big wedding feast is laid on.

The second play, Rodenburgh's *Vrou Iacoba*, similarly ends with wedding celebrations. In line with the mediaeval chronicle, the countess finally finds happiness by secretly entering into a fourth marriage, with the Zeeland nobleman Francis, Lord of Borssele, who hastens to help her out financially, invites her to an intimate dinner and romantically asks for her hand and heart in a beautifully adorned dining room.[32] After some tense political intrigue Jacqueline chooses to also renounce her last counties and her marriage can be solemnized in public, which is performed spectacularly in tableaux vivants on the Theatre's stage.[33]

The two plays examined above show how both male and female characters (Baron, Lucelle and Jacqueline) suffer from lovesickness and behave as patients whose conduct corresponds with the symptoms of the disease as described in medical handbooks. The personae are in torment, listless, by turns pale and red, restless, they go without sleep, are obsessed with their sorrow and they long for death. From a literary point of view, they are presented with a great deal of effect (stage songs, female tears) and emotional stylistic devices. Lovesick patients on stage are negative *exempla* that are to instil fear and compassion and with which audiences can identify themselves. Even we, as readers in the 21st century, can take warning from them. Meanwhile, the characters are never punished for their excessive conduct in the area of love. In the final act, Lucelle and Jacqueline are even allowed to marry the men of their dreams. Literature may hold up an image of the world to us, but that does not mean that all earthly woes need to be represented: it remains fiction.

---

32 Jacqueline's modern biographer entertains serious doubts about the historicity of this fourth marriage, which is mentioned in one late source only: ANTHEUN JANSE, *Een pion voor een dame. Jacoba van Beieren, 1401–1436*, Amsterdam 2009.

33 OLGA VAN MARION and TIM VERGEER, Gezongen emoties (see n. 21), pp. 180–181.

Bettina Noak

Pictures of Melancholia in Four Tragedies by Joost van den Vondel

1 Introduction

The subject of 'knowledge and literature' to which this volume is dedicated has experienced a large boom in research over the last few decades.[1] One important section is research into how medical concepts are mirrored in early modern literature.[2] Hereby, it is important to note that the relationship between the (medical) knowledge and the literal representation of the same is bilateral; on the one hand medical findings are added directly to literature and thereby add to an extended and widened debate. On the other hand, literature, when used as a field for experiments on human passions is predestined to induce new findings which influence the knowledge about the human form and the interaction between the body and the soul.[3] Naturally, this also applies to the genre of drama in which the physical and psychological suffering of humankind has been dealt with since antiquity.[4]

1 Cf. the volume: ROLAND BORGARDS ET AL. (eds.), *Literatur und Wissen: ein interdisziplinäres Handbuch*, Stuttgart 2013 with an overview over the research and the relevant research literature.

2 Cf. e.g. SALLY CRAWFORD and CHRISTINA LEE (eds.), *Bodies of knowledge: cultural interpretations of illness and medicine in Medieval Europe*, Oxford 2010; JAN FRANS VAN DIJKHUIZEN and KARL ENENKEL (eds.), *The Sense of Suffering. Constructions of Physical Pain in Early Modern Culture*, Leiden 2009; ROBERT JÜTTE, *Krankheit und Gesundheit in der Frühen Neuzeit*, Stuttgart 2013; STEPHEN PENDER and NANCY S. STRUEVER (eds.), *Rhetoric and Medicine in Early Modern Europe*, Farnham/Burlington 2012; MARC PRIEWE, *Textualizing Illness: Medicine and Culture in New England 1620–1730*, Heidelberg 2014; JENNIFER C. VAUGHT (ed.), *Rhetorics of Bodily Disease and Health in Medieval and Early Modern England*, Farnham/Burlington 2010.

3 Cf. for the genreal relationship between illness and literature CARSTEN ZELLE, 'Medizin', in: ROLAND BORGARDS ET AL. (eds.), *Literatur und Wissen: ein interdisziplinäres Handbuch*, Stuttgart 2013, pp. 85–95; HARALD NEUMEYER, 'Medizin und Literatur', in: ANSGAR NÜNNING (ed.), *Metzler Lexikon Literatur- und Kulturtheorie: Ansätze – Personen – Grundbegriffe*. 5e editie. Stuttgart 2013, pp. 504–505.

4 Cf. JONATHAN GIL HARRIS, *Sick Economies. Drama, Mercantilism, and Disease in Shakespeare's England*, Pennsylvania 2003; ALLISON P. HOBGOOD, *Passionate Playgoing in Early*

Lately in the research on the tragedies of Joost van den Vondel (1587–1679), a debate has been established to shed light on the anthropological side of his tragedies. This then caused the expansion of older approaches and research frameworks, which wanted to see the poet's works as a part of the early modern dramatic theoretic development – between Senecan-Scaligerian and Aristotelian Drama – ; of his religious meaning – from moderate Protestantism to Catholicism – or in terms of his political implications – fight for freedom of belief and class-oriented rights.[5] This article has been explicitly written in connection with this research. In regards to the question of the reflection of aspects of early modern concepts of melancholia in Vondel's works, hopefully a further aspect of the discussion on the anthropological question will be added to the research.

Traditionally, historical and literary works were seen as case studies when describing melancholia. Since the early modern period, Shakespeare's (1564–1616) figure *Hamlet* (1603) was seen as a prototype of the melancholic character in drama.[6] In research, attention was paid to a connection between mania, obsession and theatricality. B.P. Levack, for example, refers to the performative nature of obsession which describes almost a 'theatrical disease'.[7] The common denominator between the theatre and the manifestation of mania is the recourse to the imagination, the pathological disturbance of which can be seen as a symptom of melancholia. The source of these fantasies was the cause of heavy debate in the early modern period: are they caused by natural disturbances in the circulation of natural bodily fluids and the Pneumatic household in the body, or are they caused by the influence of spirits or demons who take command of the soul of the 'obsessed'.

Modern England, Cambridge 2014; Jan Konst, *Woedende wraakghierigheidt en vruchtelooze weeklachten: de hartstochten in de Nederlandse tragedie van de zeventiende eeuw*, Assen 1993.

5 Cf. Freya Sierhuis, 'Therapeutic tragedy: compassion, remorse, and reconciliation in the Joseph plays of Joost van den Vondel (1635–1640)', in: *European Review of History: Revue europeenne d'histoire* 17 (2010), pp. 27–51; Kristine Steenbergh, 'Compassion and the Creation of an Affective Community in the Theatre. Vondel's *Mary Stuart, or Martyred Majesty* (1646)', in: *BMGN – Low Countries Historical Review* 129 (2014), pp. 90–112. On the Vondel-research see Riet Schenkeveld-van der Dussen, 'Vondel's Works for the Stage Read and Studied over Centuries', in: Jan Bloemendal and Frans-Willem Korsten (eds.), *Joost van den Vondel (1587–1679). Dutch Playwright in the Golden Age*, Leiden/Boston 2012, pp. 7–22. For general information on Vondel's dramas cf. W.A.P. Smit, *Van Pascha tot Noah. Een verkenning van Vondel's drama's naar continuïteit en ontwikkeling in hun grondmotief en structuur*, 3 vols. 2nd edition, Zwolle, 1970; Jan Bloemendal and Frans-Willem Korsten (eds.), *Joost van den Vondel (1587–1679). Dutch Playwright in the Golden Age*, Leiden/Boston 2012.

6 On Shakespeare and melancholy cf. Douglas Trevor, *The poetics of melancholy in early modern England*, Cambridge 2004, pp. 63–86.

7 Cf. Brian P. Levack, *The Devil Within. Possession and Exorcism in the Christian West*, New Haven/London 2013, pp. 29–30. See also Jan Frans van Dijkhuizen, *Devil Theatre. Demonic Possession and Exorcism in English Renaissance Drama, 1558–1642*, Cambridge 2007.

Vondel's relationship to melancholia and melancholics in light of contemporary medical theories is to be in the forefront of this article. Four tragedies will provide the basis for this contribution: *Palamedes* (1625); *Maeghden* (*Maidens*, 1639); *Peter en Pauwels* (1641) and *Maria Stuart* (1646).[8] The connection between tragic drama and the doctrine of melancholia can already be seen in Walter Benjamin's book *Ursprung des deutschen Trauerspiels* (*The Origin of German Tragic Drama*, 1928).[9] In Benjamin's study, the centre stage is taken by the tyrant, the very antithesis of the martyr. His power doesn't correspond to his creatural existence, making him a victim of constant fear, which ultimately drives him mad. As will become apparent in this article, even the martyr can become a victim of melancholia in its diverse manifestations.

Until now, research has occasionally made a connection between Vondel's dramas and a (temporary) mania: his model tragedy *Jeptha* (1659) shows the hero suffering from cognitive disturbance after he committed the in his eyes unavoidable sacrifice by killing his daughter. However, *Jeptha's* wife remained unable to free herself from her mania caused by the immeasurable grief of losing her child.[10] Another female figure who falls prey to deterioration of the mind after a traumatic event is Rispe in Vondel's drama *Gebroeders* (*Brothers*, 1640).[11] It would though be premature to claim that Vondel only portrayed women as the victims of madness, as was done in the discourse on hysteria in 18th and 19th century.[12] In the case of Ursula in *Maeghden* or Maria Stuart in the play of the

8 For a chronological overview of Vondel's dramas see Eddy Grootes and Riet Schenkeveld-van der Dussen, 'Vondel's Dramas: A Chronological Survey', in: Jan Bloemendal and Frans-Willem Korsten (eds.), *Joost van den Vondel* (see n. 5), 1–6. I used the following edition of Vondel's dramas: Joost van den Vondel, *De werken. Volledige en geïllustreerde tekstuitgave*, ed. by J.F.M. Sterck et. al. 10 vols., Amsterdam 1927–1937 (= *WB*). Cf. http://www.dbnl.org/titels/titel.php?id=vond001dewe00 [last retrieved on March 3, 2015].

9 Cf. Walter Benjamin, *The origin of German tragic drama*, transl. by John Osborne. 2. impr., London 1990. For an analysis of Benjamin's tragedy book cf. Bettina Menke, *Das Trauerspiel-Buch. Der Souverän – das Trauerspiel – Konstellationen – Ruinen*, Bielefeld 2010.

10 Cf. for Vondel's 'model tragedy' *Jeptha*: W.A.P. Smit, *Van Pascha tot Noah* (see n. 5), vol. 2, pp. 240–379. For the interpretation of the protagonist Jeptha and his wife Filopaie see the discussion between Konst en Korsten: Jan Konst, "Geen kinderhaet verruckt u tot dees daet': de schuldconceptie in Vondels *Jeptha, Koning David herstelt* en *Faëton*', in: *Spiegel der letteren* 39 (1997), pp. 263–284 and the reaction by Frans-Willem Korsten, 'Waartoe hij zijn dochter slachtte: *Enargeia* in een moderne retorische benadering van Vondels *Jeptha*', in: *Tijdschrift voor Nederlandse Taal- en Letterkunde* 115 (1999), pp. 315–333 and the replica Jan Konst, 'De motivatie van het offer van Ifis: Een reactie op de *Jeptha*-interpretatie van F.-W. Korsten', in: *Tijdschrift voor Nederlandse Taal- en Letterkunde* 116 (2000), pp. 153–169. Cf. F.-W. Korsten, *Sovereignty as Inviolability. Vondel's theatrical Explorations in the Dutch Republic*, Hilversum 2009, particul. pp. 69–89.

11 Cf. For *Brothers* W.A.P. Smit, *Van Pascha tot Noah* (see n. 5), vol. 1, pp. 265–302.

12 Cf. Franziska Lamott, *Die vermessene Frau. Hysterien um 1900*, München 2001; Sabine Arnaud, *L'invention de l'hystérie au temps des Lumières (1670–1820)*, Paris 2014.

same name, the poet shows female figures who, by virtue of their psychological strength, can withstand melancholia.

The following article will research how Vondel treated the different appearances of melancholia. In doing so, I shall attempt to adhere to two different forms: as created in the dichotomous structure of Vondel's drama, there is the melancholia of the believers, the martyrs on the one hand; on the other there is the melancholia of those who do not believe in the Christian god, the non-believers and the tyrants. In this regard Vondel's works repeat the double view of the philosophical and medical theories of the renaissance, which on the one hand sees melancholia as an illness with natural and supernatural causes; on the other hand as proof of a certain kind of intellectual and moral divine election. This contribution is to be based on four motives for analysis: firstly, the imaginations of *conscience* which causes the ruin of the tyrant figures; secondly the figures of the cannibalistic *incorporation* which Vondel connected to religious mania; thirdly, the *ego impoverishment* of the melancholic and lastly, the chances for therapy as a *breakthrough* in the melancholic disposition.[13]

2 Melancholia in the Early Modern Period

If, in the early 20th Century, the medical world understood melancholia to be a type of depression, for example as shown in Sigmund Freud's small study *Trauer und Melancholie* (*Mourning and Melancholia*, 1917); from antiquity to well into 18th century, it was seen as a form of mania. In his *Handbuch der Pathologie* (*Handbook of Pathology*, 1799), Wilhelm Friedrich Dreyßig stated e.g. that: 'Under Melancholia, I understand a partial mania, or partial fault in judgement and ability to draw conclusions which is then limited to a certain object or to certain objects.'[14] The beginnings of the medical philosophical occupation with melancholia can be traced by to antiquity. The term was first used in the *Corpus Hippocraticum* in the essay *On Airs, Waters and Places* (written in the last third of 5th century BCE).[15] In later writings, melancholia is connected to the doctrine of humours usual at the time (humoralism).[16] The creation of melancholia was seen

13 The term 'ego impoverishment' ('Ichverarmung') can be found in Sigmund Freud's essay *Trauer und Melancholie* (*Mourning and Melancholia*, 1917). Sigmund Freud, 'Mourning and Melancholia', in: *The Standard Edition of the Complete Psychological Works of Sigmund Freud*, ed. by James Strachey et al. vol. XIV, reprint London 1963, pp. 243–258.

14 Wilhelm Friedrich Dreyßig, *Handbuch der Pathologie der sogenannten chronischen Krankheiten*, vol. 2, Leipzig 1799, p. 605 (translation by the translator of the article).

15 Cf. Hellmut Flashar, *Melancholie und Melancholiker in den medizinischen Theorien der Antike*, Berlin 1966, p. 21 et. seq.

16 For the following paragraphs see in general Roy Porter, *A social history of madness: stories of the insane*, London 1987; Wolfgang Uwe Eckhart, 'Vom Wahn zum Wahnsinn', in:

to be an excess of black bile (Greek mélas: black, cholē: bile), which gave the illness its name. Galen describes the illness as a suffering of the conscious mind, symptomised by a deep sadness and the tendency to withdraw from societal life. At the same time, even in antiquity a second way of seeing melancholia emerged. Under the influence of the pseudo-Aristotelian *Problems* (*Fragment XXX, 1*), melancholic people were assigned extraordinary mental abilities. Under this school of thought, probably from 9th Century Arabic sources, melancholia was now given an astrological association; the melancholic temperament was seen to be under the influence of the planet Saturn.

During the middle ages, for example, Constantinus Africanus (1017–1087) emphasised the manic character of melancholia. For him, melancholia is a result of the evaporations of black bile, which rise to the brain and cause manic hallucinations: 'The general symptoms of all kinds are constant, for example despondency, fear of things for which one need not fear, pondering on unimportant matters, perceiving awful things which are not there, unreal sensations. The sufferers see before their eyes horrible black creatures and similar.'[17] Also, melancholia was connected to the 'monk's illness' of the *acedia*. This constant deep sadness was counted to the seven deadly sins. The manic hallucinations of the sufferers connect melancholia with the problems of obsession. Fear and the spectre of terror were often described as the influence of the devil or certain demons in the early modern period, whereby there was also constant criticism of this view, for example from Johan Wier (1515/16–1588).[18]

Both schools of thought on melancholia were cultivated since the renaissance. On the one hand, the opinion regarding mania and impaired judgement remained. On the other hand, Marsilio Ficino (1433–1499) founded a new, more positive, view of melancholia in his book *De triplici vita* (*Three Books on Life*, 1489).[19] He saw melancholia as being influenced by psychological genius and

---

Silke Leopold and Agnes Speck (eds.), *Hysterie und Wahnsinn*, Heidelberg 2000, pp. 10–30; Wolfgang Uwe Eckart, 'Wahn', in: Bettina von Jagow and Florian Steger, *Literatur und Medizin: ein Lexikon*, Göttingen 2005, pp. 842–851; William G. Naphy and Angelika Dworzak, 'Melancholie', in: *Enzyklopädie der Neuzeit*, ed. by Friedrich Jaeger, vol. 8, Stuttgart 2008, pp. 317–319. Further studies: Raymond Klibansky, Erwin Panofsky and Fritz Saxl, *Saturn and melancholy: studies in the history of natural philosophy, religion and art*, London, 1964; Johann Anselm Steiger, *Melancholie, Diätetik und Trost. Konzepte der Melancholie-Therapie im 16. und 17. Jahrhundert*, Heidelberg 1996; Julia Kristeva, *Schwarze Sonne. Depression und Melancholie*, Suhrkamp, Frankfurt/M. 1998; Burkhart Brückner, *Delirium und Wahn. I. Band: Vom Altertum bis zur Aufklärung*, Hürtgenwald 2007; Andrea Sieber (ed.), *Melancholie zwischen Attitüde und Diskurs. Konzepte in Mittelalter und Früher Neuzeit*, Göttingen 2009.

17 Quoted from Wolfgang Uwe Eckart, 'Wahn', in: *Literatur und Medizin* (see n. 16), p. 844.

18 Cf. the article by Hans de Waardt in this volume.

19 For an English edition see Marsilius Ficinus, *Three books on life*, a crit. ed. and transl. with introd. and notes by Carol V. Kaske, Binghamton/New York 1989.

divine inspiration. One of the most important works of the early modern period on melancholia is Robert Burton's (1577–1640) *The Anatomy of Melancholy* (first edition in 1621).[20] Under the pseudonym Democritus Junior, he wrote a humanistic treatise on the subject, based on diverse sources on the subject available at the time and in which he analysed the different causes and forms of melancholia. For Burton, physical and genetic (hereditary) causes of the condition are as possible as demonic or divine punishment or the influence of witchcraft and astrology. In the style of Erasmus' (1466/69–1536), *Moriae encomium* (*In Praise of Folly*, 1511) he represents the world in its entirety as a victim of mania or melancholia.

3 Melancholia in Johan van Beverwijck

Melancholia also played an important role in the medical discourse of the early modern Dutch republic. The physician and humanist Johan van Beverwijck (1594–1647) can be seen here as an exemplary author in this field.[21] He became famous, above all, through two works, namely *Schat der gesontheyt* (*Treasure of Health*, 1636, 1671 and 1674) and *Schat der ongesontheyt* (*Treasure of Illness*, 1643, 1671 and 1674), which appeared in various new editions and were translated into German by Philipp von Zesen (1619–1689). Van Beverwijck defined melancholia as follows:

> *Melancholye*, is onder de sieckten, die, gelijck *Galenus* schrijft, haren naem hebben van de oorsaeck: te weten, de Melancholijcke vochtigheyt. Maer wy noemen de selvige nae haer werckinge, *Swaermoedigheyt*, is een krancksinnigheydt, meestendeel vermengt met schrick, en benaeutheyt van herten, selden met vreught, en vermaeck, sonder Koortsche, ontstaende uyt een vaste en verkeerde inbeeldinge. En gelijck in andere soorten van *Rasernye*, soo wert oock alhier de *Inbeeldinghe* en *'t Verstant* beschadight: maer insonderheyt de inbeeldinge. Want het *Oordeel* der Melancholijken staet dickwils een dingh de verkeerde inbeeldinge toe, en de Melancholijken nemen voor waer aen,

20 *The Anatomy of Melancholy* is available via Project Gutenberg: http://www.gutenberg.org/files/10800/10800-h/10800-h.htm [last retrieved on March 3, 2015]. Cf. for research Angus Gowland, *The Worlds of Renaissance Melancholy. Robert Burton in Context*, Cambridge 2006.

21 Cf. regarding Van Beverwijck: Gerrit Arie Lindeboom, *Geschiedenis van de medische wetenschap in Nederland*, 2nd edition, Haarlem 1981, pp. 44, 75–75; Lia van Gemert, 'Johan van Beverwijck als instituut', in: *De zeventiende eeuw* 8 (1992), pp. 99–106; Lia van Gemert, 'Severing what was joined together: debates about pain in the seventeenth-century Dutch Republic', in: Jan Frans van Dijkhuizen and Karel Enenkel (eds.), *The Sense of Suffering. Constructions of Physical Pain in Early Modern Culture*, Leiden/Boston 2009, pp. 443–468; Bettina Noak, 'Samen und Worte – sprachliche und natürliche Zeugung bei Johan van Beverwijck und Jacob Cats', in: Lydia Bauer and Antje Wittstock (eds.), *Text-Körper. Anfänge – Spuren – Überschreitungen*, Berlin 2014, pp. 35–57.

dat valsch is, daer sy in andere saken (het welck *Vives* niet sonder reeden vremt en dunckt) wel en wijslijck oordeelen.[22]

According to Van Beverwijck, the manifestation of melancholia depends on the world which the melancholic inhabits, therefore, there are innumerable different types.[23] This connects melancholia with dreams, since the melancholic is nothing other than a person living a waking dream.[24] Although Hippocrates associated melancholia with fear and terror, Van Beverwijck stresses that the illness can also occur as a form of despondency and occasionally as merriness. In other words, it can happen to the crying Heraclitus and the laughing Democritus.[25] Robert Burton also saw the world – and often himself – under the mask of Democritus (Junior).

Van Beverwijck poses, as a cause for melancholia, an illness in the brain which is also closely connected to an illness in the heart, because changes of mood directly affect the heart and vice versa. The reason for this would be an imbalance in the humours (*pneumata*). If the temperate constitution of the heart is spoiled, the constitution of the brain is also spoiled; thus, an illness in the *spiritus vitalis* in the heart has a direct negative effect on the *spiritus animalis* in the brain.[26] As a consequence, he differentiates between four types of melancholia according to where the damaging humours, which cause the illness, gather: 1. Melancholia of the brain, 2. Melancholia of the heart, 3. Melancholia of the Organs, also known as Hypochondria, 4. Melancholia of the Uterus. Furthermore, Van Beverwijck attributes lovesickness (*Dulle Liefde*) to melancholia and differentiates ultimately between mania (*Dulligheydt*) as an especially severed form of melancholia and obsession (*Frenesye ofte Uytsinnigheyt*) as a mania caused by a fever. As it will become apparent, some of these concepts can be found in Vondel's dramas.

22 '*Melancholia* is among the illnesses, which, according to Galen, have been named by their cause. According to his theory, the illness was named after the melancholic humidity. However, we call it by its effect. Therefore, *Depression* is a mental illness that usually accompanies fear and terror in the heart, however, seldom with happiness or excitement. It appears without a fever and comes from a firm and inverted imagination. As in the other kinds of *Mania*, here the *imagination* and *reason* are infringed upon, above all the imagination. The melancholiac's *judgement* is often subject to an inverted imagination and they see the truth in what in reality is false, whereby they are correct in other areas and can make sensible decisions (which *Vives* does not see as curious without reason)'. Van Beverwijck, *Schat der ongesontheyt*, II, I, VI, 38. I used the edition: Johan van Beverwijck, *Wercken der Geneeskonste, bestaende in den Schat der Gesontheyt, Schat der Ongesontheyt, Heel-konste etc.*, Amsterdam 1680.

23 For the following paragraphs cf. Van Beverwijck, Schat der ongesontheyt (see n. 22), pp. 33–56.

24 Cf. Van Beverwijck, Schat der ongesontheyt (see n. 22), p. 39.

25 Cf. Van Beverwijck, Schat der ongesontheyt (see n. 22), p. 43.

26 Cf. Van Beverwijck, Schat der ongesontheyt (see n. 22), p. 43.

4 Melancholia under Tyrants – Conscience

The connection between the baroque sovereign and melancholia has been researched since Walter Benjamin's book on tragedy. Benjamin emphasised that a significant characteristic of the baroque tragedy was the conflict between 'absolute sovereignty and poorness of human nature'. For this reason, the martyr figure and the tyrant are complimentary: the tyrant, often seen as a sovereign with absolute power, is also a martyr of his political position. Or, as Benjamin said: 'In the baroque the tyrant and the martyr are but the two faces of the monarch'.[27]

In his drama, *Peter en Pauwels*, Vondel shows Emperor Nero as the prototype of a tyrant on stage and describes his insanity in an impressive way. Vondel uses this to reflect the connection between theatre and melancholia. Nero used to play the role of Orestes, who is chased by the goddesses of vengeance; after a while he is unable to distinguish reality from the illusoriness of the play. He becomes Orestes, whom Erinyes as a personification of his plaguing conscience hunt and cause him to feel fear, which directly leads to the delusional transformation of his imagination.

Vondel depicts in detail the symptoms of mania that Nero suffers. His confidant Agrippa describes how the illness manifested itself: a fever raged in his spoiled blood and consumes his life force. The patient gasps for breath. His voice becomes hoarsely, his tongue can barely form words. His face alters from pale to a blue colour and becomes patchy in some areas. Soon the emperor is spirited and soon becomes despondent. He shies away from the most innocent of sounds and then stares about himself with a look that is as 'red as fire and blood'. His hair is on end, he trembles, he breaks out into a cold sweat and cries out for help. His imagined fear does not leave him any peace:

De Vorst, die onlangs speelde Orestes, droef en dol,
En vlughtigh voor de wraeck, speelt nu zijn eige rol;
Maer in der daet, en niet in schijn, van schrick gedreven,
Druckt uit, hoe veel de schijn en 't veinzen scheelt van 't leven.
De vlam, in 't rotte bloet ontsprongen, knaeght het vleesch.
Hy hijght naer zijnen aêm. de spraeck luit schor, en heesch.
De tong slaet yzerklanck, en slibbert onder 't spreken.
Al 't aengezicht, gelijck met dootverf overstreken,
Ziet bleeck, en blaeuw, als loot, en hier en daer gevlackt.
Nu steeckt hy 't hooft om hoogh. nu hangt het hooft, en zackt
Zwaermoedigh naer beneên, tot dat hy raeckt aen 't schricken,
Om 't kraecken van een deur; en opschiet, en twee blicken,
Zoo root als vier en bloet, aen alle zyden slaet,

27 Cf. Walter Benjamin, The origin of German tragic drama (see n. 9), p. 69.

En opspalckt; en al 't hair recht op te berge staet,
Om zijn verbeeldingen. dan tsidderen de leden,
Het koude zweet breeckt uit, en, van zijn schim bereden,
Verdaeght al 't hofgezin te hoop, met ope keel.
Hoe schichtigh is dit hof gedraeit, als een tooneel!
Hoe 's Vorsten staet verkeert! wat wil die plaegh beduien?
Daer komt hy weder aen, en heeft het hooft vol buien.
(Peter en Pauwels: 1383–1402)[28]

Here, Nero's visions bear a striking resemblance to the manic hallucinations already described by Constantinus Africanus. Although Nero, as opposed to Vondel's Christian heroes, does not know any fear of sin, he is still followed by the goddesses of vengeance as the voice of his conscience. In early modern drama, the ghosts of the dead can appear – a famous example would be *Hamlet* – to threaten the living or to directly represent their conscience and repressed guilt.

This is also the case in Vondel's *Maeghden*, where Attila and his counsels are subject to the violence of their conscience. Attila, whose outer ugliness is also a picture of his mania, is subject to two kinds of insanity in Vondel's drama.[29] His love for Ursul knows no bounds; he is ready to sacrifice all his political advantages for her. This then gives the Hun leader all the requirements for melancholia caused by love as described in medical literature of early modern times. Ursul's rejection turns this love into hate: the murder on the steadfast princess is the (futile) attempt, once again, to gain power over her. However, the leader of the Huns fails at this and becomes a victim of tyrannical melancholia.

---

28 'The prince who played the grieving and manic Orestes, who fled away from revenge, now plays his own role: however, he really is ruled by fear and does not just seem to be. He shows how different appearance and hypocrisy is from life itself. The flame, borne of corrupted blood eats at the flesh. He is gasping for breath and his voice is croaky and hoarse. His tongue strikes sparks and rolls while he was talking. His entire face, as if he were dead, is pale and blue and spotted here and there like lead. Presently, he raises his head, and then he sinks his head depressed. This continues as long as he is held by fear from a slamming door and he startles and looks sideways with two eyes as red as fire and blood. His eyes fly open, his hair is on end because of what is in his imagination. He shivers, he breaks out in a cold sweat and, possessed by his spirit, he screams at the top of his voice so that his entire court comes running to his aid. How suddenly this court has changed, like a theatre stage. How this prince's life has changed! What is the meaning of this torture? He returns and is full of delusions'.

29 In *Maeghden* Ursul impressively describes Attila's ugliness in verses 673–682. Cf. for research on this drama Elida Maria Szarota, 'Die Ursulagestalt in Vondels Maeghden', in: *De nieuwe taalgids* 59 (1966), pp. 73–89 and recently Olga van Marion, 'De Amsterdamse Ursula: een Keulse martelares in Vondels 'Maeghden' (1639) en preken van vader Marius (1633)', in: *Nederlandse letterkunde* 17 (2012), pp. 92–108; Bettina Noak, 'Vondel as a Dramatist: The Representation of Language and Body', in: Jan Bloemendal and Frans-Willem Korsten (eds.), Joost van den Vondel (see n. 5), pp. 115–138.

How powerfully Ursul's spirit controls Attila's conscience can be seen in his delusional visions of a 'Christian Army of Amazons' at the end of the tragedy, which, answering their prayers, comes to rescue the Christians:

Op dat gebed, helaes! verscheenme strax mijn Min,
Met haer doorschote borst. die schoone Koningin
Verscheen met dees quetzuur, die versch noch deerlijck bloede.
Hoe werd mijn hart zoo bang, dat strax zoo grimmigh woede!
De standerd zeegh, en viel, met eenen viel de moed. (Maeghden: 1543–1547)[30]

The sight of the murdered Ursula with the bowshot in her breast leaves Atilla confused and discouraged, his fighting spirit seems broken forever. The blood of the martyr seems to have a special power. Its sight causes tyrants to question their conscience, which can cause them to go mad. The trauma of the violence therefore also does not only affect the victim, but also has an effect on the perpetrators in a special way, because they cannot release themselves from their guilt. In this way, the dead martyrs are able to directly confuse the spirits of the perpetrators.

The power of blood also becomes clear in Vondel's *Maria Stuart*. After Maria's death, her confessor threatens Queen Elizabeth with the pangs of guilt felt by a tyrant: 'Dit Martelbloet roept wraeck, en houdt niet op van tergen'. (Maria Stuart: 1656)[31] According to Maria's confessor, Elizabeth acted like Herodias and the price she has to pay for that would be the transformation to a raging fury:

Het knagend hart will haer ten brein, ten kop uitroocken.
Bezwalcken al het hair met bang en bloedigh zweet.
Zy zal by naere nacht verbaest, met kreet op kreet
Verschricken hofgezin en hof en kamenieren,
En, als een Razerny, door zael en kamer zwieren. (Maria Stuart: 1665–1669)[32]

The pangs of guilt from the heart are transformed into morbid vapours that damage the brain and then dissipate. The consequences of questioning the conscience are therefore physical, too; the spirit and the body affect each other directly. Here also the physical characteristics of mania can be seen: hair becomes covered in a bloody sweat from fear and Elizabeth becomes unable to sleep and runs through the palace at night screaming for fear like a fury. At this

30 'Due to this prayer – unfortunately – my love appeared to me with a shot wound in her breast. The beautiful queen appeared before me with this wound that was fresh and still bleeding. My heart was full of fear, which a short time before was so angry. The banner sank and with it sank my courage'.

31 'This blood of the martyr cries for revenge and does not stop threatening'.

32 'The tormenting heart wants to leave its brain, steaming from its head, covering the hair with fearful and bloody sweat. She will run through shivering during a fearful night screaming and screaming to her court, scaring her court and her courtiers and, like a fury, she will run through the halls and rooms'.

point, the sounds of doctrine from antiquity regarding madness can be seen clearly; the furies have always been seen as the embodiment of mania.

This then places Vondel's works on the same side as the traditional discourse of melancholia. The illness is caused by a disturbance in the humours of the body and the life forces (*pneumata*) which affect the brain from the heart. However, Nero's rage, in connection with a hot fever, probably goes beyond melancholia and moves towards the concept of obsession described by Van Beverwijck (*Frenesye ofte Uytsinnigheyt*). Atilla also shows typical signs of lovesickness (*Dulle Liefde*).[33]

In the early modern descriptions of melancholia, the influence of damaging imaginations on the process of the illness is stressed over and over again. In Vondel's work, these imaginations are represented by visions which are directly connected with the theatrical field. So Nero plays Orestes, Attila sees himself as being surrounded by Amazons and Elizabeth of England turns into Herodias chased by furies. In *Palamedes*, it is Sisyphus and Megeer (Megaira) who represent the traumatic history and the weighted conscience and who spur on Ulysses in his plot against Palamedes. Under further analysis, it shall become apparent how Vondel expands the discourse by adding the cannibalism motive, the 'ego impoverishment' and the chances for therapy as a breakthrough in the melancholic disposition.

5 Religious Mania and the Insanity of the People – Incorporation

In Vondel's 'political' drama Palamedes, one can see different forms of insanity.[34] Reference should be made to the figure of Ulysses, who had to be shown as the shrewd Greek in full possession of his capacities. However, Ulysses hates Palamedes, because Palamedes exposed him while he feigned psychological illness while ploughing to avoid fighting in the Trojan war. Palamedes put little Telemachus in the furrow and made Ulysses stop the plough, showing everyone that he was feigning illness. Ulysses bears a heavy grudge against Palamedes for revealing his trickery.[35] The feeling of irreparable animosity makes his soul

33 Cf. VAN BEVERWIJCK, Schat der ongesontheyt (see n. 22), II, I, IV–V, pp. 26–37 and VII, pp. 48–53. On lovesickness cf. the contribution by OLGA VAN MARION in this volume.

34 Cf. on the political interpretation of *Palamedes* recently MIKE KEIRSBILCK, *Om de vorst zijn' moedwil te besnoeien. Governementele verkenningen in Vondels Palamedes (1625), Gysbreght van Aemstel (1637) en Lucifer (1654)*, Diss. Gent 2013, pp. 67–141.

35 Cf. Palamedes: 203–208.

vulnerable to the influence of evil spirits who are represented here as Sisyphus and Megeer. Ulysses is literally 'obsessed' with hate.[36]

In addition to this, a specific form of mania deserves mention: religious mania, in connection with superstition. Different forms of religious mania were prominently shown in Burton's *Anatomy of Melancholy.* English history, especially the period of the Puritan civil war, seems to have been especially predestined for this kind of disturbed perception. However, this motive can be found in Dutch history as well, in the bloody period of religious battles and persecution of heretics during the reign of Charles V (1500–1558). The humanist author Dirck Volckerstz Coornhert (1522–1590) compared religious fundamentalism with mania and demanded a free practice of religion guided by common sense.[37] Vondel saw the religious zeal of the Counter-Remonstrants, i.e. the orthodox Calvinists, who were responsible for the execution of the Grand Pensionary Johan van Oldenbarnevelt (1547–1619), as the embodiment of the same nonsensical, obsessed religious fanaticism. In this light, *Palamedes* can be seen as the climax of a debate which troubled the poet for many years and was possibly responsible for his later conversion to Catholicism.[38]

In Vondel's tragedies, the motive of cannibalism is strikingly present. The tyrants are always prepared not only to draw the blood of the heroes, but also to drink it. They want to consume, to incorporate their nemeses. Here, the poet speaks of that specific type of mania which removes the maniac from every part of humane society, and denies them any kind of interaction with human culture. In *Palamedes* just the description of the religious insanity of the priests served this goal, making it one of the most memorable parts in Vondel's dramas. At the beginning, Ulysses says that no crime is too great that the cloak of religion cannot cover it: patricide in the sanctuary, the rape of his own sister, even blasphemy against the highest of gods by abusing his wife or his favourite, Ganymed – it all remains unnoticed, if done under an altar cloth.[39]

---

36 Also in light of the imminent civil war, which will be caused by Ulysses' actions, Vondel still speaks of possession. The war is de-glorified and degenerated into a mad slaughter. Cf. Palamedes: 358–386.

37 Cf. on Coornhert's vision of mental illness Bettina Noak, 'Concepts of illness and health in the *Zedekunst dat is Wellevenskunste* (*Ethics, or the Art of Living Well*, 1586) by Dirck Volckertszoon Coornhert (1522–1590)', in: Anne Eusterschulte et. al. (ed.), *Anthropological Reformations – Anthropology in the Era of Reformation*, Göttingen 2015 (forthcoming). On his plea for toleration see Jaap Gruppelaar and Gerlof Verwey, *D.V. Coornhert (1522–1590): polemist en vredezoeker: bijdragen tot plaatsbepaling en herwaardering*, Amsterdam 2010.

38 Cf. on his religious attitude Judith Pollmann, 'Vondel's Religion', in: Jan Bloemendal and Frans-Willem Korsten (eds.), Joost van den Vondel (see n. 5), pp. 85–100.

39 'Al hebtge 't hayligdom met vadermoord bevleckt: / V susters schaemt ontbloot, int aensicht van u swager: / Ia self den blixem drigh gekroont tot hoorendrager, / Verkraght syn eegemael,

At the end of the second act, the chorus of Peloponnesers and Ithakoysen sings of the insurmountable power of fate. Their prayer first addresses Hecate, the threefold, changeable Goddess of the Moon, who – as goddess of the underworld and magic – could also be made responsible for obsession. In a second step, the chorus turns its attentions to the immutable fate that controls the earth. As in euphoria, the chorus lists the crimes for which destiny is responsible: Saturn, who castrates his father and from the blood of whom and the foam of the sea, Venus the unchaste is born; Zeus' unchastity; Bacchus' rage; Mars' war lust; the cannibalism of the Africans, who feed on human flesh, drink human blood and wear human skin. The motive of cannibalism is expanded with Tantalus, who served the gods the flesh of his son.[40]

In the fifth act, the play describes how Palamedes becomes a victim of a raging mob. The mania of the religious priests and leaders was transferred to the people who stoned their victim to death. Just like Orpheus becomes the victim of a hoard of ferocious maenads; Palamedes is also cut in pieces by being stoned.[41] The reference to Orpheus also contains a reference to the subject of mania, because Orpheus – like King David – was able to bring unbalanced souls into balance again. At another point, another cannibalistic motive can be found here, because the rabble dip sweaty cloths in the blood of the martyr and drink his blood mixed with wine.[42]

The cannibalistic motive can be connected to mania in different ways. Vondel's portrayal of the 'prayer' of the chorus in Peloponnesers and Ithakoysen, which is addressed to the Goddess of Destiny, shows that they follow a religion which is far removed from any common sense or moral compass. As when presenting the 'wild peoples', who practice cannibalism, the followers of Hecate put themselves outside of any civilisation. Vondel's exclusion of the religious maniacs from human society is thereby complete.

The motive of 'devouring' in cannibalism can be seen in another connection. It's Satan, who according to Christian teaching 'devours' humans, even destroys them completely. This complete destruction can also be seen by the martyr Palamedes, when his body is destroyed by the rabble who then literally drink his blood. One could also speak here of a reversed Eucharist – where the last supper serves to strengthen the believers, in Catholicism symbolises the unity created between the body of Christ and the believer; the wine and blood of Palamedes serves here a more hellish ritual that also further proves the obsession of his

en schencker Ganimeed: / Ten word niet eens gemerckt, als maer een outerkleed / Die grouwelen bedeckt, ten strecken dan geen sonden'. Palamedes: 530–535.

40 Palamedes: 677–724.

41 Palamedes: 1972–1984.

42 Palamedes: 1985–1994.

adversaries. This then gives the mania in *Palamedes* shown as religious rage, a very dark form.

6 The Tears of St. Peter – Ego Impoverishment

If Walter Benjamin saw the tyrant as also a martyr surrounded by deep despair; in Vondel's dramas, it seems that also the martyrs are not free from the evils of melancholia.[43] In *Palamedes* itself, the hero's monologue shows how much he suffers at the hands of society's deficiency.[44] Grief for the nonsensical nature of the world and doubt on its positive nature befits the educated melancholic, as can be seen in the case of the famous painting by Dürer, *Melancholia I* (1514).[45] Therefore, the second part of this article will address melancholia in martyrs. It is, in certain ways, the classical form of this illness, since – as Van Beverwijck describes – it has been ascribed to the more ingenious and spiritual figures of history since the days of Aristoteles.[46] Most of the time, this illness is seen as a male illness, Vondel, however, also includes his heroin Maria Stuart in this discourse.

In Vondel's Drama *Peter en Pauwels*, the two apostles are surrounded by deep melancholia. In the first scene where they appear, in the dungeon at night, Peter cannot stop crying.[47] He is plagued by memories of the betrayal of his Lord. Peter suffers from a desperation that, quite literally, breaks his heart. As a sign of his suffering, he loses the ability to speak clearly:

> O Paeschlam, ick holp u verraden,
> In 't onweêr van die wreede schaer.
> De kusser van 's verzoeners wangen
> Verriet maer eens der menschen zoen:
> Mijn mont, na dat hy was gevangen,
> Verriet, helaes! hem driemael; toen
> Hy vast bespot wiert, en bespogen.

43 Cf. about the figure of early modern martyr in general: ELIDA MARIA SZAROTA, *Künstler, Grübler und Rebellen. Studien zum europäischen Märtyrerdrama des 17. Jahrhunderts*, Bern/München 1967; PETER BURSCHEL, *Sterben und Unsterblichkeit: zur Kultur des Martyriums in der frühen Neuzeit*, München 2004; SUSANNAH BRIETZ MONTA, *Martyrdom and literature in early modern England*, Cambridge 2005; ANDREAS KRASS (ed.), *Tinte und Blut: Politik, Erotik und Poetik des Martyriums*, Frankfurt/M. 2006.

44 Palamedes: 1–166. The monologue opens the drama.

45 Cf. the famous study about Dürer and the early modern melancholy by RAYMOND KLIBANSKY and ERWIN PANOFSKY/FRITZ SAXL, Saturn and melancholy (see n. 16).

46 Cf. VAN BEVERWIJCK, Schat der ongesontheyt (see n. 22), p. 38.

47 The 'Lacrimae Petri' are also a motive in early modern music and pictorial art. Cf. e.g. Orlando di Lasso's 'Lagrime di San Pietro'.

Erbarm u myner: zie om laegh:
Alziende Waerheit, straf mijn logen:
Verzwaer de ketens, die ick draegh.
Wat woorden liet ick my ontslippen!
Verzaeckte ick zoo mijn' Godt, mijn' heer!
Wat lastren schonden deze lippen!
Ick nock, ick berst, ick kan niet meer.
Mijn geest bezwijckt. ick zijgh ter neêr.
Och och och och och och och och. (Peter en Pauwels: 305–320)[48]

Peter does not seem able to carry the guilt of the betrayal. He reacts to St. Paul's attempts to comfort him by describing his sorrows: whether he actually hears the cockerel crowing, or whether it is just in his mind has direct physical consequences. It reminds the saint of his betrayal. This then causes a narrowing sensation in his arteries which almost threaten to burst. Blood re-enters the body, drop for drop at first, but then gushing forth in rivers. Only the simultaneous flow of tears protects Peter's heart, overflown from this flood, from ceasing to work.[49]

The scene of betrayal is constantly in a traumatic repetition before Peter's inner eyes: when Caiaphas' maid recognises him as a follower of Jesus in the yard of Caiaphas' palace, Peter denounces his lord and then the cockerel crows. It is a turning point that pushes Peter into the depths of despair: Jesus looks at him punitively and in that moment, he sees his mistake and it never again lets him rest:[50]

48 'Oh agnus dei, I helped to betray you in the storms of this brutal hoards. The kisser of the cheek of the saviour only once betrayed the son of man. However, my mouth, after being imprisoned, betrayed him three times while he was being mocked and spat on. Have mercy on me, look down, oh omnicognisant truth and punish my lies. Weigh down the chains I carry. What words did I allow myself to utter! That is how I betrayed my God, my Lord! What sacrileges shamed my lips! I shake, I break, I can't stand it any longer. My spirit expires. I sink to the ground. Oh, oh, oh, oh, oh, oh, oh, oh'.

49 'Mijn amptgenoot, ick weet, ick reck u taey gedult / Te lang, door 't moeielijck vernieuwen van mijn schult; / Zoo menighmael de haen aan 't sluimrigh hart komt kloppen. / Wat raêt? mijn hartaêr berst, in 't eerst allengs by droppen, / Dan korter, drop op drop; dan gietze beecken uit: / En schrey ick niet, zoo is 't alleens of 't hart my sluit. / Ay medebroeder, laet mijn tranen ruim gaen weien. / Laet my mijn dootvergrijp ophalen. laet my schreien.' (Peter en Pauwels: 331–338). 'My fellow, I know that I have tried your patience for too long by gratingly renewing my debt, whenever the call of the cockerel tears at the strings of my sleeping heart. But what to do? My veins burst, slowly at first but then quicker, drop follows drop and then it flows in rivers. If I were to cease crying, my heart would close itself to the outside. Oh Brother, let my tears flow, let me refresh my unforgivable crime again and again. Let me weep'.

50 The concept of 'repetition compulsion' ('Wiederholungszwang') can also be found in Freud, in his article *Erinnern, Wiederholen und Durcharbeiten* ('Remembering, Repeating and Working-Through'). Just as we can see in the example of Peter, Freud emphasises that the patient doesn't really remember the traumatic incident, but *acts* it over and over again.

> Een meisken, dat my, in de voorzael, zitten vont,
> Stoof op: dit's oock van 't slagh, die twist en oproer zoecken.
> Ick schrik, verzaek mijn' heer, verdoem mijn ziel met vloeken,
> Noch eenmael, en nog eens; en daetlijck kraeit de haen;
> En Jesus ziet my stijf met straffende oogen aen,
> Die dringen in de ziel. waer was ick toe gekomen!
> Het hart wou op de tong, die liet zich naulix toomen,
> Wee my, ellendigh man! erbarm u mijns! o heer.
> Och och och och och och. (Peter en Pauwels: 364–372)[51]

In his work mentioned above, *Mourning and Melancholia*, Sigmund Freud shows melancholia as a state of absolute 'ego impoverishment'. Peter was in this state. His entire ego disappears behind his profound grief and perpetual guilt, a guilt which is constantly re-enacted. On this impoverishment, Freud writes:

> The melancholic displays something else besides which is lacking in mourning – an extraordinary diminution in his self-regard, in impoverishment of his ego on a grand scale. In mourning it is the world which has become poor and empty; in melancholia it is the ego itself. The patient represents his ego to us as worthless, incapable of any achievement and morally despicable; he reproaches himself, vilifies himself and expects to be cast out and punished. He abases himself before everyone and commiserates with his own relatives for being connected with anyone so unworthy. He is not of the opinion that a change has taken place in him, but extends his self-criticism back over the past; he declares that he was never any better.[52]

This analysis can be applied to the figure of St. Peter. During his incarceration, he is almost solely obsessed with thinking about his past, and it does not show him any positive reason to come back to life. Any attempt to save him made by his Christian friends is doomed to failure. Only a martyr's death can release Peter from his situation. His martyrdom is therefore passive, it releases him from the temporality, however does not change anything in regard to his melancholic nature.

SIGMUND FREUD, 'Remembering, Repeating and Working Through', in: *The Standard Edition* (see n. 13), vol. 12, London 1958, pp. 147–156.

51 'A maiden, who saw me sitting before the court, jumped up: he belongs to those who are always looking for hassle and trouble. I got scared, betrayed my Lord, damned my soul with oaths, again and again; and suddenly the cockerel crows. And Jesus stares at me with punishing eyes that penetrate my soul! Whither did I go! My heart wanted to speak and cannot be tamed. Woe is me, I am a miserable man! Have mercy on me! Oh God. Oh, oh, oh, oh, oh, oh'.

52 FREUD, Mourning and Melancholia (see n. 13), p. 246.

7 Maria Stuart – Numbness and Breakthrough

If Peter's longing for death results from a deep melancholic despair; Maria Stuart's martyr's death is her victory over melancholia. Vondel's *Maria Stuart* shows us a new type of martyr. Ursul is shown as a strong, confident woman who almost effortlessly conquers insane Attila and completely incorporates the power of her belief; she does not suffer from self-doubt. Palamedes, however, is not free of the kind of melancholia, which suffers from the delusion of time and sees every rational deed in a certain light as nonsensical. Peter takes the place of the desperate man, almost paralysed by the knowledge of his sins, who sees the only way to escape his illness in sacrificing his own life. Maria Stuart shows, how a Christian martyr can progress from a state of illness to a state of health.

At the beginning the main character in Vondel's *Maria Stuart* significantly displays the classic symptoms of melancholia in its medical manifestation. Maria's personal physician, Burgon, explains how her psychological suffering led to an impairment of the heart and a constant fever and ultimately to a dropsy in her whole body. Although this fevered state had given way, the dropsy still remained.[53] The reason for this dropsy is an impairment of spleen and liver. The first is responsible for the formation of blood; the second is responsible for detoxification and neither work properly anymore. Therefore, the harsh and humid fluids remain in the body and rise to the brain which they overshadow and they consequently destroy the noble common sense:

Want milt en lever (dees de winckel van het bloet,
En die het vuylnisvat des lijfs, te lang misvoedt)
Zijn beide schier verslenst, bedorven, overstreden
Door overvloet van raeuwe en koude vochtigheden,
Die (d'oirsprongk van dit quaet) met vuilen damp op damp
Bezwalcken 't edel brein; benevelen de lamp
Van 't kloeck vernuft, ja zelf door 't beckeneel geslagen,
'T gezalfde hair met sneeuw bedecken voor zijn dagen:
En wie verwondert zich, die op haer jammer ziet?
Des kerckers eeuwigheit, en 't nypende verdriet,
Verdruckten de natuur, die al te noode aen 't wijcken,
Ten leste eens onder 't pack der rampen most bezwijcken. (Maria Stuart: 211–222)[54]

53 Maria Stuart: 198–210.

54 'The spleen and the liver (the first responsible to store the blood, the latter container of decay of the body that has been fed incorrectly for too long) are both completely worn out, rotted and overwhelmed by the abundance of harsh and cold fluids. These (the cause of this ill) fog the noble brain with damaging vapours; they darken the lamp of intelligent reason and, when they penetrate through to the skull, they cover the anointed hair with snow before its season. And who is surprised, when he considers her suffering? The eternity of imprisonment, the

For Van Beverwijck, damaging fluids that accumulate due to an overload of the heart were a reason for melancholia as well. Maria's confessor confirms the physician's diagnosis. In his opinion, although the queen has a stable character, her body cannot resist the power of the degenerate humours, especially considering her weak female constitution. Maria Stuart also has hereditary problems. Her cousin, Maria the Catholic also suffered from dropsy, caused by an upsurge of emotions, which ultimately killed her.[55]

The psychological consequences of this disorder of bodily humours are also described explicitly: Maria Stuart starts displaying characteristics of a broken woman, 'sickness of spirit and body and melting like snow in the sun', as she characterises herself.[56] Using a picture of the emblematic literature, she describes herself as a ship that has given way to the fickle waves of the sea. Like the all-consuming surge of the sea, the devouring masses can drag this ship down.[57] The people, here, are the representatives of the English puritanism, who constantly strive after the life of Maria and would also – again in the metaphor of devouring – have her annihilated completely. Maria's personal physician, Burgon, and the chorus of ladies in waiting (Rey van Staetjofferen) are very worried about the queen. The chorus refers to Christ in his role as *Christus Medicus*, who can bring peace to the soul and thereby the body, to comfort the queen.[58]

This constellation changes as the drama progresses. Maria Stuart's strength of mind becomes more intense thanks to the pressure that the English lords put her under. Within a short period of time, it is she who teaches her private physician. The succession of Christ can bring her to teach her entourage about the correct guidance of the soul. The closer the unfair punishment comes, the stronger Maria seems to become. At the start of the fourth act, the reader experiences her *agnitio:* for the first time, her soul longs for the shores of peace after suffering the stormy waves of the sea. Her ship is sailing towards this port with sails held high. Where it was just craving peace, her soul is now actively striving towards release and tranquillity.[59] Here, however, it is the 'juichende gemoedt', as Vondel describes the life-giving, mental pneuma that flows through the blood in the veins to the brain, to feed the immortal soul, while Maria's body is doomed to perishableness:

> Het juichende gemoedt
> Begeert naer zulck een prijs te rennen door het bloedt

tortuous worry suppress nature, which fights against it and ultimately succumbs to the strokes of fate'.

55 Maria Stuart: 225–241.

56 Maria Stuart: 594.

57 Maria Stuart: 472–477.

58 Maria Stuart: 309–318.

59 Maria Stuart: 1214–1224.

Der adren, en om hoogh t' aenschouwen, vol genoegen,
Hoe hier de vyanden, geknaeght en bleeck van 't wroegen,
En onverzaet van wraeck, geen vatten vinden aen
't Onsterflijck deel, de ziel, nu 't lichaem moet vergaen. (Maria Stuart: 1224–1229)[60]

Obviously, after she accepts her martyrdom, Maria's body ceases to be a hindrance to her, as opposed to the stadium of melancholia described above. Since she received redemption from the *Christus Medicus*, physical suffering will no longer impede the triumph of her soul – she has conquered her melancholia. Just as Van Beverwijck described, the *spiritus animalis* has become subject to the *spiritus vitalis:* hope and happiness now govern Maria's emotions, much to the surprise of her physician (and her confessor – as the leader of her soul) and especially her enemies, who thought to have conquered her through grief and despair.

8 Conclusion

As in general in early modern literature, Vondel gives melancholia many faces. It can be a delusional disorder, as in the case of the angry conscience of a tyrant, whose evil deeds come back to haunt them by creating manic hallucinations, which confuse the delicate balance of humours and thereby prove the existent interplay between body and soul in early modern medical discourse. Just as the tyrants devour their victims, thereby completely destroying them, they are devoured by their mania which destroys their personality. Vondel takes this finding from the individual figures and applies it to entire groups of people. Especially religious zeal causes believers to completely relinquish their rational capacities and to only live through hate. At this point, Vondel makes diverse use of the cannibalism motive: the consumption of the enemy does not leave any trace of him on earth, thereby completing his demise. At the same time, the tyrants, demagogues and the raging hoards are also consumed by mania, from which they can no longer release themselves, therefore, as individuals and as society, they are doomed to downfall.

As in antiquity, Vondel also deals with melancholia in positive figures, in this case the martyrs. Above all, he portrayed two martyr heroes: one was of St. Peter, completely destroyed by grief, who could not release himself from the chains of his past, who had lost every sense of self-worth and who drew the consequences

60 'The joyful soul desires, seeking such a price [salvation B.N.], to run through the blood in the veins and from above sees with splendid satisfaction how our enemies here on earth, pale and weary from hard labour and unsatisfied by their revenge do not affect the immortal part, the soul, while the body perishes'.

from his 'ego impoverishment' and could not live any further. A similar numbness, a stiffness in grief is typical, at least at first, of Maria Stuart. She also sees only false decisions in her past, which put pressure on her conscience and constantly bring her to a state of heartache, which directly affects her health. However, for her, her martyrdom ultimately becomes a source of healing for her psyche. By subjecting herself to the will of Christ, she can break through the power of her despair and thereby not only gains power over her spirit, but also regains control over her body.

Ronny Spaans

Diagnosing the Poetic Inspiration: Medical Criticism of Enthusiasm in the Poetry of Jan Six van Chandelier (1620–1695)

1 Introduction

Sometime around the year 1648, the Amsterdam merchant and poet Jan Six van Chandelier (1620–1695) wrote a poem with the peculiar title: 'Verrukkinge der Sinnen, aan Joannes Hoornbeek, dr. profr., en predikant t' Uitrecht: En Simon Dilman Geneesheer'.[1] The first part of the title, 'Verrukkinge der Sinnen', means literary 'rapture of the senses', in modern English it would translate as 'ecstasy'. The rest of the title refers to the two persons, to whom the text is addressed: the preacher and professor in theology at the University of Utrecht, Johannes Hoornbeeck (1617–1666), and the physician Simon Dilman.

Jan Six van Chandelier is known in the Dutch literature as a *poeta doctus*; the poems of his collection, *Poësy* (1657), are rich in classical references and fraught with obscure puns and allusions. The same goes for this poem. In 'Ecstasy', Six imitates ode IV, II of Horace. In this poem the Roman says that he was asked by his friend Iulus to sing of Augustus' victories in a Pindaric ode. Horace declines, arguing that he lacks the talent, and requests Iulus to compose the poem himself. Six says he intends to do the same for Frederick Henry, the Prince of Orange, but as with Horace the result is quite different. In the middle of the text, Six changes his mind and, as apparent from the title, instead greets Hoornbeeck and Dilman, who both were friends of the poet. The reference to the Prince of Orange gives reason to believe that the poem is written around 1648 – that year the Peace Treaty of Münster took place, which ended the Eighty Year's War and finally made the United Netherlands independent from the Spanish Crown.

The poem is typical of Six. The Dutch Calvinist poet is famous for his realistic poetics, in opposition to the aristocratic pretentions of his fellow poets. This view on poetry is present in 'Ecstasy'; Six ridicules the genre by writing an ironic ode. It is no coincidence that the Amsterdam poet resorts to Horace when

1 The poem has the number 177 in the commented edition of Six' collection of poetry, *Poësy:* Anne Evert Jacobs, *Joannes Six van Chandelier: Gedichten*, 2 vols., Assen 1991.

intending to write a Pindaric poem. Horace (65–8 BC) is known as an advocate for modesty and temperance in the literature of Antiquity. When, throughout *Poësy*, Six points out Horace as his favourite among the classical poets, he profiles himself as the anti-aristocratic poet of the literature of the Dutch Golden Age.[2]

The Pindaric odes refer to the poems written by the Greek author Pindar (520–445 BC). His odes were panegyric texts written to state occasions, as a ruler's accession, birthday, or funeral. Of his vast corpus, only the *epinika* – odes to athletic victories – have survived in complete form. The genre is characterized by the so-called triadic form, which means that the poem consists of a strophe, followed by an anti-strophe and epode.[3] Other characteristics are an irregular metre and an elevated language, with intensity of feelings and daring imagery. As many of the classical genres, it was rediscovered in the Renaissance, and became a popular model for Renaissance poets, from Pierre de Ronsard to Joost van den Vondel. As Pindar, they used the form to lofty themes. Examples of Pindaric odes or poems influenced by the style in the Dutch literature are Vondels 'Zegesang ter eere van Frederick Henrick', ('Victory song to the honour of Frederick Henry') (1629) and 'Bouwsangh', ('Building song') (1648).[4]

The title 'Ecstasy' points to the main characteristic of the singer of the Pindaric ode, the notion of the poet as a receiver of a poetic inspiration, which leads him into a state of *furor poeticus*, 'poetic madness'. The original Greek word, *ekstasis*, literally means 'standing outside of oneself' or 'losing one self'. We should take into account both the psychological meaning of the term – 'a state of emotion so intense that a person is carried beyond rational thought and self-control' – and a religious meaning: 'a trance, frenzy, or rapture associated with mystic or prophetic exaltatio'. The last meaning points, as we shall see, to the religious origin of the *furor poeticus.*[5]

The identification of Pindar with frenzy can also be traced back to other classical sources. The Greek poet was not only famous as an author of victory odes, but also of dithyrambs. The association of Pindar with the dithyrambs comes from Horace, more precisely ode IV, II, 11–12 – the ode which Six imitates in 'Ecstasy'. The dithyramb was first and foremost known as a choral song to

2 For Six' realistic poetics, see Maria Adriana Schenkeveld-van der Dussen and Wil-lemien B. de Vries, *Zelfbeeld in Gedichten. Brieven over de poëzie van Jan Six van Chandelier (1620–1695)*, Amsterdam 2007. For the Pindaric ode in the renaissance literature, Stella P. Revard, *Pindar and the Renaissance Hymn-Ode: 1450–1700*, Arizona 2001.

3 'Keer', 'teegenkeer' and 'toesangh' in Six' vocabulary.

4 See these and others examples, Renè Veenman, 'De Thebaensche Swaen. De receptie van Pindarus in de Nederlanden', in: *Voortgang. Jaarboek voor de Neerlandistiek* XIII, 1992, pp. 65–90.

5 Christine Augner, *Gedichte der Ekstase in der Literatur des 16. und 17. Jahrhunderts*, Tübingen 2001.

Dionysus, the god of wine. The dithyramb was therefore considered as written under the influence of wine, which was thought to contain the spirit of the God, and therefore was a means to evoke the *furor poeticus*, the artistic *enthusiasmos* ('enthusiasm'); the ecstatic language of the poems made Horace believe that they were written in free verse. *Enthusiasmos* is Greek and means 'possessed by a god'. 'Where are you hurrying me, Bacchus, full as I am of you? Into what woods, what caves, am I being driven at such speed in a strange state of mind?', sings Horace in another praise poem to Emperor Augustus, ode III, 25. Enthusiasm, the notion of a mystical union with the gods, is an essential ingredient in the Pindaric poetry. The Pindaric author is not an ordinary poet; he is a prophet-poet – a *vates*, according to classical terminology.[6]

Like Vondel, Six wrote a number of texts in the Pindaric form, but as René Veenman has pointed out, Six' use of the genre is marked by irony.[7] Later in this article I will come back to a couple of other Pindaric odes by Six. There is one thing that is striking in regard to the treatment of the genre in 'Ecstasy', a feature which demonstrates that more is at stake than just parody of a turgid artistic form: namely the attention that Six pays to the physical condition of the *vates*-poet. In this essay I will examine the self-presentation of Six van Chandelier in the light of the notion of poetic madness. The two persons to whom the poem is dedicated represent three important aspects of Six' life that will be of importance. Firstly, the physician brings us to the spleen ailment of which Six suffered, secondly, the commercial activities of Six, the trade in exotic medicines. Finally, the theologian presents us to the distinct self-scrutinizing voice that demonstrates the poet's strong Calvinist belief.

2 'Ecstasy'

Before I return to Dilman and Hoornbeeck, a closer analysis of 'Ecstasy' is required. The first stanza of 'Ecstasy' is significant in regard to the ironic representation of poetic inspiration. Six present himself as a priest-prophet, pos-

6 'Quo me, Bacche, rapis tui/ plenum? quae nemora aut quos agor in specus/ velox mente nova?'. The English translation is quoted from Horace, *Odes and Epodes*, ed. and trans. Niall Rudd, Cambridge 2004, pp. 201–203. See also the discussion on *furor poeticus* by the Dutch classical scholar Gerardus Joannes Vossius (1577–1644), whom Six mentions in several texts in his collection of poetry. In his *Poeticarum institutionum libri tres* (1647) Vossius treats the divine inspiration and different types of frenzy mentioned in classical literature, as in Plato's *Ion* and *Phaedrus*. See the modern edition of his work, ed. and trans. Jan Bloemendal, 2 vols., Leiden/Boston, 2010, vol. 2. pp. 1896–1915. Cf. also J.P. Guépin, 'Het enthousiasme van dichters', in: *Bzzlletin* 144, 1987, pp. 47–64.

7 For ironic use of the genre, see also the odes of Willem Godschalck van Focquenbroch, Veenman (see n. 4).

sessed by a supernatural force, a sacred fervour, which provides him with a divinatory power to predict the future (l. 1–10):

Wat voel ik voor een seldsaam vier
Myn vadsich herssenslym ontsteeken?
Ik raak in brand, en schuimbek schier,
Als dolle lui, en weet met geen belul te spreeken.
De Poësy is soete raaserny.
De sienders, en Poeëten
Voorseggen, sonder toovery,
Niet selden, sonder van voorsegginge te weeten,
Of wat het werden zal.
Hun Godheit straalt, en leert geen dingen by geval.

(What a rare fire, I feel,
That ignites my indolent brain matter?
I catch fire, and almost foam at the mouth,
Like mad people, and do not speak with reason.
Poetry is sweet frenzy.
The seers, and Poets
Predict, without sorcery,
Not infrequently, without knowing that they are predicting,
Or knowing what is going to happen.
Their Divinity beams, and learns that nothing happens by chance.)

The ironic description of the divine mania is conspicuous. The same goes for the attention for the physical reactions the inspiration evokes. Six feels the mystical union so strongly that he almost begins to foam at his mouth! Six thus experiences the frenzy as a bodily disturbance. In a resume of the contents of the poem, I will further investigate Six' description of this bodily condition.

In the next two stanzas, Six discusses the relationship between Pindar and Horace regarding the different views on poetry they represent. Anyone who tries to follow the high-flying style of Pindar, will perish like Icarus, writes Six, referring to the Horace's famous ode IV, II. In this text Horace says, as mentioned above, he was asked to sing of Emperor Augustus' victories in the manner of Pindar, but he tells how he will never succeed in the task; the Roman poet compares himself with the mythical hero who flew too close to the sun and declined, informing us that he lacks the talent for such a sacred task. But Horace's ode is, nevertheless, strikingly Pindaric in form and structure. By applying the rhetorical figure of *praeteritio* – which implies 'a mentioning by not mentioning' – the ode after all emerges as praise to the Roman god-king. Six gives in his ode an explanation of Horace's inconsistent behaviour. Horace could not help himself from imitating Pindar, because he was blinded by the splendour of the Greek poet (l. 11–30).

Holland also has two Pindaric poets who proudly come ruffling their feathers, continues Six in the third stanza, still in ironical, hyperbolic terms; Joost van den Vondel and P.C. Hooft (l. 38–40). Six sees a parallel in the opposition Horace-Pindar and the opposition between himself and the two stars of Dutch poetry. He tries to reach the artistic level of these 'bird kings' (l. 41), but he admits that he will fall short (l. 51–56):

Maar of natuur, en dichtens kunste
Gebaart, uit tyds, en oeffninghs schoot,
My weigerden haar Heemelgunste,
Om gest te kneeden, in het brood,
Van myn niet wel gereesen brein:
Zoo zal ik met myn riemen roeijen.

(But even if nature and the art of poetry
Born out of the womb of time and exercise,
Denied me her favour of the heaven,
To knead yeast, in the bread
Of my not well risen brain:
So I shall row with my oars.)

Although he has inherited his talent from his mother, and masters poetic craftsmanship thanks to *exercitio*, he is refused heavenly inspiration. He gives his own physical condition the blame for this. He lacks an inner fire – the force required to achieve a high 'ferment'.[8] But even so, as apparent from the quote, he will make an attempt.

In the next stanza (l. 61–70), Six expresses what his intention is with the ode. He asks Apollo to fill him with his solar power, so that he – despite of his lack of poetic imagination – may be able to compose a hymn to the marriage between Astrea (the goddess of justice) and the Dutch Peace Prince, Frederick Henry of Orange. The prince of Orange thus emerges as Six' equivalent to Horace's Augustus. Speaking in allegorical language Six refers to the significance that Frederick Henry meant for the Peace Treaty of Münster.[9] If Apollo will help him

8 Six is possible referring to the theories of early modern iatrochemy. The fermentation was created by a mysterious life force, the so-called 'archeus', a spiritual entity lodged in the human body, according to Joan Baptista van Helmont, see H.A.M. Snelders, *De geschiedenis van de scheikunde in Nederland. Van alchemie tot chemie en chemische industrie rond 1900*, Delft 1993, pp. 31–32. This reference would be understood by the physician to whom Six address the poem, but also by the theologian Hoornbeeck; Hoornbeeck was married to a niece of Franciscus de le Boë Sylvius, a famous chemist in Six' Amsterdam. Many of Sylvius writings were in Hoornbeecks' library, see E.D. Baumann, *Francois dele Boë Sylvius*, Leiden 1949, pp. 47–48. Hoornbeeck also used Sylvius as doctor, see T. Briemen, *Johannes Hoornbeeck (1617–1666): Eminent geleerde en pastoraal theoloog*, Goudriaan 2008, p. 83.

9 Frederick Henry died before the Peace of Münster, but Dutch poets celebrate him as one of the

in this, he will be filled with divine power, so that 'vuur vloeije, uit een diamante pen, / Op dichtende papieren' ('fire [will] flow out of a diamond pen, / On poeticizing papers') (l. 65–66).

The lofty theme of the text, the planned celebration of the Peace Prince, is, however, soon abandoned. The intention proves to be neither an apotheosis of a mighty person or a celebration of a public event. With his Pindaric ode Six has no higher intention than to greet two dear friends (l. 71–74):

Met sulken pen, o Haarlem, wil
Ik Hoorenbeek uw soon vereeren,
Die, met syn daagen in April,
Een vruchthoorn meededeilt, van goude soomerpeeren.

(With such a pen, o Haarlem, I
Will honour your son, Hoornbeeck,
Who, with his [birth in these] days in April,
Presents a horn of fruit, of golden summer pears.)

So much for the omniscient pretentions of the divine *vates!* The high poetic flight ends with an anti-climax: congratulation to his friend Johannes Hoornbeeck for his new-born son in April that year. The content of the following and final stanza (l. 81–90) is equally prosaic; Six expresses his admiration for the medical skills of Simon Dilman.

The function of the poem as a critic on the high-flown literary style of his fellow poets is obvious. I already mentioned Vondel as producer of Pindaric poems, and as we just have seen, Six identifies Hooft and Vondel with Pindar. But there is more to be said about the poem. A study of Six' literary work shows that the anti-aristocratic poetics of the Dutch Calvinist is not as consistent, when it comes to the crunch. In 1648, Six published the pamphlet *Vreughde-Zangen* [...] (*Songs of Joy* [...]), which he dedicated to the Peace Treaty of Münster.[10] In this collection of panegyric odes, Six does what he said he was not able to do in 'Ecstasy': he assumes the role of the inspired prophet-poet and worships Frederick Henry as a deity. The following year the eleven poems of the pamphlet were included in the anthology *Olyf-Krans Der Vreede* [...] (*Olive-garland of Peace* [...]), where among others Vondel contributed. The Dutch poets in the collection celebrate the Frederick Henry as one of the precursors to the peace,

precursors to the peace, see SIPKO MELISSEN, 'De heedendaagse Goude-eeuw', in: *Spektator*, 1981/1982, pp. 30–60, here pp. 37–38.

10 I.S.V.C. [JAN SIX VAN CHANDELIER], *Vreughde-Zangen Over den eeuwigen Vreede, Tusschen Spangien En de Vereenighde Nederlanden: Daar by noch andere invallingen van den Rijmer, voor en ontrent 't sluyten der selver Vreede*, Amsterdam 1648.

comparing him to Augustus, and the new period of peace in the Dutch Republic with Augustus' introduction of a new Golden Age in the Roman Empire.[11]

Six' pamphlet contains, nevertheless, stanzas where a reservation against the role as priest-prophet is visible. The opening text of the cycle, 'Toewydinge aan de Vreegodinne' ('Devotion to the Peace Goddess'), is actually just as ironic as 'Ecstasy'.[12] Here, Six opposes the priest-prophets who claim divine inspiration, by setting up a contrast between two types of poets, the 'nachtegaalen' ('nightingales') – *vates*-poets, who are in cosmic harmony with Pax, the Peace Goddess, so that they are able to write divine poetry – versus the 'bastaardvoogels' ('bastard birds') – rhymesters who are denied celestial insight and therefore have to seek inspiration elsewhere. 'En dierhalve gevoelende in my risen een krachtige gest van Nieuwen Triaakel, gelyk ik daagelyks handel', ('and therefore I feel a powerful yeast of new theriac rising in me, [a product] in which I daily trade'), says Six, informing us that his *furor poeticus* is of a more worldly origin. By presenting himself as a poet intoxicated on theriac – an expensive, medical concoction with opium as one of its main ingredients – Six identifies himself with the last group. At the end of the text, the irony is unmistakable. Six presents his pamphlet as incense that will befog the heavenly throne of the Peace Goddess and fill her nostrils with vapour.[13]

The similarities between 'Devotion to the Peace Goddess' and 'Ecstasy' are conspicuous. This makes it plausible that 'Ecstasy' is not just meant as a parody on Vondel and other Dutch Golden Age authors, but also as an ironic comment on his own role as author of divine poetry. Some elements in 'Devotion to the Peace Goddess' underline an important feature of Six' treatment of the *furor poeticus*, which I will discuss further in this article: the material aspects of the poetic inspiration. As already mentioned in relation to the dithyramb, wine was considered a means to evoke the *furor poeticus.* The so-called 'Parnassus language' of the Dutch renaissance authors, especially Joost van den Vondel, and his imitators, as Jan Vos and Reyer Anslo, is in this regard of interest. The 'Parnassus language' is imbued with references to the sacraments and sacrifices of classical

11 See Sipko Melissen, De heedendaagse Goude-eeuw (see n. 9).

12 Text number 218 in Jacobs, Joannes Six van Chandelier (see n. 1).

13 Six' profiling as a 'bastard bird' is based on several poetological statements in classical and early modern literature. Firstly, we recognise an allusion to Persius' famous self-presentation as a 'semi-clansman', who never drank from the sources of the Muses, in the prologue of his *Satires.* Secondly, Six ridicules Ronsards destinction in *Preface sur la Franciade* between the authentic Poet and the rhymester, a difference that is akin to the difference between a venerable prophet and a quack peddling theriac, according to the French poet. For these allusions and other poems of Six where he speaks of an opposition between 'rymer' ('rhymester') and 'poëet' ('poet'), see Maria Adriana Schenkeveld-van der Dussen, 'De anti-idealistische poëtica van een christen-burger, Joannes Six van Chandelier', in: *De nieuwe taalgids* 76 (1983), 4, pp. 291–316.

mythology, such as incense, gems, perfumes and ambrosia.[14] In 'Ecstasy', Six spoke, as we saw, of a 'diamond pen', fraught with divine power, while in 'Devotion to the Peace Goddess' of incense and theriac. This observation points to Six' commercial activities.

3 Ecstasy as a danger to physical health

I now return to the friends of Six, first to Simon Dilman. What is the reason for addressing a Pindaric ode to a physician? To answer this question we need to go to the person Six. As already mentioned, the Amsterdam poet suffered from a spleen ailment. At the same time we have to consider Six' occupation: Six was a prosperous drug merchant. As a wholesaler, he imported exotic spices, fruit and minerals, which he sold to physicians and hospitals in Amsterdam. Six thus had two reasons for contacting Dilman, firstly as patient, secondly as drug seller.

Six' collection of poems, *Poësy*, confirms this. Surprisingly, many poems are addressed to the physician. There are even poems addressed to his family members. One almost gets the impression that Six served as a house poet for the family. In addition, Dilman's son, Jacob Dilman, was an apprentice in Six' drug store, 'De vergulde Eenhoorn' ('The gilded Unicorn') in Amsterdam. No doubt a friendship had developed between the families, but Six visited Dilman finally because of his spleen disease. Most poems between them are formed as a conversation between a patient and his doctor.

The role that the commodities of 'The golden Unicorn' play in Six' life is complex and of relevance regarding the relationship between Dilman and Six. In the seventeenth century, there were discussions on the medical, social and political dangers of foreign drugs. An important work in this context is the polemic pamphlet *Inleydinge tot de Hollandtsche genees-middelen* [...] (*Introduction to the Dutch medicines* [...]) (1642) by the famous Dutch physician Johan van Beverwijck. Here, plants and herbs from the local environment are defined as more consistent with the bodily disposition of the Dutch people than exotic drugs, which Van Beverwijck associates with a number of negative phenomena; luxury, adulteration, illness etc. Six seems to be influenced be these ideas. In many of his poems, he sees his disease in relation to consumption of exotic merchandise.[15] This is the case with one of Six' poems to Dilman: 'Dankdicht aan

14 For the 'Parnassus language', see KAREL PORTEMAN and MIEKE B. SMITS-VELDT, *Een nieuw vaderland voor de muzen. Geschiedenis van de Nederlandse literatuur 1560–1700*, Amsterdam 2008, p. 403.

15 See my PhD thesis, *Godenbloed te koop. Exotica, extase en verboden kennis in de poëzie van Jan Six van Chandelier (1620–1695)*, Oslo 2014. For the discussion on local versus foreign

Simon Dilman, geneesheer', ('Thank poem to physician Simon Dilman').[16] Here, Six expresses his gratitude for advises on diet and ethical life conduct, which he has received from his doctor. In the early modern period, disease was a matter of moral behaviour, and Six expresses in his poem that he is conscious of the dangers which '[a]mbar of een kostelyker prys', ('ambergris, or a [drug of a] more costly price') (l. 40) carry. Apart from its use as a perfume, ambergris was used as a medicine in the early modern period.

Interesting in this context is the clinical picture Six gives of a body exposed to foreign culinary and medicinal luxuries: Gluttony not only causes blockage in the stomach, but – given the great importance that the Galenic physiology gave to the digestive system in early modern time – also blockage in central body processes, so that undigested spirits rise and fill the brain with vapour. The result is various disorders such as confusion and weakening of the judgment, which result in a surrender to other desires (l. 29–32).[17]

A similar expounding of the dangers of consumption of exotic drugs and its consequences for bodily health and moral conduct can be found in 'Dankoffer, aan gesondheit', ('Thanks offering, to health').[18] The text contains a record of a rather heavy medical treatment, which Six underwent, and which included blood-letting, that provoked hallucinations with the patient. The poem is marked by an allegorical interpretation of the treatment. According to the title, the text forms a thank offering to the goddess of health, Hygeia. In addition the 'naaneeven' ('cousins') (l. 24) of the goddess, are mentioned. Six is possibly referring to Simon Dilman and his college physicians. Relevant for us is the fact that Six not only includes culinary excess, but also excess related to other pleasures, such as luxury buildings, precious merchandise, furniture and music ('Musentoon', ['tone of the Muses']), (l. 39–52). A refrain in Six' poetry is his adherence to a neo-stoic ideal, i.e. with the classical dicta 'know thyself' and 'nothing in excess'. This ideal is mirrored in Six' self-critical examination of the use of exotic drugs in various spheres of society, and the linking of them to different desires, such as lust, avarice, recklessness and curiosity.[19]

From this, it is not a long way to the hubris of the Pindaric poet. In this context, Six would be aware of the excess of the *furor poeticus*. One son of Dilman, Johannes Dilman, actually obtained his doctorate on the topic frenzy.

---

drugs, see Alix Cooper, *Inventing the Indigenous. Local Knowledge and Natural History in Early Modern Europe*, Cambridge 2007.

16 Poem number 142 in: Jacobs, Joannes Six van Chandelier (see n. 1).

17 For a study on Galenic medicine and early modern poetry, see Michael Schoenfeldt, *Bodies and Selves in Early Modern England: Physiology and Inwardness in Spenser, Shakespeare, Herbert, and Milton*, Cambridge 1999.

18 Poem number 184 in: Jacobs, Joannes Six van Chandelier (see n. 1).

19 See Spaans, Godenbloed te koop (see n. 15).

Six wrote a poem for the occasion: 'Welkomst, aan Joannes Dilman, van Leiden, naa hy geneesheer was gemaakt, alvooren hebbende beweert, wat raasernye was' ('Welcome to Johannes Dilman, from Leiden, after he was made physician, having shown what frenzy was').[20] It might therefore be that Six had discussions with the Dilman family about the 'soete raaserny' ('sweet frenzy') of poetry and possible medical explanations into the phenomenon.

Early modern medical theories give us further proof of Six' awareness of the pathological dangers of frenzy. In the chapter 'diseases of the head' in his medical reference book, *Schat der Ongesontheyt* (1656), Johan van Beverwijck discusses different forms of 'raasernije'.[21] Unfortunately, Van Beverwijck does not mention frenzy in relation to poetic inspiration, but he touches on an interesting point in relation to Six van Chandelier: the effects of exotic drugs on the human body. In the section on the 'drunkenness', a subcategory to frenzy, Van Beverwijck emphasizes that not only wine, but also aromatic drugs, such as nutmeg, tobacco and opium make you 'drunken'. Here, as with gluttony, the physician talks about undigested spirits which rise to the brain and disturb our rational capacities, so that the disposition of the body is changed. Consumption of hot, foreign drugs will change the innate modesty of the Dutchman to lustfulness and arrogance.

'Ecstasy' can be seen as a medical self-fashioning in the same way as 'Thank poem to physician Simon Dilman'. Six proves that he is aware of the dangers of poetic excess. He demonstrates that his innate Dutch sobriety is incompatible with the presumptuous artistic style that he was planning to follow. Six lacks, after all, the inner fire required to achieve the high 'ferment' of prophet-poet. And for the matter of the poetic madness of 'Devotion to the Peace Goddess', by relating it to the consumption of a hallucinogenic drug, Six criticizes the notion of divine inspiration by defining it as drunkenness.

4 The healthy, Christian ecstasy

I then turn to Johannes Hoornbeeck, the preacher and theologian. Where Dilman would have been interested in the concept of *furor poeticus* from a medical point of view, as frenzy; Hoornbeeck would have approached the concept from a theological perspective, in relation to the notion of religious ecstasy, *enthousiasmos.*

Johannes Hoornbeeck needs further presentation. The same goes for Hoornbeeck, who was a distant cousin of Six, as for Dilman: Surprisingly many

20 Poem number 381 in: Jacobs, Joannes Six van Chandelier (see n. 1).
21 Johan van Beverwijck, *Schat der ongesontheyt*, Amsterdam 1656, pp. 87–114.

poems in *Poësy* are addressed to the theologian. The texts treat both personal and religious matters. Hoornbeeck, on the other hand, sends him his theological works, for which Six expresses his gratitude in poems. Hoornbeeck occupied an important position in the intellectual circuit of the Dutch Republic. The professor of theology at the University of Utrecht, who knew thirteen languages and wrote a number of theological works before his untimely death, was known as one of the main figures of the so-called Further Reformation, a Dutch version of the Puritanism.[22] Where Dilman acts as a medical supervisor for Six on his way to health, Hoornbeeck seems to have the role as a spiritual leader for the merchant poet in his search for salvation. Considering the fact that church history and the Old Testament were Hoornbeeck's academic specialities, he had the best qualifications to understand the obscure poetic language of Six, full of references to gods and religious practices of Antiquity.

The reason for addressing 'Ecstasy' to Hoornbeeck is thus already clear to us: To a Christian, the notion of a mystical union with pagan gods presents a problem. By addressing an imitation of a pagan poem to the theologian, Six demonstrates his struggle with the pagan inspiration. Six wants to prove himself a true Christian. Hoornbeeck is in this respect the right man. In the chapter 'Enthusiastis et libertinis' in his magnum opus, *Summa Controversiarum Religionis* (1658), the theologian discusses different concepts of *enthusiasmos.*[23] Here, he distinguishes between positive and negative enthusiasm. These two are again divided into two subcategories: one ordinary and one extraordinary. With regard to the good, extraordinary enthusiasm – which refers to the direct divine inspiration of the prophets and the authors of the Bible – Hoornbeeck is advocate of the strict Protestant position: miracles and prophecies do not occur after Biblical time. The good, ordinary enthusiasm is the power of the Holy Spirit which inspires the community of true believers. The negative enthusiasm, on the other hand, is either of a diabolical character or is based on illusions, such as false revelations, visions and oracles.

Hoornbeeck examines the concept primarily in the light of various religious groups and cults, from false prophets in biblical times to mystics of his own time, such as the Rosicrucians. But as Michael Heyd stresses, Hoornbeeck and other Reformed theologians who treat the problem of enthusiasm, do not always have an explicit sect in mind, but refer to different groups who lay claim to esoteric knowledge (prophecy, prediction capability, etc.), or individuals whose psy-

---

22 Briemen, Johannes Hoornbeeck (see n. 8).

23 Six may already have read Hoornbeeck's discussion on enthusiasm in the *Paradoxis et Heterodoxis Weigelianis Commentarius ubi et de Swencfeldo aliisque similis indolis*, Utrecht 1646, which was entirely included in *Summa Controversiarum Religionis*. For a discussion on Hoornbeecks treatment of the enthusiasm, see Michael Heyd, *Be Sober and Reasonable: The Critique of Enthusiasm in the Seventeenth and Early Eighteenth Centuries*, Leiden 1995.

chological behaviour (ecstasies, convulsions, etc.) are associated with enthusiasm.[24] At the same time, Hoornbeeck's treatment of the problem does not only refer to inspiration in the modern sense of the word, but acquisition of all kinds of knowledge and science. According to Hoornbeeck, complete knowledge is impossible for the human being. This brings us to two other poems of Six. As with 'Ecstasy' these two texts problematize the pagan poetry of Antiquity as a source for knowledge.

We turn first to a poem called 'Verrukkinge van Sinnen', 'Ecstasy' – the same title thus as the main text of this article.[25] This fact makes it likely that Johannes Hoornbeeck was the intended reader of this poem. The text is an imitation of Horace's ode III, I, where Horace asks the uninitiated vulgus to be silent and calls attention to his lofty inspired poetry. As in 'Ecstasy', Horace in this poem comes forward as a Pindaric *vates.* Six does the same in his imitation; he presents himself as the priest of the Muses. Encouraged by holy inspiration, Six writes, he dares to ask some existential questions: What did God do before He created the universe and the earth, and why did He create the world? (l. 6–10). Six then describes how he through metempsychosis, a transmigration of the soul, is brought to a wilderness full of diamonds and other precious stones (l. 16–18). But this time, as well, the ecstasy fails to produce a prophetic revelation. The poem ends in an anti-climax. A snow white sheet with crimson letters descends from the heaven. On it the answers to Six' questions are written: God has 'a rod of fire […] for such ungodly questions' (l. 27–28).[26] Six associates the *furor poeticus* with a dangerous curiosity, a desire for forbidden knowledge. This brings us to the epistemological dilemma of Hoornbeecks discussions of different types of enthusiasm. Hoornbeeck links the position of the divine *vates* to an enthusiasm that has a diabolical origin.

The following text is a poem letter addressed to the theologian: 'Brief, aan Joannes Hoornbeek, te Uitrecht', 'Letter, to Johannes Hoonbeeck, at Utrecht'.[27] In this text too, a situation where Six is tempted away from the Christian belief, is at the centre. The text of Six is formed as a moral test: which literary source, the Psalms of David or the poetry of Horace is the most trustworthy when it comes to interpreting nature? The text presents Six with a choice between two kinds of poetic inspirations, an antique pagan versus a Christian one. The poem has a narrative structure. Six is on a travel trip in France, and while riding through a rocky terrain in Anjou, his Psalter falls unnoticed out of his pocket. The other

24 Heyd, Be Sober and Reasonable (see n. 23), p. 22.
25 Poem number 401 in: Jacobs, Joannes Six van Chandelier (see n. 1).
26 Cf. Acts 11:5–6.
27 Poem number 236 in: Jacobs, Joannes Six van Chandelier (see n. 1).

book that he brought on his journey, Horace, is in his hand, because, when sensing the beauty of the nature, he felt such an urge to read the pagan Roman.

But in his letter to the theologian, Six opts for a deeper, spiritual explanation of the prioritization of Horace above David: The devil – 'd' Onsichtbre Onkruidenier' (l. 50), 'the Invisible Merchant of Poison' – sat behind him on the horse, took the book out of his pocket and threw it away. 'Merchant of Poison' is obviously chosen as a counterpart to early modern iconographic depictions of Christ as a pharmacist. This topos goes back to the concept of Christ as a Healer as well as Saviour, and the exegetical interpretation of the numerous references to incense, perfumes and oils in the Old Testament – according to the exegesis these should not be read literary, but as symbols of the divine, fragrant blood and body of Christ, who has sacrificed himself for our sins, or as symbols of the Holy Spirit.[28] But the metaphor 'Merchant of Poison' also refers to Six's own identity as a drug merchant. Six thus wants to show that he is conscious of the fact that the medical oils and spices of his drugstore, just as his favourite poet, have a pagan background.

The awareness of standing before a choice between idolatry and Christianity, is stressed in the characteristic which Six uses on Hoornbeeck; he calls the preacher a 'Priester van Apollon, / De Kriste Orakelgod, te Sion', ('Priest of Apollo, / the Christian Oracle God of Sion') (l. 57–58). Hoornbeeck, not Horace, is the right *vates.* Six promises at the end of the poem that he in the future will distinguish better between Christian and pagan inspiration.

In this context, I wish to turn our attention to a poem Six wrote to another preacher, which underlines Six' struggle with the associations his literary and commercial enterprises evoke to idolatry. This text, 'Troost aan Sirikzee, oover 't verlies van Pieter Wittewrongel, Kerkenleeraar, hier beroepen' ('Comfort to Zierikzee over the loss of Petrus Wittewrongel, Doctor of the Church, who has received a call to come to here [Amsterdam]') treats a similar contrast between a pagan and Christian enthusiasm, and moreover, the text contains interesting references to medical drugs.[29] The text speaks to the inhabitants of Zierikzee, telling them not to lament the fact that the famous Petrus Wittewrongel has moved from their home town to Amsterdam, informing them that they will still be able hear his wise words, because his sermons have been published in book form. As in the case of Hoornbeeck, Six addresses the Reformed preacher as a

---

28 Both 'Christ' and 'Messias' are derived from Greek and Hebrew words for 'anoint'. 'Onkruid' literally means 'weed'. I have translated it as 'poision', in accordance to the early modern definition of 'onkruid'. Biblical fragrance and incense as symbol for the words of preachers were popular in the early modern culture, e. g. Cornelis van Niel, *Een Welrieckende ende Hertsterckende Balsem, Vloeijende uyt den Heylsamen Boom des Levens* […], Amsterdam 1683.

29 Poem number 123 in: Jacobs, Joannes Six van Chandelier (see n. 1).

'Kristen Apollo' (r. 70), and through a play on the name of the preacher – where the original meaning of 'Wittewrongel' is activated, 'curdled milk' – Six praises the physical qualities of his words; this 'curd' surpasses 'nectar' and 'ambrosia' (l. 29–36), the drink and food of the pagan gods. Six underlines further that Wittewrongel's Christian 'raasen' ('frenzy') (l. 59) is preferable to the madness of the Muses.[30] His 'frenzy' has in fact a surprising therapeutic impact, (r. 63–68):

> Ghy raakt ons ingewand, zoo krachtigh,
> Dat wy schier Kristus neemen an.
> Metaale tongh, doordringh uw spraaken,
> Uit saalicheits verborgen licht,
> Wie voelt syn nierenvet niet blaaken?
> My parst ghe tot dit waare dicht.
>
> (You touch our intestines, so powerfully,
> That we almost assume [the presence of] Christ.
> Metal tongue permeates your speeches,
> From the hidden light of the salvation,
> Who does not feel his kidney fat glow?
> You press me to this truthful poem.)

The passage is remarkable. It reveals again how the pharmaceutical background of Six van Chandelier leaves its mark on his poetry. The drug merchant describes the tongue of Wittewrongel as an exceptional specimen of a mineral remedy. This 'metal tongue' has a special purging effect: as Wittewrongel preaches, the audience feel their kidneys glow. According to early modern pathology the kidneys purify the blood for contaminated substances.[31]

Let us go back to 'Ecstasy' and the recipients of the poem. While the demonstration of a physical incompatibility with poetic excess would have been at the centre of the attention of Simon Dilman, the proof of an awareness of the danger of a pagan ecstasy would be important to Johannes Hoornbeeck. For Six, the right enthusiasm comes from a Christian source, and it has a non-material origin, in contrast to the ointments, incense and precious stones of paganism. But that does not take away the notion that the Christian grace has a physical impact; Six' pharmaceutical description of the language of Reformed preachers is, as we have seen, striking. Considering that there are no theological arguments in 'Ecstasy', Hoornbeeck would also have appreciated that Six sought to distance himself from pagan inspiration by defining it as a bodily disturbance. This is in line with the shift Michael Heyd observes, taking place in the views of the

30 Cf. also Petrus Wittewrongel's discussions on a healthy versus a unhealthy 'drunkenness' in his *Oeconomia christiana. Christelicke huys-houdinge*. 2 vols., Amsterdam 1661, vol. 2, pp. 1094–1096 and 1105.

31 Van Beverwijck, *Schat der ongesontheyt*, 1656, p. 148.

enthusiasm in the early modern period. Where sixteenth-century theologians identify enthusiasm with demonic forces, divines of the seventeenth and eighteenth centuries explain the phenomenon by means of medical theories.[32]

5 Defectiveness as evidence of humanness

In 'Ecstasy', Six delivers a medical critique on the notion of *furor poeticus*. Six tells us that the poetic mania contains no divine revelation, but hallucinations produced by medical drugs. We have to understand Six' self-presentation as a sober 'rhymester' in the light of the social context of the poet.[33] As a member of Calvinist, bourgeois society, Six wants to distance himself from all kinds of excess. The notion of divine inspiration in the poetry of Six is, as we have seen, linked to exotic and luxurious drugs: Incense, oils and gems which were considered to be spiritual agents, both in his own days – in the Catholic Mass and in the pagan religions of other people which the Dutch learned to know in their trade travels to foreign worlds – and in the religious ceremonies of Antiquity, a part of the artistic arsenal of the literature of renaissance Europe. In addition, the idea of drugs carrying secret and astral powers was not limited to the sphere of religion, but widespread among Paracelsian chemists in Six' days, who sought to isolate the 'life force' of materials through the art of distillation.

For Six, the Horatian modesty means health, while Pindaric excess illness. In this sense, it is possible to connect Six to an important mental shift in the early modern culture, the rise of the age of reason – a paradigm shift which is expressed in scholarly works as Michael Heyd's *Be Sober and Reasonable: The Critique of Enthusiasm in the Seventeenth and Early Eighteenth Centuries* (1995). By diagnosing the divine inspiration as 'drunkenness', Six blurs the boundary between pathological and supernatural mania. This movement thus attests to the modern character of Six' poetry – it is marked by a de-spiritualization of the world.

We could then conclude that, when Six defines poetic frenzy as an illness, he empties the notion of its pre-modern, positive meanings.[34] In the end we should

32 As earlier mentioned, Hoornbeeck was in contact with the chemist Franciscus de le Boë Sylvius, see n. 8. Cf. also the theologian Gisbertus Voetius' interest for scientific explanation of magical phenomena: M.J. van Lieburg, 'Voetius en de geneeskunde', in: J. van Oort, e. a. (ed.), *De onbekende Voetius: Voordrachten Wetenschappelijk Symposium Utrecht 3 maart 1989*, Kampen 1989, pp. 168–180.

33 See Maria Adriana Schenkeveld-van der Dussen, De anti-idealistische poëtica van een christen-burger, Joannes Six van Chandelier (see n. 13).

34 Intoxication as positive, artistic force, see Marty Roth, *Drunk the Night Before. An Anatomy of Intoxication*, Minneapolis 2005.

however stress that the notion of illness is more complex than that in Six' poetry. What is at stake in Six' criticism of *furor poeticus*, is not so much a contrasting of rationality and health versus irrationality and illness, as an acceptance of one's humanness versus pretentions on divinity. In this context pathological reactions are actually given a positive meaning. When Six in 'Ecstasy' emphasizes that he lacks an inner fire and is not capable of high divine flights, he gives proof of his status as a fallible human being. Defectiveness is thus attributed a positive value, while the perfect and divine a negative value.

In the end, we should not underestimate Six as the witty and playful poet, that he was. At the same time as he criticizes the notion of a *furor poeticus*, denying that he is able to fly like the 'bird kings' of the Dutch poetry, he does the same trick as Horace deed with Iulus. By applying the rhetorical figure of *praeteritio*, Six actually uses much space to describe the Pindaric flight and the divine speech, that were irreconcilable with his modest nature. His two friends, both learned academics, would have understood the trick and laughed at Six' subtle way of honouring them.

Helmer Helmers

Illness as Metaphor: The Sick Body Politic and Its Cures*

1 Introduction

The body politic is possibly the oldest, and certainly one of the most tenacious metaphors in political thought. Political philosophers ranging from Plato to John of Salisbury to Thomas Hobbes conceived of the state as analogous to the human body. Throughout the Middle Ages and the early modern period, the corporeal metaphor pervaded the literary tradition in Europe, inspiring a rich political vocabulary that was both anatomical and medical.[1]

If many of these terms, including 'corporation', 'member', 'head of state', and 'crisis' (originally a medical term) are still widely used today, they are – for most of us, at least – dead metaphors, disconnected from the intricate web of associations and beliefs of which they were originally part. Even a spin-doctor, a very explicit modern variant of an essentially early modern image, is not commonly associated with a medical practitioner. For early modern authors, by contrast, the language of the body politic was imbued with significance. Informed by the Neoplatonist conception of a mystic, but nevertheless very real correspondence between macrocosm and microcosm, the analogy between body and state was, for many, part of the texture of God's Creation. But even for those in whom the belief in the actual correspondence between body and state was lacking or weak, the human body, and the anatomical and medical knowledge that informed it, functioned as a heuristic device, as a means to achieve and report knowledge of good statecraft. Early modern

* This article was written with the support of a Veni-grant by the The Netherlands Organisation for Scientific Research (NWO). I thank Frans-Willem Korsten for his comments on a draft version.

1 Paul Archambault, 'The Analogy of the 'Body' in Renaissance Political Literature', in: *Bibliotèque d'humanisme et renaissance* 29 (1967), pp. 21–53; David Hale, *The Body Politic: A Political Metaphor in Renaissance English Literature*, The Hague 1971; David Hale, 'Analogy of the Body Politic', in: Philip Wiener (ed.), *Dictionary of the History of Ideas* I, New York 1973, pp. 68–70.

political discourses and debates were therefore fundamentally shaped by an ever-contested, ever-evolving biological language.

Central to this language was the idea that the body politic, like the natural body, could be wounded, suffer from disease, and die. Susan Sontag, whose title I have borrowed, has shown how potent and misleading a metaphor illness is in modern literature.[2] Infused by the idea of the body politic, it was no less potent and no less misleading in the early modern period.[3] Especially in the context of the religious wars and the rise of absolutism in the sixteenth and seventeenth centuries, when the quest to end the endemic conflicts that affected the European states was at its most intense, political thought was, in Jonathan Gill Harris' words, deeply concerned with 'social pathology' and therefore parallel to, and partly overlapping with, medicine.[4] In *The Prince*, Machiavelli famously stated that princes should be like doctors because both have to diagnose illnesses before they become too serious, and find the right cure.[5] Simultaneously, as Jake Soll has shown, medical knowledge came to be valued by rulers for its political implications. At the French court, doctors were increasingly called upon to diagnose the state. Similarly, Jean Bodin consulted the great medical works of Hippocrates and Galen when he wrote his own universal political theory, which he himself regarded as a 'therapy for the social body'.[6] In view of this changing appreciation, medical professionals therefore increasingly claimed expertise in matters of social sickness.[7] In the Dutch Republic, doctors such as Johan van Beverwijck did not only write medical treatises, but also political pamphlets, thus applying their skills of diagnosis to the body politic. Other doctors, such as Nicolaes Tulp, assumed political power themselves.[8]

This chapter analyses and contextualizes the political uses of illness in the Dutch Republic. Whereas the language (in the Pocockian sense) of the diseased body politic has been extensively researched for the English, and, to a lesser extent, for the French context, Dutch uses of the metaphor have not yet been analysed. This is unfortunate, because potentially, the Dutch Republic offers an

2 Susan Sontag, *Illness as Metaphor and AIDS and Its Metaphors*, New York 2001.

3 Margaret Healy, *Fictions of Disease in Early Modern England: Bodies, Plagues and Politics*, Houndsmill 2001; Jennifer Vaught (ed.), *Rhetorics of Bodily Disease and Health in Medieval and Early Modern England*, Farnham 2013.

4 Jonathan Gil Harris, *Foreign Bodies and the Body Politic Discourses of Social Pathology in Early Modern England*, Cambridge 2006.

5 Niccolò Machiavelli, *The Prince*, Translated and edited by Peter Bondanella, introduced by Maurizio Viroli, Oxford 2005, p. 8, 94.

6 Jacob Soll, 'Healing the Body Politic: French Royal Doctors, History, and the Birth of a Nation 1560–1634', in: *Renaissance Quarterly* 55:4 (2002), pp. 1259–1286, here pp. 1264–1265.

7 Roy Porter, *Bodies Politic: Disease, Death and Doctors in Britain, 1650–1900*, London 2001, ch. 9.

8 I thank Michiel van Groesen for the suggestion.

interesting contrast to the monarchies that surrounded it. One might expect this new, Republican state, with its complicated constitution, its advanced medical science, and its highly developed culture of political debate, to develop its own variants to European themes. Indeed, the culture that brought forth Rembrandt's *Anatomical lesson*, one should think, would be especially apt in dissecting the functions and dysfunctions of the body politic as well.

My purpose is therefore to situate the Dutch discourse of political illness in an international tradition, and to define its main currents. In many ways, I will show, Dutch uses of the metaphor conform to conservative European trends. Perhaps surprisingly, even the topoi of the natural, single-headed body politic and monarchical doctoring were echoed in Dutch sources, although the claims were often slightly softened to apply to the stadholders. It was mainly with respect to the role of communication that the Dutch seem to have developed a distinctly Dutch etiology.

2 The body in crisis

The frontispiece of Thomas Hobbes' *Leviathan* is arguably the most famous representation of the body politic (fig. 1). Hobbes' book sported an engraving depicting a tremendous body towering over the land, dominating the countryside, whilst supported on left and right by columns symbolizing civil and ecclesiastical authority. Composed of a multitude of subjects, it possesses only one, crowned head (looking slightly like Charles II). The image thus brilliantly captures Hobbes' novel absolutist philosophy, showing that a human corporation thrives, and the country is pacified, when it subjects itself to a single ruler who subordinates the state and the church.[9] Concord and harmony make up the health of Hobbes' body politic.

Hobbes' frontispiece is so well-known that it may well be the first image that comes to mind when the body politic is mentioned. Yet Hobbes' unnatural, 'artificial' corporation, with its monstrous name, in some ways constitutes a departure from more traditional representations of the body politic, which emphasized its naturalness. Rather than a multitude, they represent a single figure such as the monarch, whose body was mystically natural and political. Indeed, one of the sources of inspiration for Hobbes' frontispiece may be a Dutch image of this kind (fig. 2). Designed by Crispin van der Passe for Gabriel Rollenhagen's *Nucleus Emblemata* (which appeared in Dutch in 1615), the emblem showed a monarchical

9 For a brilliant analysis of the frontispiece, see: Quentin Springer, *Hobbes and Republican Liberty*, Cambridge 2008, pp. 185–198.

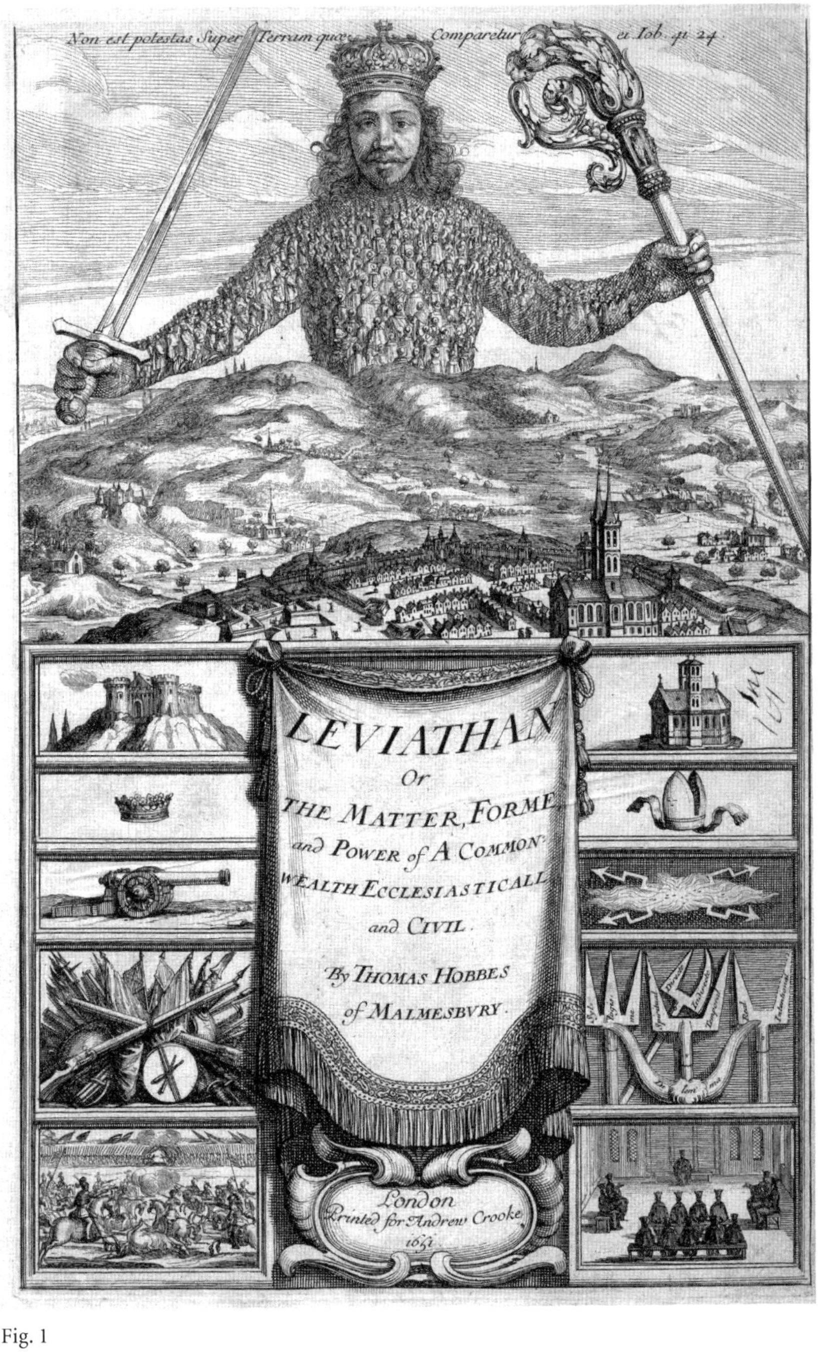
Non est potestas Super Terram quæ Comparetur ei. Iob. 41. 24.
LEVIATHAN
Or
THE MATTER, FORME and POWER of A COMMON-WEALTH ECCLESIASTICALL and CIVIL.
By THOMAS HOBBES of MALMESBVRY.
London
Printed for Andrew Crooke
1651

Fig. 1

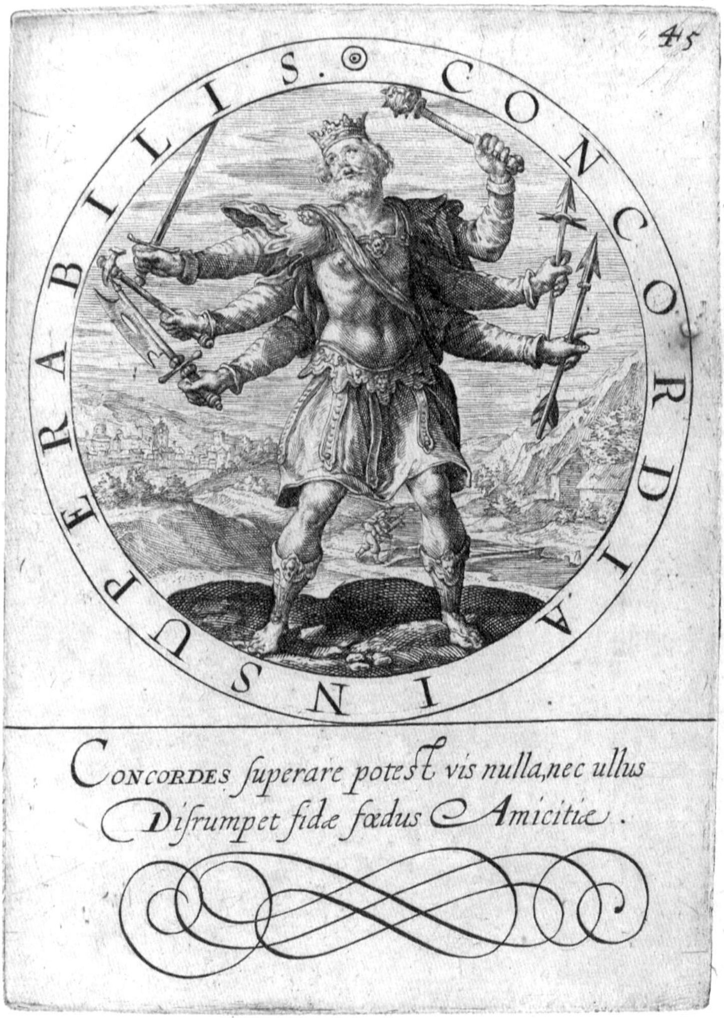

Fig. 2

body politic with six arms.[10] Like Hobbes' corporation, it dominated a peaceful landscape, and illustrated the power of concord. Here, however, the figure is clearly that of the monarch alone, whose powers are increased by the invisible people behind him who act in concord with him.

More frequent still are the images of (heraldic) animals that symbolize certain nations: the Dutch Lion, the French Cock, and the German Eagle are well-known

10 Gabriel Rollenhagen, *Nucleus Emblemata selectissimorum, quae Itali vulgo Impresas vacant*, Arnhem 1615, p. 93.

examples, omnipresent in seventeenth-century political print. Of course, such images often functioned in the context of hostile political fables. The Dutch lion, Marijke Spies has shown, had long been used as an image of the Spanish enemy before it was gradually appropriated by the emerging Dutch state.[11] By the time Claes Jansz Visscher published his famous *Leo Belgicus* (1609) the lion had become a symbol of the viable Northern provinces. Like a monarchical figure, such animal figures were natural political bodies representing a healthy, functional, organic unity of several parts. As Hans Nadler's famous *Quaterionenadler* illustrates, they especially suited the more complex political confederations (fig. 3).

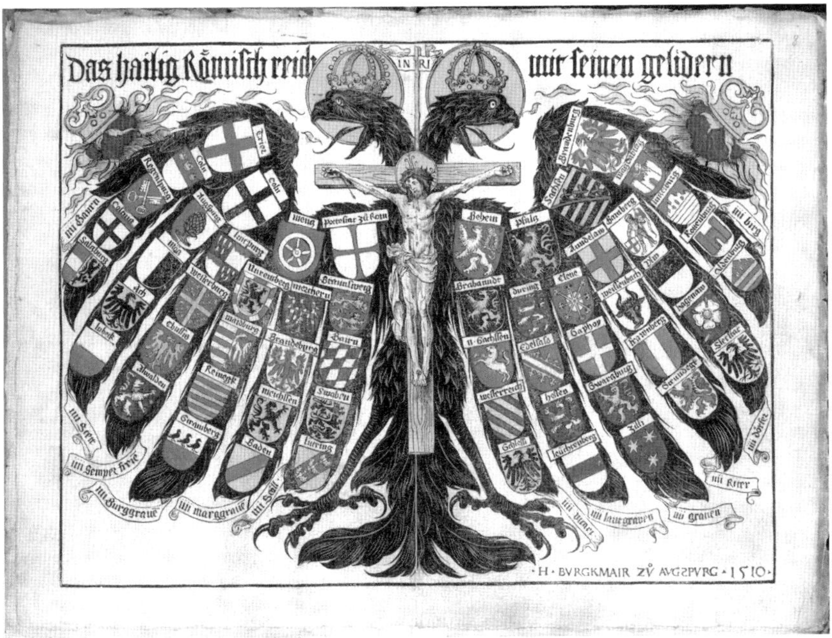

Fig. 3

However different in appearance, in one sense, these three modes of representing the body politic were all alike: they imposed and required concord. Sickness, the implication was, was a lack of unity. Indeed, Hobbes explicitly states that sedition was the body politic's disease, and civil war its death.[12] A similar idea of sickness can be found in numerous political pamphlets such as

11 Marijke Spies, 'Verbeeldingen van vrijheid. David en Mozes, Burgerhart en Bato, Brutus en Cato', in: *De Zeventiende Eeuw* 10 (1994), pp. 141–155, here pp. 146–148.

12 Thomas Hobbes, *Leviathan*, C. B. Macpherson (ed.), London 1985, p. 81. On the 'birth defects', 'infirmities' and diseases of the Commonwealth, see also pp. 363–376.

Den Krancken Gier (*The Sick Vulture*), a satire of the Holy Roman Empire during the early Thirty Years War (fig. 4) showing Nadler's proud German eagle perverted and incapacitated by civil strife, Catholicism and the ambitious House of Habsburg, and attended by an incapable Spanish doctor.[13]

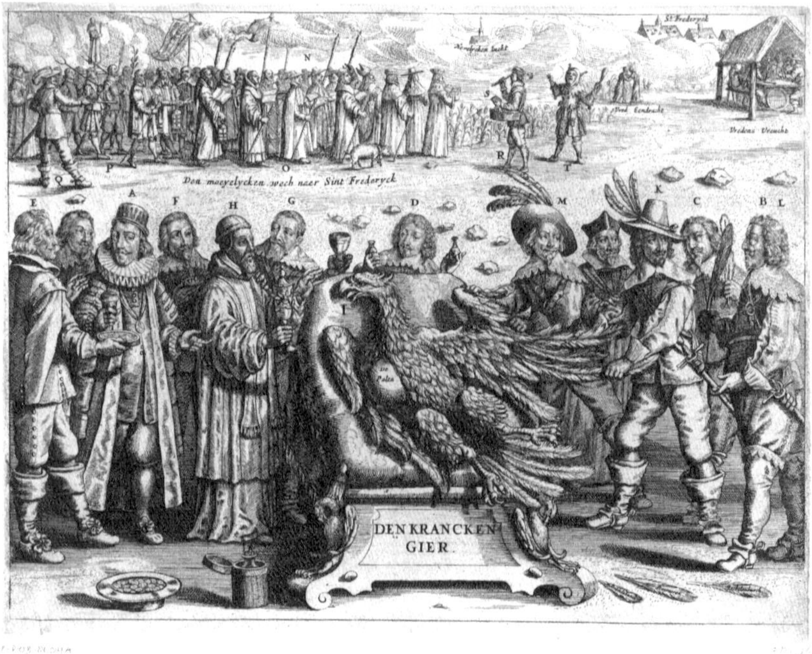

Fig. 4

The early modern state plagued by civil war and religious violence was as a body in disarray, even monstrous. Augustine considered a community without a head to be a trunk, incapable of action.[14] Although that is perhaps the most common image of political monstrosity, Republics might also be represented as hydra's with many heads.[15] When Samuel Pufendorf tried to explain and remedy the violence and instability that had troubled the Holy Roman Empire, he, possibly inspired by Nadler's complex, two-headed eagle, diagnosed the problem in terms of the body, famously stating that the German Empire was an 'irregular and monstrous body' ('irregolare aliquod corpus et monstro simile'),

13 Crispijn van der Passe (II), *Den krancken gier* [*The sick vulture*], Amsterdam 1622, FMH 1476.

14 Archambault, 'The Analogy' (see n. 1), p. 35.

15 On the discourse of political monstrosity, see: Laura Knoppers and Joan Landes (eds.), *Monstrous Bodies/Political Monstrosities in Early Modern Europe*, Ithaca/London 2004.

deformed because it had a flawed constitution (pun intended).[16] Arguing for a standing army paid for by all the German states and the depolitization of religion, Pufendorf's solution for the Empire's 'disease' in a way anticipated the German nation state. Like Hobbes, he considered the absolute rule of a dynasty (albeit different from the Austrian Habsburgs, whom he despised) to be the best cure against its deformities: a body must have a head.

Such widespread ideas about the dysfunctional body politic rooted in Plato's *Timaeus* and his *Republic.* Plato described a well-ordered polis as analogous to the human body: its rationality resides in the philosopher-king, who is sustained by the passionate 'heart' of the auxiliary class, and the appetitive organs of workers and peasants.[17] This formulation of the ideal political body had a major influence on later thinkers. It presented many a monarchist with an excellent metaphor, because it allowed the single, ruling head of state to be represented as a natural phenomenon. Dante, in *De Monarchia*, pleads for a single monarch in the Empire, because this type of rule occurs in all 'natural' organizations, human body, family, and tribe alike.[18] In early modern political thought, which grappled with the chronic (religious) violence and civil wars between estates and princes, such ideas of order had an undiminished appeal. Many sought to explain the disruption of contemporary European experience by pointing out the deviations from a natural situation corresponding in its tripartite organisation to the human body.

The main literary source of the disorderly body politic is Aesop's fable of the belly. In its simplest, third century form, Aesop's tale is about an argument between the belly and the feet about who was the most important; the stomach argues its precedence because it provides the body with the nourishment that keeps it alive, the feet argue that the belly would be nothing if it had no feet to carry it. When the belly stops digesting, the feet soon lose their energy and recognize their mistake. In itself, the fable of the belly was not explicitly political. From the earliest reworkings by Livy and Cassius Dio, however, political language was introduced to it, the debate becoming a 'rebellion', in Livy, or a 'strike', in Cassius Dio. The morale of such reworkings was conservative. Livy describes how Menenius Agrippa successfully uses the tale in a public speech meant to prevent a rebellion. Agrippa convinces his hungry, plebeian audience that the patricians use the resources at their disposal for the benefit of the entire commonwealth; they are rich and well-fed to maintain the community. Medieval and early modern authors provided similar applications to instill obedience to Popes

16 Horst Denzer, 'Samuel Pufendorf', in: Horst Denzer and Hans Maier (eds.), *Klassiker des Politischen Denkens. Zweiter Band: Von Locke bis Max Weber,* München 2007, pp. 27–52, here p. 29.
17 Eugene Thacker, 'Nomos, Nosos and Bios', in: *Culture Machine* 7 (2005), Online resource.
18 Archambault, 'The Analogy' (see n. 1), p. 30.

and princes in their readers.[19] For them, the corporeal metaphor of the state was mostly a conservative one, declaring a given situation to be natural.

Although that natural order often implied Plato's head of state, Aesop's tale of intestine disruptions was also applied by those who opposed royal rule. In his *Apology*, William of Orange referred to the fable of the belly extensively, yet he used it to spur the States General to action and support his revolt against the king. William urged the States to protect the 'beautiful' body of the state, which was being deformed by the king, and to make sure that 'the stomach, which is the Council you shall ordain', would 'digest' all the food first, and send 'medicines' wherever in the body a 'disease' would manifest itself.[20] For William, the king had upset the body politic by violating ancient rights, thereby upsetting the natural order. In this sense, his application of Aesop's fable was perfectly conservative. It was fully in line with the Aristotelian idea prominent in medieval literature that the Prince, being the head of the body, depends on his subjects as much as they depend upon his direction.

A particularly amusing variant of the motive of bodily competition in Dutch seventeenth-century literature is Adriaen Stikke's *Battle of the Body Members* (*Leedenstryt*, w. 1627, p. 1630).[21] Beginning his poem rather conventionally with a debate between various body parts, including the Eye, the Nose, the Hand and the Foot, Stikke takes the genre to its ludicrous consequences by introducing 'another member', 'a straight stem', 'a ruler of kings and gods', who has brought together 'nun and papist', 'maiden and menial' and fills the world with people. After a monologue from this anonymous lower body member, the carnivalesque tone reaches its greatest height when the Ass 'bursts out' impatiently to assert its own prominence. When she is prevented from speaking by the other members, however, she takes her revenge, and 'shuts her doors'. Soon the body is plagued by the terrible consequences of constipation: the 'stomach shrank, the bowels became stiff', and the body quickly deteriorates. No medicine avails, the 'gates remained closed', and as a result, a 'strange mist of vapours' ascends to the head, causing 'cold fearful sweat and rising hairs'. The other body parts, 'lame and half-dead', forget their former pride, and succumb to all the demands of the slighted Ass.[22] Farcical and burlesque, Stikke's bodily disarray still has strong

19 David Hale, 'Intestine Sedition. The Fable of the Belly', in: *Comparative Literary Studies* 5/4 (1968), pp. 377–388, passim.

20 Pieter Cornelisz. Hooft, *Apologie, ofte Verantwoordinge des doorluchtigen ende hoogh-geboren vorsts ende heers, Wilhelm … Prince van Orangien … Teghen den ban ofte edict, by forme van proscriptie tegen hen ghepubliceert by den Coningh van Spangien*, Leeuwarden 1746, p. 185.

21 Adriaen Stikke, *Leedenstrydt*, The Hague 1630; I have used the copy of Leiden University Library, sig. BKNOOG 300. Available online through: http://www.let.leidenuniv.nl/Dutch/Renaissance/Facsimiles/Leedenstrydt1630/index.htm [last retrieved on March 3, 2015].

22 Stikke, Leedenstrydt (see n. 21), sig. C2v-C4r.

political overtones, and ends with an admonition to those in power: 'Thus everybody should behold, that even a minor power, / Is often raised as soon as it is despised'.[23]

Although Stikke's tone contrasts sharply with William the Silent's grave rhetoric, his politics speak directly to the *Apology.* Stikke, who wrote his poem when the Dutch war against Spain was going particularly well, probably had the Low Countries in mind when he chose to assert the power of the lower body parts (Shakespeare, too, made the pun in *2 Henry IV*). Equating their stubborn fight for their privileges against the high and mighty king of Spain to the Ass' strike, the *Leedenstryt* was first and foremost an allegory of the Revolt. Yet given Stikke's comic mode and his egalitarian lesson at the end, it is not altogether surprising that not everybody read the poem in this way.

When Pieter Baerdt adapted the *Leedenstryt* for republication ten years later, he turned it into a political plea for democratic rule. Baerdt used Stikke's text to argue that a political body needs all its members to be active and speak up for its interests in order for it to function. For Baerdt, democracy instead of monarchy was the most natural form of government: 'For who in the world could ordain a better established Republic than the one thus established by our High and Mighty Creator?'[24] Baerdt's advocacy of popular democracy was exceptional even in the Dutch Republic,[25] but it is telling that even this unorthodox author considered it useful to couch his message in the language of bodily harmony – thus presenting his favoured political order as natural. His strategy was markedly less radical than that pursued by the French revolutionaries one and a half century later. As Antoine de Baecque has shown, they used the image of the body politic to describe the degeneration of the nobility; if the state was a body, they argued, it was able to age and die.[26]

Although ideological applications of the metaphor of crises in the body politic ranged widely in the Dutch Republic, all authors are functionalists who abhor dissent and dictated that intestine disorders should be avoided and remedied at all costs. They argued or implied that such disorders can be remedied by constitutional means: adopting a 'natural' organization of government provided protection against, or remedied, rebellion. This classically inspired representation of the body politic promoted a sense of unity and coherence and

---

23 Stikke, Leedenstrydt (see n. 21), sig. D2v.

24 Pieter Baerdt, *Democratia corporis humani; dat is, Leden-stemminghe des menschelijcken lichaems; gevoegt op een democratike regieringe sommiger republijcken*, Leeuwarden: Fonteyne 1640; I use Weststeijn's translation (see n. 25 below).

25 Arthur Weststeijn, *Commercial Republicanism in the Dutch Golden Age*, Leiden 2012, p. 271.

26 Antoine de Baecque, *Le corps de l'histoire: métaphores et politique (1770–1800)*, Paris 1993.

foregrounded mutual responsibilities within the state. Yet of course, the body politic could also be upset by exterior causes.

3 The xenobiotic other

Jonathan Gil Harris has argued that along with the development and spread of the new Paracelsian paradigm, that came to vie with the Galenic model, the Renaissance saw a shift in the conception of social illnesses as well. In contrast to the disruptions within the body represented by the variants of Aesop's fable, Paracelsian medicine emphasized that disease was caused by malignant, exterior 'foreign bodies'. In political discourse, too, Harris described a new emphasis on foreign agents of disease.[27] Rather than disciplining dysfunctional or dissatisfied members of the body, the language of infection required their removal, through surgery, violent medicines, or purging. Raising the fear of the xenobiotic other, this medical discourse was an integral part of early modern nationbuilding, in which the permeability of the body was a central concern, because it idealized the nation as a functional whole.

As the religious wars of the sixteenth century had raised the awareness of the danger religious dissidents might pose to the state, the most feared xenobiotic element in the state was the religious other. In the Dutch Republic, like in Protestant England, the medical language of infection was often employed against the pestilence of Catholicism – which became a notable topos in the pamphlet literature. As the Catholic powers retrieved ever more territory in Europe during the seventeenth century, the fear of infiltration and the resulting paralysis or death of the state ran deep in Protestant states. In his *Corrosive against the cankering pestilence of popery* (*Corrosiif. Teghens de in-etende pest-kole van't pausdom*), the Zeeland Puritan Willem Teellinck, for example, inventorized the reasons why a Reformed government should ban all Catholic practices from its territory. Importantly, Teellinck employed the language of purification; the 'pestilence' needed to be removed in order for the body politic to become unpoluted, thereby regaining its health.[28]

Evidently, the religious infection of the body politic in Teellinck's sense was not necessarily the result of foreign immigration – many religious dissidents were simply locals. They were constructed to be foreign to the body politic rather than the land. However, in the case of the Catholics, the connections to Catholic states and the allegiance to Rome opened up the body for foreign intrusions, for

27 Harris, Foreign Bodies (see n. 4), pp. 9–16 and passim.

28 Willem Teellinck, *Corrosiif. Teghens de in-etende pest-kole van't pausdom. Ofte Grondigh ondersoeck, of het wel geoorloft is de paepsche superstitien te dulden*, s.l. 1620, Kn. 4449.

example by ambassadors, or worse, Jesuits. These internationally operating figures could change even a mild sore into a festering wound. By contrast, especially in the first half of the century, reformed Protestants, even if they lived as far away as Hungary, were even often seen as part or extensions of the Dutch politico-religious body in Teellinck's time. When foreign Protestants were persecuted, Reformed pamphleteers such as Voetius spoke of the pains done to 'our body', and throughout the seventeenth century, Dutch politicians saw it as their task to connect with and to care for foreign Protestants.

Other religious minorities, such as Jews, sectarians and gypsies, were seen as infectious and various authors advised remedies against them. That a removal of the foreign infection might require violence, as Teellinck requested, was defended with reference to medical analogy. Thus, in his *Politica*, Justus Lipsius – who, in contrast to Teelinck, was a Catholic – argued that religious dissidents were like infected members, and advised his readers to 'burn' and 'cut' them away, 'in order that some member perishes rather than the whole body'.[29] The phrase, taken from Cicero's *Philippics*, circulated widely in early modern Europe, and its tenor seems to have been accepted by authorities of various ideological backgrounds. And yet, analogizing statecraft to surgery (undoubtedly the most aggressive and painful form of bodily treatment before the invention of anaesthetics) was rather more radical than traditional ideas about curing the body politic. The logic of amputation therefore did not please everybody. Dirck Volckertsz. Coornhert, the great proponent of religious toleration, was one of the readers who took the metaphor literally and accused Lipsius of promoting cruel prosecution. Lipsius later defended himself by denying that all dissenters should be burned and cut in a literal sense, but his defence did not amount to a huge shift in either position or logic. 'The meaning of the phrase', Lipsius explained, 'is to use a strong medicine (…) I punish some disturbers with fines, others with exile and a rare few with death'. For Coornhert and other more liberal thinkers, the surgical thrust in political thought was dangerous and silly, but Lipsius was far from alone in presenting the religious other as the most hurtful disease, which required strong medication.

Another form of forcibly removing the foreign element from a body politic can be found in texts reflecting on hostile conquest. The pamphlet *The Duke of Bavaria's Illness and Emetic* (*De sieckte ende braeck-dranck vanden hertogh van Beieren*), (re)published in several languages in 1632 on the occasion of Gustavus Adolphus' spectacular series of victories in Germany, presented several doctors 'from a variety of countries' quarreling over the Duke of Bavaria's afflictions

29 This paragraph is based on: Jan Waszink, 'Introduction', in: Justus Lipsius, *Politica. Six Books of Politics or Political Instruction*, Jan Waszink (ed.), Assen 2004, pp. 1–198, here pp. 71–72.

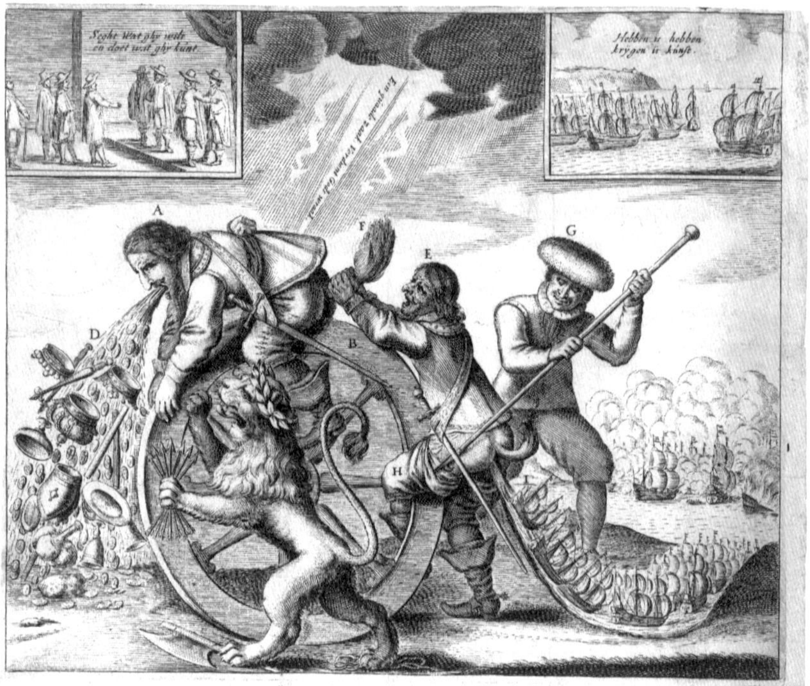

Voorſpookkend Zinne-beeld, op den Staat der Engelſche en Nederlanders.

DE Staat-zucht trok'et Koor-kleed aan,
En liet de Schotſe Trommel ſlaan,
Om d'oude Trouw de nek te breekken:
De Nikker blies een voor de wind;
En wiſt de Teems, puur doof en blind,
Dit voor wat Hailigs in te preekken.
Mit kreeg de Britze Troon een krak.
De Deugd gaf voort de leſte ſnak,
En look, op 't Moord-tooneel, 'er oogen.
De Roof, verzien met Bus en Swaard,
Sprong daadlik op'et dolſte Paard,
En ſtal al 't Koningklik vermoogen.
De (a) Liſt, verguld met ſulk een Schat,
Klom vaardig booven op'et (b) Rad
Van Avondtuur; en ſloeg zen blikken
Op STUARTS Na-zaadt, zo verwoed,
Dat d'Onderdaan van 'sKonings Bloed,
Helaas! geen enig woord dorſt kikken.
Dus wierd hy, als een God, gevreeſt.
Tot dat, na'et voorſpook van mijn Geeſt,
Een (c) fiere Leeuw, met krulde lokken,
En ſtark van pooten, lang gehoont,
In 't Vecht-parck, om zijn Deugd gekroont,
Quam loeren op zijn goude brokken.

Getergde Wraak ſprong na de Kruk;
En deed'et Rad, met eene ruk,
Meer dan een groote hand breed draayen:
De Staart-man wierd'et Hoofd te ſwaar:
Hy riep en kreet, met ſulck misbaar,
Dat Meeſter TOM hem niet kon paayen.
De quaalikheid ſloeg voort na'et Hart.
Hy gaf, van angſt en vrees benart,
Met eene gulp, zijn (d) Rijkdom over.
De Leeuw, vol moedts, deê noch een ruk;
Mit greep, doch tot zijn ongeluk
Een (e) Gier de (f) Staart van d'opper Roover.
Zit vaſt, Lord OLEF, zit doch vaſt,
Of 't Schip verſeilt op Bijl en Baſt,
Zo riep de Zee-haan, groot van ſpooren:
Hy ſloeg zen beenen om 'et Rad,
En kreet, en beet als Martens Kat:
Maar al den handel was verlooren.
Want, eer hy om zag hoe 't 'er ging,
Streek een (g) Matroos, ô wonder ding!
De (h) Plunder-broek hem op de hielen:
Dit Hollands Deuntje klonck te wreet;
Des (i) ſcheet de Vraat, met eene ſcheet,
Wel vijftig wel beſeilde Kielen.

Dus keerde zich op 't leſt de kans:
De dolle Staart-man moeſt zen Swans
An 't Dreumelt-mutsjen over geeven:
Hier hilp geen huilen als een Hond;
Geen karmen, noch geen vuille mond:
Geen Judas, Kus voor 't eerloos leeven.
Het hailig Recht verſchoont geen Moord
Of Roovery, gants ongehoord
Gepleegt an Vriende en Bont-genooten;
Het gaat zen gang, en ziet niet aan:
Het Bloed-Rijk moet in Bloed vergaan,
Al ſchijnt'et weelig opgeſchootten.
Verheug u dan, Doorluchtig Volck,
Dat dus lang voor de wreetſten Dolck,
In ballingſchap, uw hail moeſt derven:
De fiere Leeuw verbijt den Dog:
Het Rad draait om: Hy zal 't Bedrog
Wel haaſt den Kop an ſtukken kerven.
Ik droom! wat ydelheyd is dit?
De Leeuw ſchijnt krachtloos van gebit;
Des krimt my 'tHart. Och bitre ſlaagen!
Hoe dus mijn Ziel? zijt wel gemoedt.
Al 't geen de Geeſt hier ſpookkend doet,
Daar van ſal 't haeſt in Holland waagen.

Fig. 5

during the Thirty Years War. The doctors, who include Christan Bravo, a reference to the fierce Protestant paladine Christian of Brunswick, and a Spanish doctor, presumably the general Ambrogio Spinola, agree on the cause of the archduke's sufferings: Bavaria had overeaten by incorporating the lands of the exiled Elector Palatine Frederick V in 1622, and had never managed to digest them properly. As a result, the duke suffered from a severe case of flatulence. Although the doctors disagree over the proper treatment, the medicin eventually chosen is a bitter emetic that will cause him to disgorge all the xenobiotic cities and lands devoured earlier.[30] At the moment of publication, in 1632, the implication of the *Braeck-dranck* was clear: the prescribed emetic was the Swedish army, which had invaded Bavaria in the previous spring. The satire adopts the metaphor of the sick body politic to legitimize and celebrate Gustavus Adolphus' retributive war. Its effectiveness hinges on the idea that contemporary European states were stable, separate bodies, who could not cannibalize each other without risking disease. The logic employed could be called Paracelsian: the toxic medicine of war was required to restore the European bodies politic to their pure and 'natural' state.

In a comparable way to the *Braeck-dranck*, a Dutch print published during the First Anglo-Dutch War (1652–1654) described the war effort as a purgative, which was vividly illustrated by an engraving that showed Dutch sailors forcing the illegitimate conquests from Oliver Cromwell's body (see fig. 5).[31] In both satires, the language of the body politic functioned to express a distinct conservative as well as essentialist agenda: presenting a given order as natural, it was used to reject not only revolution, but also conquest. In this seventeenth-century vision, the personification of the states of Europe in political print is taken to its logical conclusion: that they are well-prescribed bodies that resist foreign elements and cannibalism.

4 The Princely Healer

The concern with infection in the period of religious war and nation-building also reinforced age-old beliefs in the healing power of the sovereign. In 1612, James I, king of England, published a *Declaration*, printed in English and in Dutch, in which he defended his opposition against the appointment of Conrad Vorstius to the chair of theology in Leiden. In it, James offered a non-religious explanation for his meddling in Dutch religious affairs. 'Were Leiden to be contaminated with [the heresies of Vorstius]', he wrote, 'then England would soon be infected too'.[32] While showing himself equally aware of the danger of

30 *De sieckte ende braeck-dranck vanden hertogh van Beieren*, s.l. 1632, Kn. 4200. The original, German pamphlet was *Bayerische Kranckheit beneben Geschwulst deß Magens*, Prague 1632.

31 *Voorspookkend Zinne-beeld, op den Staat der Engelsche en Nederlanders*, s.l. 1652, FM 2040.

32 The *Declaration* was first printed in Holland in French, and, according to Winwood in a letter to Cecil, also translated into Dutch (the Dutch version is not in the STCN and may be lost). The English title is *James I, His Majesties Declaration concerning his Proceedings with the States generall of the United Provinces of the Low Countries, in the matter of D. Conradus*

religious infection in two countries as proximate as England and the Dutch Republic as Lipsius, James took a different approach to religious dissidents, preferring profylactic measures to surgery. At the same time, he presented himself as England's physician, who guarded the health of his country.

Shakespeare's *Macbeth*, written at the beginning of James' reign, is an instructive example of how this particular royal physician was constructed.[33] The play, as many critics have noted, is pervaded with the language of disease. After Macbeth has murdered Duncan and usurped the crown, Scotland itself is described as bleeding, and each new day, Malcolm says, 'a gash / Is added to her wounds' (4.3.40–41). As desperation takes possession of Macbeth, the king turns to his doctor to 'cast the water of my land' and 'purge it to a sound and pristine health' (5.3.50–52). Of course, the Scottish doctor is unable to help. As Shakespeare's audiences knew all too well, the only way to 'purge' the land would be to remove the usurper Macbeth himself, who unwittingly constitutes the disease he seeks to have cured.

The only person in the play whose healing abilities are effective is Edward, the king of England. 'Such sanctity hath heaven given to his hand', the English doctor asserts, that the king of England is able to cure 'a crew of wretched souls' (4.3.160–6). As Marjorie Garber has emphasized, the language of disease and healing helps to shape and foreground a crucial opposition: whereas 'Macbeth's bloody hand brings death; Edward's holy hand brings life and healing'.[34] Importantly, it is the same Edward who defeats Macbeth in battle and restores order in Scotland. The king of England's healing power applies both to the natural bodies of his subjects and to the body politic of Scotland, which is purged from sick-making tyranny by a lawful holy ruler.

The idea that monarchs possessed remedial powers was deeply rooted in European culture. The analogy between a king and a doctor, which we have already encountered in Machiavelli, was extremely old. In *De principis instructione* (c. 1217), Geraldus Cambrensis, had already emphasized that the Prince administering justice was like a surgeon guarding the health of state. Cambrensis, however, saw the analogy in terms of duty, arguing that the prince should be prudent in punishing his subjects: it was preferable to cure sick members of the kingdom than to amputate them altogether and thus weaken the body.[35] *Macbeth*, by contrast, suggests a more mystical reading of the king's healing power. As Marc Bloch has famously shown, the kings of England and

Vorstius, London 1612. Cited in: ANTHONY MILTON, *Catholic and Reformed: The Roman and Protestant Churches in English Protestant Thought, 1600–1640*, Cambridge 2002, p. 405.

33 I have used the Arden Shakespeare edition: WILLIAM SHAKESPEARE, *Macbeth*, KENNETH MUIR (ed.), London 2005.

34 MARJORIE GARBER, *Shakespeare After All*, New York 2004, pp. 718–719.

35 ARCHAMBAUD, The Analogy (see n. 1), 29.

France were long believed to possess the 'Royal Touch', which was presumed to cure scrofula, the king's disease. Until the late seventeenth century, the kings of England performed healing ceremonies that drew huge audiences, suggesting that many believed in the literal healing powers of royalty. This belief in the efficacy of the royal touch also applied to the royal blood, which was often believed to be therapeutic as well.[36] Even in the Dutch Republic, where magical beliefs are often presumed to have lost their appeal by the early seventeenth century, hundreds of people flocked to such ceremonies, and handkerchiefs with royal blood were sold on the streets.[37]

Shakespeare's play exemplifies that this magical belief was deeply intertwined with the belief in the sacredness of true royal rule – as opposed to usurped royal power. The healing of human bodies and the body politic were two aspects of the same source of power, and as such they were closely related to, and probably derived from, the 'political theology' of the king's two bodies.[38] If the king's natural body possessed a healing power to natural bodies, his body politic could heal the natural corporation of the state. Obviously, this belief in the thaumaturgic powers of royalty rooting in their divine status was weak, implicit or simply absent in many texts that invoked the image of the physician-king. For many political thinkers, foremost Machiavelli, the analogy between prince and doctor functioned mainly as a heuristic and didactic instrument. Yet the belief did much to energize rhetoric and logic of the diseased body politic, and few explicitly rejected it.

The idea of the prince as healer of the body politic was especially urgent in times of civil unrest, when the head could impose order on the rest of the body. During the English civil wars various pamphlets appeared that reported the healing miracles performed by Charles I,[39] implying that he was wholesome to the body politic as well. When the king had been executed, the state, too, was decapitated and could be healed only by restoring the House of Stuart to the throne. By contrast, according to one pamphlet circulating widely both in England and the Dutch Republic, the only doctors which the English Republic could muster in an attempt to heal the dismembered body politic were 'Selfishness', 'Ambition', 'Distrust' and 'Inquisitiveness', who evidently inflicted only more damage to the dying patient.[40]

36 Marc Bloch, *The Royal Touch. Sacred Monarchy and Scrofula in England and France*, London 1973.

37 Helmer J. Helmers, *The Royalist Republic. Literature, Politics and Religion in the Anglo-Dutch Public Sphere*, Cambridge 2015, pp. 133–137.

38 Ernst H. Kantorowicz, *The King's Two Bodies: A Study in Mediaeval Political Theology. With a new preface by William Chester Jordan*, Princeton 1998.

39 Andrew Lacey, *The Cult of King Charles the Martyr*, Woodbridge 2003, pp. 62–64.

40 *Engelse Anatomy*, s.l. 1649, Kn. 6447.

As in the English Civil Wars, Dutch civil unrest invariably led to cries for a princely physician. During the First Anglo-Dutch War, for example, when panic reigned the streets after the disastrous battle of Portland, *The Discovery of the Dutch Cancer, With which the entire body of our state is grievously infected* (*Ontdeckinghe van den Nederlandtschen cancker. Waer mede 't gheheele lichaem van onsen staet deerlijck is besmet*, 1653) identified the 'overflowing sins of the land' as the disease of the Dutch Republic, and the main cause of the disastrous development of the war with English. This sinfulness, however, is largely facilitated and expressed by the rule of the ungodly regents, 'who use religion only as a pretext for their designs'. The Prince of Orange, as the protector of the reformed religion, is presented as the medicine who will restore the country to its former pious and therefore prosperous condition.[41]

Frequently, such political satires depict the country as passive, fragile and feminine, in need of a strong, male infusion. The traditional personification of Dutch political bodies, the allegorical virgin, provided a suitable image for Orangist pamphleteers. In 1672, when the Dutch Republic was overrun by the French forces of Louis XIV, Crispin van der Passe published a print showing the ill Dutch Virgin attended by a doctor, who diagnoses that the cause of her ailments is the headless rule of the regents, who, being only interested in 'Mammon', have unsettled her body. As medicin, he prescribes 'William', the 'head' who had instituted Dutch unity and whose 'name will heal all pain'.[42] This time, the dominant wholesome quality of the prince resides not in his religion, but in his protection of the common good in the spirit of the father of the fatherland, and in the fact that he was to be the single head of state, which was the only natural form of government.[43]

The Orangist medicine of 1672 advertised by Van der Passe and pamphlets such as *Medicine for the Dutch ailments* (*Genees-middelen voor Hollants-Qualen*) also suggested the need for surgery along the line of Lipsius' advise.[44] As Michel Reinders has shown, the violent murder of the De Witt brothers, later that year, aimed at healing the nation by removing the Wittian disease. The terrible mutilations that the De Witt bodies suffered (fig. 6) were not only produced by crazed panic, but were also seen as justified imitations of the damage they themselves had done to the Dutch body politic. Thus, one pamphleteer sug-

41 *Ontdeckinghe van den Nederlandtschen cancker. Waer mede 't gheheele lichaem van onsen staet deerlijck is besmet*, 'Heylstad' 1653, Kn. 7441, A2r-A2v.

42 *Sinne-beeld. Ter eeren van Sijn Doorluchtighste Hoogheyt Willem de III. Prins van Oraenjen*, &c, Amsterdam 1665/72, FM 2306, plano.

43 Michel Reinders, *Printed Pandemonium. Popular Print and Politics in the Netherlands, 1650–1672*, Leiden 2013, pp. 176–179.

44 *Genees-middelen voor Hollants-Qualen. Vertoonende de quade regeringe der Loevesteinse factie*, Antwerpen (false imprint), 1672, Kn. 10376.

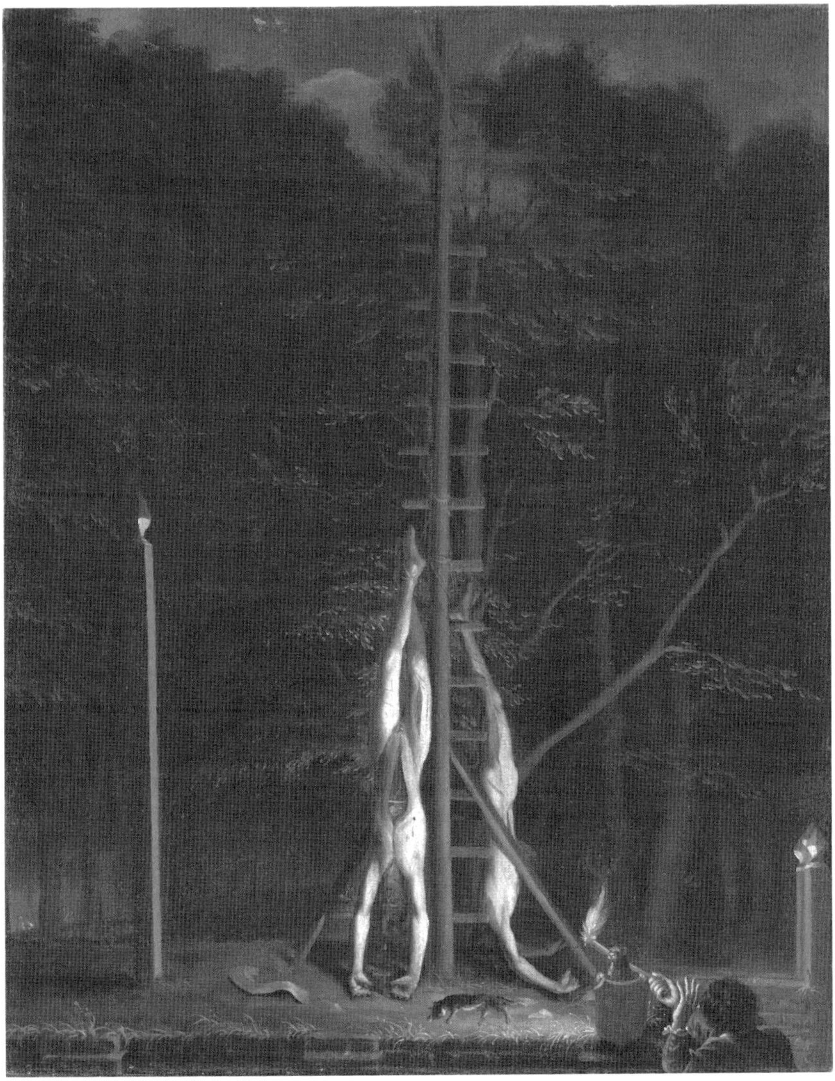

Fig. 6

gested, the flesh had been 'squeezed from their bodies' in the same way as the citizenry had been squeezed by the war.[45]

This Orangist use of medicinal language would prove extremely persistent – it was still used a century later, in the 1780s, when civil war loomed again. It is striking that in contrast to their colleagues in neighbouring kingdoms, Dutch

45 Reinders, Printed Pandemonium (see n. 43), pp. 166–168.

authors seem to refrain from representing the Prince of Orange as a doctor. In all the instances of the trope of the healing ruler I found, as in the examples above, they present him as a cure. That the Prince was, by implication, a passive object administered by a third-party doctor rather than the doctor himself is significant, and peculiar to the nature of Dutch Orangism, which predominantly saw the prince not as the absolute power, but as the servant of the state.[46] Rather than the prince, the implied doctor in this pamphlet was the pamphleteer himself. This points to a final, to my knowledge unrecognized corrollary of the political discourse of disease and infection of the body politic: political print.

5 Print as disease and medicine

When we speak of a tweet going 'viral', the metaphor will only rarely summon up images of mediated communication as a sickmaking agent that will affect the body social. Instead, it is usually meant only to convey the speedy, multidirectional, and non-hierarchical replication of information. Rather than sickening, tweeting and engaging in other forms of public communication are, in the West at least, predominantly seen as wholesome activities, a connotation that stands in sharp contrast with the biological vehicle that is employed to describe them. In early modern Europe, the virus – discovered first by Dmitri Ivanovsky in 1892 – was not yet known, but language of sickness was as eagerly applied to the media as it is today. Media, as we shall see, were alternately condemned as infectious diseases or praised as effective medicines.

That print was capable of seriously disturbing the body politic was a commonplace in early modern Europe ever since Luther's reformation. The insight was soon integrated into traditional representations of the body politic. One interesting example of this integration is offered by Lambert van den Bosch's allegorical comedy *Lingua: ofte Strijd tusschen de tong en de vyf zinnen, om de heerschappy* (*Lingua, or the Combat of the Tongue and the Five Senses for Superiority*). This play, a translation of Thomas Tomkis' eponymous university play, is set in the 'little world', or the microcosm of the human body, and depicted the attempts of 'Speech, a lady' to become the sixth and ruling sense with the help of 'Lie, her page'. The five (male) senses resist the efforts of the 'idle prating dame', as 'Hearing' calls her. They accuse her of upsetting rightful hierarchy in the microcosm by playing towards 'the Prophane eares' of the vulgar; they issue

46 Jill Stern, *Orangism in the Dutch Republic in Word and Image, 1650–1675*, Manchester 2010; Arthur Weststeijn, 'Why the Dutch Didn't Read Harrington: Anglo-Dutch Republican Exchanges, c. 1650–1670', in: G. Mahlberg and D. Wiemann (eds.), *Contexts for English Republicanism*, London 2013.

a petition, in which they denounce both her and her followers, amongst whom are 'foggers' (low-class lawyers), 'bawds', and, significantly, 'News-carriers'. In the end, they lock her up 'in Gustus his house', behing white bars and two strong doors.[47]

Although Tomkis' original text and Van den Bosch's translation do not differ much, there is one crucial difference between the two plays. Unlike its source, Van den Bosch' *Lingua* appeared in the context of the great upheaval of the English civil wars, in which, after years of fighting, Parliament had gained the upper hand over its king, Charles I. This evidently changed the way in which the play on the revolt in microcosm was read. It is no coincidence that rumours were circulating in the 1650s that Oliver Cromwell, the great Parliamentary leader, had been inspired to revolt against his king when he played a role in a school performance of *Lingua* at the tender age of four. These rumours, which were brought into circulation by the printer Simon Miller, are probably false.[48] But whether true or not, they do show that the association between the rebellion of the tongue and the rebellion of Parliament was easily made. It was made, moreover, in circles very close to Van den Bosch: Simon Miller was the printer of his own English work.[49]

Van den Bosch's translation, then, associates Tomkis' warning against the unsettling, revolutionary effects of unruly language on the body politic with the civil wars in England. This was highly appropriate and in itself hardly original. The English civil wars had seen the collapse of royal censorship, which had unleashed an unprecedented outburst of political debate: the 'bawds' and 'news-carriers' referred to in the play were thriving and, like 'Madam Tongue', unafraid to deny the authority of those in power. The explosion of political print and opinion had often been deplored by English commentators, but ironically, such commentators had considered it to be part of the 'Amsterdamnification' of England.[50] Van den Bosch seems to return the compliment by suggesting that the English 'Madam Tongue' should now be silenced.[51]

Tomkis' and Van den Bosch's 'Madam Tongue' evidently stands in the long

47 Lambert van den Bosch, *Lingva: ofte Strijd tusschen de tong en de vyf zinnen, om de heerschappy*, Amsterdam 1648, passim.

48 Sidney Lee, 'Tomkis, or Tomkys, Thomas (fl. 1614), Dramatist', in: *Oxford Dictionary of National Biography* [www.oxforddnb.com; last retrieved on March 3, 2015].

49 See e.g. Lambert van den Bosch, *Florus Anglicus: or, an Exact history of England from the Raign of William the Conquerour to the death of the late King*, London 1657. The rumour was picked up in the Dutch pamphlet Kn. 8236, *Hervadte beestespraeck* (1660).

50 Reinders, Printed Pandemonium (see n. 43), p. 19.

51 He probably did so because Parliamentary agents had sought to sway Dutch public opinion with translated pamphlets in the past decade, and English politics, as a result, had become a source of unrest in the Dutch Republic as well. See: Helmers, The Royalist Republic (see n. 37), pp. 27–61.

tradition of Aesop's fable, but it alerts us to a phenomenon unknown to the classical and medieval writers that had preceded them: the role of political print in disrupting the bodily humours. In Van den Bosch's Galenic allegory, the Tongue incites the passions and upsets the humours of the microcosmic body. More frequently, and arguably more aptly, print was targeted in Dutch pamphlets as an infectant. Thus, in the early 1780s, when civil war loomed again in the Republic, an Orangist author presented an 'antidotum' to the 'pestilence' spread by revolutionary pamphleteers. As ever so often, the prescription was simple: the Prince of Orange would quickly heal the sick body politic of the Dutch Republic.[52] This time, the prince, as the ultimate authority, was expected to 'moderate' or 'temper' the passions of the body politic that had been aroused by print, as early modern authorities were often supposed to.[53]

Of course, the representation of print as a bringer of disease was not uncontested.[54] Indeed, nearly all the great intestine conflicts produced a debate on the issue. The religious dispute between Remonstrants and Contraremonstrants of 1612–1619 was such a conflict. Numerous pamphlets in favour of both religious groups appeared during this years, contributing to the violent mood that took over the Dutch Republic. At the height of this conflict, a pamphlet appeared with the curious title, *Reuck-appel af-ghevende den lieffelijcken geur vande daden des [...] vorsts, den prince van Orangien (Pomander, spreading the lovely scent of the deeds of the Prince of Orange)*. In it, the Remonstrant polemicist Jacobus Taurinus used a variety of historical arguments to argue that the Prince of Orange was bound to maintain religious freedom in the Dutch Republic (which was contrary to the Contraremonstrant position, and not soon after proved contrary to Maurice's intentions as well).[55] Since the pomander was a ball of herbs that early modern people wore around their neck as a protection against contagious diseases (which were supposed to be spread by foul air), the title presented the historical argument as a remedy against the infectious lies spread by Contraremonstrant pamphlets. Taurinus' assertion that history – even in a pamphlet – was a potent cure to the body politic was in line with the Protestant

52 *Antidotum voor de pest, welke een drietal fameuze schryvers [...] hebben getracht te verspreiden*, Amsterdam 1780, Kn. 19428.

53 On the discourse of moderation and authority, see: ETHAN H. SHAGAN, *The Rule of Moderation. Violence, Religion and the Politics of Restraint in Early Modern England*, Cambridge 2011.

54 The author of the *The Duke of Bavaria's Illness*, for example, called himself 'The physician from the Parnassos', implying that his political publications were capable to remedy the Germany's illnesses.

55 JACOBUS TAURINUS, *Reuck-appel, af-ghevende den lieffelijcken geur vande daden des [...] vorsts, den prince van Orangien [...]: teghen de quade lucht, onlanghs [...] veroorsaeckt, door het op-doen ende aenwijsen van een valsche, fenijnighe Spore, tot verdedingh vande op-rechte Na-sporingh*, s.l. 1618, Kn. 2562.

tradition that pleaded for religious freedom. The anti-absolutist Huguenot Francois Hotman also considered his own history *Francogallia* (1573) to be a remedy to the bodily discord troubling France during the wars of religion.[56]

Despite this illustrous predecessor and the Dutch history of Protestant political print, Taurinus' *Pomander* was soon rebuked in the language of infection. The Contraremonstrant reply, *Den Orangien-appel (The Orange-Apple)*, accused Taurinus of being a 'depraved pharmacist', a 'quack', whose 'foul-smelling' pamphlet contained too many 'harmful' ingredients and spread 'vitriolic fumes'. The 'unmixed' airs of the *Orange-Apple* provided an antidote to its poisonous predecessor, and an aid against faint-heartedness.[57] Rather than to the text of the pamphlet, the title in this case referred to Prince Maurice himself: he was the perfume that would cure the land. It is probably no coincidence that the association between Maurice and a pomander echoes a familiar monarchist trope. Rulers such as Elizabeth I were often depicted with pomander, which was not just a precious jewel signifying their wealth, but also a metonymical reminder of their own healing qualities.

The conflict between the healing qualities of print and prince runs through a subgenre of the pamphlet literature, the so-called alarum pamphlets. Whereas the monarch was supposed to heal the body politic by tempering the passions political print aroused, alarum pamphlets claimed to heal it exactly by arousing the passions. Thus the bilingual pamphlet *Den Coninckljcke Morgen-wecker / Kingly Cocke* (1636), which appeared in the context of the debate on the English participation to the Thirty Years War, represented the non-intervening king of England as suffering from an unnatural sleep caused by the poisonous misinformation administered by foreign diplomats (see fig. 7). The pamphlet itself was the healthful antidote.[58] Similarly, when the Dutch truce with Spain was about to expire, the *Morning Alarm to the Old and Loyal Batavers* was advertised to contain 'a cure against their sleeping sickness'.[59] In the Dutch Republic, it was not the sovereign who needed to be awakened. Therefore, the sleeping body politic in such pamphlets, which originate in the Revolt, was usually a lion.[60] The message of all alarums, however, is the same: a healthy body is always vigilant, always alert to outward danger that might polute and weaken it. Print, they suggest, helps to keep it so and cures unnatural slothfulness.

56 Soll, 'Healing the body politic' (see n. 6), pp. 1259–1260.
57 *Orangien appel*, s.l. 1618, Kn. 2568, pp. 12, 93.
58 Crispijn van de Passe, *Coninckljcke Morgen-wecker / Kingly Cocke*, s.l. 1636, BM Satires 133.
59 Henricus Slatius, *Morgenvvecker, aen de oude ende ghetrouwe Batavieren, met een remedie teghen haere slaep-sieckte*, Amsterdam 1620, Kn. 3087.
60 Johannes Wierix, *Den Slapende Leeu*, s.l. 1578, FM 524aa.

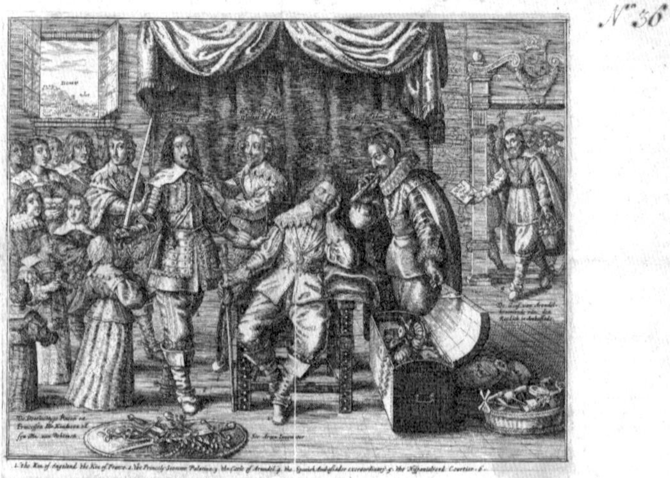

Den Coninckliicken Morgen-Wecker.

Haer Maj. van Engelant.

Haer Maj. van Francrijck.

De Spaenschen Ambassadeur.

Den Engelschen Favorit van de Koninck van Hispanjen.

Graef van Arundel comende van den Rycxdach van Regensburch.

The Kingly Cocke.

The King of Engeland.

MIne eyes are charm'd with these melodious straines
And sleepe my sences binds with silken chaines,
To rest I must betake mee; and whilest Mars
Displaies his bloodie colours, so that scarce
One neighbouring land is free from sword and fire
Devouring their faire cities, I desire
To hold the peace I have, warre is by God
Sent on a Land to plague it, 'tis his rod.
My Land is happie through this golden peace
Flowe & o'r flowe it doth with great increase
Of people, cattle, corne, oh no good thing
It wants; in arts & science flourishing.
Yea, I with peace (the time though long and late)
Hope to regaine the lost palatinate.

The King of France.

AWake, awake, sleepe hath too long possest
Your slumb'ring eies you haue tooke too long rest.
Drawe forth your Kingly sword; the man that spies
His neighbours house on fire, and yet lies
Secure in his owne may with the flame
Be scorch'd & burne & die with greife & shame.
Your eares are chain'd too fast vnto the aire
Of this impostors fluite, who will en snare
You Argos like in his spred net of gold
As other Princes he in thraldome hold.
Looke on your owne deare blood, these branches faire
Who through this tirants rage as exiles are,
And neuer more shal repossess their land
By peace, as you doe dreame, but by strong hand.
I Lodowicke, euen I firnam'd the iust
Whose faithfulnes you may beleiue and trust
Doe sweare, I will for these sweet children fight
To set them in their patrimoniall right.
Now, Prince, rowse vp, now, Brother, joyne in feild
With mee by armes to make this tyrant yeild,
No longer listen to this Pipers fluite
Nor be no longer cheated with his fruite.
They are but apples pluck'd from Pluto's garden
Accursed poisonous fruite doe not regard them.
As fore (they say) you haue; by which o'rsight
Your dearest nephews Land is ruin'd quite,
And they as exiles without Land lament
You did no sooner this hells fruite resent.

The English favorite to the King of Spain.

HOlla, french King, who taught you be so rude
So neare our King who sleepes thus to intrude?
Awake him with alarmes? your plot is knowne,
To set our Land in vproares like your owne.
Our land is now in rest, in peace, in quiet
Away with warre, warre is not for our diet.
What is your meaning, trowe, to make resort
With all these Princes to the English court?
Had not their Father to Bohemias crowne
Aspir'd, they had in quiet held their owne.
Who willing burnes his bodie, must be sure
The paines of swelling blisters to endure.
What troubles haue we had? what legates gone
(But all in vaine) for RESTITVTION?
'Tis better dance, be merrie, joviall still,
With Spanish Pistolets our purses fill,
Better with pictures gaie to feed our sight
Than naked corpses gor'd with blood in fight,
In hunting spend our time than all in vaine
With losse of men & monie warre with spaine.

The Spanish Ambassador Extraordinarie.

THis tune, I see, did not well please the King
I must another to his humour sing.
That Lodowicke did from his sleepe awake him,
Was to my masters hurt, a vengeance take him.
Well to't I must, and trie my vtmost skill
To help all this, else all I'ue dene is ill,
Else Flanders for the Paltz I see must goe
And pleasant Brabant is in perill too,
The Hollander will also not be slacke
On this occasion to fal on our backe;
No, no, a daintie aire I will invent,
That all these evills, I may soone prevent,
Then shall we ouerrun the Monsieurs Land
And James shall of himself come in our hand.

The Earle of Arundel returning from the diat holden at Regensburgh.

WHat? sleepes the King? Great God him keepe & blisse
Behold I bring him news, strange news it is,
I bring his sacred Majestie a blanke
For which I thinke his Highnes wil not thanke
The scorne full Diet for, when I propounded
His Majesties demand on reasons grounded,
They one with t'other laughing and in sport
My King derided and his seruant for't,
Rake hell, said they, & aske the devills there
Of RESTITVTION if they once did heare.
As for the letters pictures that I bare him
Cæsar saies thus, dumbe showes cannot feare him.
Send next the churlish brazen poste that stand
On Tower wharfe, he'l not pray, but command.
It is our Cannon and the martiall wight
That exercis'd in warre is, lord or knight,
Who knowes to lead an armie, that must get
Better content than any Legate yet.
Take out of every towne one man of ten
And with these well train'd well arm'd English men
Invade we Flanders, this is the way I tender
To make them on good termes the Paltz surrender.

Ghemaeckt door een Lief-hebber des Cheur Palts.

Fig. 7

6 Conclusion

The main characteristic of the incredibly rich political language of illness is undoubtedly its pliability. Whereas medieval authors employed it to express a feudal hierarchy in which the people and the prince were mutually dependent, William of Orange used it to justify the Dutch Revolt, Pieter Baerdt to promote democracy, and Thomas Hobbes to argue the necessity of absolutist rule. To a considerable extent, the commonplace metaphor of the sick body politic was a floating signifier, and as such the object of fierce ideological contest.

Despite this pliability, certain constants have emerged in the analysis of Dutch political literature presented above. As elsewhere in Europe, the rhetoric tended mostly (but not exclusively) towards conservative values, and towards idealizing one-headed rule as natural and even magically wholesome. In the seventeenth century, foreigners and especially religious others were increasingly identified as xenobiotic, sickmaking agents. In response to the wars of religion and the increased mobility of people and political information, the sick body politic that in classical and medieval literature had been applied almost exclusively to questions of domestic hierarchy, was increasingly employed to construct otherness, thereby helping to shape essentialist notions of national purity and autonomy.

Being a travelling commodity that did much to spread infectious subversive ideas on both a national and an international level, political print was frequently seen as an infectant too, which, like religious dissidents, could upset the passions of the corporate community. In the light of the main strands of the discourse, the prince was the logical antidote and moderator to the distempers it caused. Yet representations of the healing prince were invariably contested, and frequently, in what may be an ultimate Paracelsian gesture, countered by representations of print as medicine to the diseases it had caused itself.

Rick Honings and Steven Honings

The Poet as Patient: The Curious Case of Willem Bilderdijk: A Retrospective Approach[1]

1 Myth and the melancholy man

'Life, for as far back as I can remember, has been for me a painful, troublesome and vacuous proposition.' This is how the elderly Bilderdijk chose to start an autobiographical sketch. He reports never having experienced a second of satisfaction in his life, and having suffered much mental anguish. He felt that he did not belong on this earth.[2] Of all the many facets of his life and work, the poet Bilderdijk is best known for this, his melancholy. He himself was responsible for this image, for time and again he fervently proclaimed his pessimistic outlook on life.

Literary, history views Willem Bilderdijk (1756–1831) as being one of the few romantics – and indeed one of the most eccentric – that the Netherlands ever brought forth. He established a name for himself in the second half of the eighteenth century, the era of literary societies. Later in life, he distanced himself from these organisations in his didactic poem *De kunst der poëzy* (*The Art of Poetry* 1809) in which he claims that poems are not the product of literary societies; writing poetry is an individual undertaking. True poetry, to Bilderdijk, is the intuitive and spontaneous effusion of feeling, without aim, akin to laughing or crying: 'The pouring out of a feeling that demands air, that must expand, that

1 The authors would like to thank Eep Francken, Karin Hohmann, Manfred Horstmanshoff and Gwynne van Zonneveld (translation) and Peter van Zonneveld. This article was written as part of the NWO Veni-project *The Poet as Pop Star. Literary Celebrity in the Netherlands 1780–1900*. It is a revised version of the previously published article Rick Honings and Steven Honings, 'Voer voor psychiaters. Willem Bilderdijk als patiënt', *Tijdschrift voor Nederlandse Taal en Letterkunde* 130 (2014), pp. 281–303.

2 Willem Bilderdijk, *Geschiedenis des vaderlands*, vol. 13., Amsterdam 1853, p. 29. On Bilderdijk's life: Rick Honings and Peter van Zonneveld, *De gefnuikte arend. Het leven van Willem Bilderdijk (1756–1831)*, Amsterdam 2013. On Bilderdijk's literary, theological and philosophical ideas: Joris van Eijnatten, *Hogere sferen. De ideeënwereld van Willem Bilderdijk (1756–1831)*, Hilversum 1998.

must express itself and proliferate, lest the heart burst.'[3] These words bring to mind William Wordsworth's definition of poetry as 'the spontaneous overflow of powerful feelings'[4] in his preface to *Lyrical Ballads* (1798).

Bilderdijk is also known for his keenly articulated death wish. Where did this originate? There can be no doubt that the poet felt unhappy quite often throughout his lifetime, and for this he had every reason. As a child of five, he contracted *periostitis*, an infection of the connective tissue around bone, after a neighbour boy had kicked him in his left foot. A wrong diagnosis combined with the wrong treatment left him crippled, forcing him to bring a great deal of his childhood alone indoors, hobbling about on a painful clubfoot. This, in turn, made him shy and unsociable, while simultaneously encouraging him to study excessively, whereby he acquired his exceptional breadth of knowledge. He was further burdened by the loss of many loved ones in adulthood: he lost ten children from his two marriages, not including his second wife's numerous miscarriages. Adding insult to injury, Bilderdijk's most fervent wish – a professorship – was to remain unfulfilled, even though he lived to a respectable old age.

Bilderdijk's melancholy, however, is not to be explained solely with arguments based on events from his life. Upon reading his letters, one cannot help but conclude that it is, at least partially, a product of *self-fashioning*. By cultivating melancholy as part of his public image, he implicitly reinforced his status as an exceptional human being. In doing so, he placed himself in a long literary tradition. Melancholy, and the bemoaning of physical and mental ailments, imaginary or otherwise, had served as a mark of genius since the late eighteenth century.[5] By that time, the idea that madness, melancholy and genius go hand in hand had become widely accepted.[6] In his study *The Mad Genius Controversy* (1978), the German sociologist George Becker, formulated it this way: 'The aura of 'mania' endowed the genius with mystical and inexplicable quality that served to differentiate him from the typical man, the bourgeois, the philistine, and, quite importantly, the 'mere' man of talent; it established him as the modern heir of the ancient Greek poet and seer and, like his classical counterpart, enabled

3 Willem Bilderdijk, 'Over dichterlijke geestdrift en dweepery', in: W. Bilderdijk, *Taal- en dichtkundige verscheidenheden*, vol. 1, Rotterdam 1820, p. 7.

4 William Wordsworth, *Lyrical ballads, with other poems*, vol. 1. 2th edition, London 1800, p. xiv.

5 Leo Braudy, *The Frenzy of Renown. Fame & its History.* New York [etc.] 1986, p. 420. Cf. Wilhelm Lange-Eichbaum, *Genie, Irrsinn und Ruhm. Eine Pathographie des Genies*, 5th edition, München [etc.] 1961.

6 Cf. Maria-Theresia Leuker, *Künstler als Helden und Heilige. Nationale und konfessionelle Mythologie im Werk J. A. Alberdingk Thijms (1820–1889) und seiner Zeitgenossen*, Münster [etc.] 2001, p. 172 et sqq.

him to claim some of the powers and privileges granted to the 'divinely possessed' and 'inspired".[7]

Bilderdijk was undoubtedly acquainted with examples of melancholic figures from history.[8] Whether or not he owned the classic work *Anatomy of Melancholy* (1621) by Robert Burton is not known, though it is probable he had knowledge of it. It offers page upon page of examples of melancholy, and discusses its causes and cures. We do know for a fact that Bilderdijk read the Latin work of the melancholic scholar Caspar Barlaeus[9], as well as the seventeenth-century Dutch playwright Joost van den Vondel, who was also known to have been a melancholic figure: Vondel's biographer, Geeraardt Brandt, typified him in 1682 as being tormented by 'melancholia hypochondriaca'.[10] Nineteenth-century writers were quick to point out parallels with Bilderdijk. The Amsterdam author Jeronimo de Vries, a friend of Bilderdijk's, wrote, for example:

> Vondel had a profound intellect and refined taste, but an extremely irritable, melancholic disposition. This he had in common with the only Phoenix of our age. It rendered both at times sharp and bitter.[11]

Only once, in his didactic poem *De Ziekte der Geleerden* (*The Illness of the Scholars* 1807), did Bilderdijk write explicitly about melancholy.[12] In its three thousand lines, he elucidates the numerous physical and mental afflictions to which scholars are prone. Excessive studying, he claims, leads to overstimulation of the body, to insomnia and to the wasting of bodily humours. Yet Bilderdijk also interpreted sickness in the light of his religious beliefs: he was

---

7 Quoted to Kay Redfield Jamison, *Touched With Fire. Manic-depressive Illness and the Artistic Temperament*, New York [etc.] 1996, p. 4. On the same subject cf. A. Hankir, 'Bipolar disorder and poetic genius', in: *Psychiatria Danubina* 23 (2011), pp. 62–68.

8 Cf. Marius J. van Lieburg, 'De geneeskunde in de boekerij van Willem Bilderdijk', in: M. van Hattum and J. Zwaan (eds.), *Bilderdijks boekenwijsheid. Symposium 28–29 april 1988. Bijdragen over de veilingcatalogi van Bilderdijks bibliotheek*, Amsterdam 1989, pp. 69–82.

9 Frans F. Blok (ed.), *Caspar Barlaeus. From the Correspondence of a Melancholic*, Assen [etc.] 1976.

10 Geeraert Brandt, *Het leven van Joost van den Vondel*, A.J.E. Harmsen (ed.). DBNL 2000, p. 25.

11 Jeronimo de Vries, 'Verhandeling over het nationale in onze dichtkunst', in: *Vaderlandsche Letteroefeningen* (1839), p. 636. On Bilderdijk/Vondel: Rick Honings, 'Een ruwe diamant, maar van het eerste water'. Het Vondelbeeld in de eerste helft van de negentiende eeuw', in: *De Zeventiende Eeuw* 28 (2012), pp. 176–195.

12 Joris van Eijnatten, 'Hypochondrische ziel. Lichaam en geest in *De ziekte der geleerden* (1807) van Willem Bilderdijk', *De Negentiende Eeuw* 22 (1998), pp. 185–205; P. Gerbrandy, 'Tussen de oren van Willem Bilderdijk', Piet Gerbrandy and M. van Hattum (eds.), *Wie leert 't krekeltjen zijn lied? De poëtische oorspronkelijkheid van Bilderdijk. Negen beschouwingen over gedichten van Bilderdijk*, Groningen 2000, pp. 23–38; M. Dekker, "De ziekte der geleerden' door Willem Bilderdijk', in: *Geschiedenis der Geneeskunde* 11 (2007), pp. 295–301.

absolutely convinced that all illness was a direct consequence of the fall of man, which had permanently disrupted the divine order in the human body (the body being *pars pro toto* for all of creation).

The link made in the eighteenth century between genius and melancholy, is in fact based on a much older tradition. In the fourth-century B.C. text *On Melancholy*, generally ascribed to Aristotle, the author asks, 'Why is it that all those who have gained eminence in philosophy or politics or poetry or the arts, are so clearly melancholics?'.[13] The author attributes melancholia to a disturbance in the four bodily humours. This view corresponds with Hippocrates, who posited that in every human being there is normally a balance between blood, phlegm, yellow bile and black bile. Later in the Middle Ages, the four humours were to form the basis for the theory of the four temperaments: the sanguine, phlegmatic, choleric, and melancholic. The melancholic temperament was then thought to be caused by an excess of black bile.[14] The author of *On Melancholy* concludes that geniuses run the risk of sinking down into the marsh of melancholy, while that same state of mind is a prerequisite for exceptional artistic achievement.

In the eighteenth century, the Aristotelian connection between melancholy and genius was taken one step further: melancholy became a fashionable affliction, seen as a 'mark of both superior social and intellectual status and accomplishments'.[15] In the view of Joris van Eijnatten, it was a phenomenon that fitted well into the stratified eighteenth-century social class system: to be a member of the scholarly class was to suffer from this typically scholarly illness.[16] It is against this backdrop that one must interpret Bilderdijk's depression. The theory of the four temperaments and the notion of a melancholy disposition continued to be influential until deep in the nineteenth century. Although in the early nineteenth century the belief in black bile was no longer so wide-spread, Bilderdijk appears to have held on to it. In a passage from 1780, he points to black bile as the cause of the 'suffocation' in his chest.[17]

From his childhood onwards, Bilderdijk seemed to glorify melancholy. Practically all his letters open with an enumeration of physical and mental complaints. One moment he's suffering from 'buzzings' in his head, feels short of

13 Aristoteles, *Over melancholie*, Groningen 2001, p. 28.

14 Philip van der Eijk, 'Inleiding', in: Aristoteles, *Over melancholie*, Groningen 2001, pp. 6–25; M. Kemperink, *Gedeelde kennis. Literatuur en wetenschap in Nederland van Darwin tot Einstein (1860–1920)*, Antwerpen 2011, p. 119 et sqq.

15 On melancholy as a fashionable disease in the eighteenth century: C. Lawlor, 'Fashionable Melancholy', in: Allan Ingram, Stuart Sim, Clark Lawlor a.o., *Melancholy Experience in Literature of the Long Eighteenth Century*, Basingstoke [etc.] 2011, pp. 25–53.

16 Van Eijnatten, Hypochondrische ziel (see n. 12), p. 186.

17 Willem Bilderdijk, *De Dichtwerken*, vol. 6, Haarlem 1856–1859, p. 249.

breath, is dizzy or confused, and complains about the weakening of his brain. The next he reports insomnia, rheumatism, coughing, spitting up blood or a variety of pains. This he follows up with page upon page of erudite reflections. It seems as though he wanted to impress his friends by demonstrating what, in spite of everything, he was capable of. In this way he presented himself as an exceptional human being – in short, a true poet.

To describe his melancholy, Bilderdijk continually sought and found new metaphors. One time he is a soldier, whose stiff members prevent him from following the flag. Then he is a crippled horse, or a cat which has fallen from a high wall. His attitude toward life he compares to a dog bite full of wasps rooting about in it. From his dissatisfaction with life stemmed his legendary death wish, which he expressed in grandiloquent lines like 'For me, for me, is nought to crave / In this punishing life, except the grave'.[18] In his work he enthusiastically glorified his image as the dying poet right at death's door.[19] There can be no doubt: Willem Bilderdijk was no stranger to a bit of melancholic posturing!

2 A Retrospective Approach

In this study, however, we choose to approach Bilderdijk from a different angle. What do we stand to learn, if we do not view him as someone flaunting his depression, but rather take his symptoms seriously? It is a well-known fact that Bilderdijk was a hypochondriac, and not one to eschew exaggeration. Yet what would happen if we avoid interpreting Bilderijk's melancholia as part and parcel of his public image,[20] and regarded him as a patient instead? How would a psychiatrist assess his state of being, and what would the diagnosis then be? In this article, several of Bilderdijk's physical and mental symptoms will undergo scrutiny. We will put him on the psychiatrist's couch, and, using modern insights, will study the poet as a psychiatric patient. Of course it would also be possible to diagnose Bilderdijk in accordance with eighteenth- and nineteenth-century insights.[21] For this, one would need to take into account protestant views

18 Bilderdijk, De Dichtwerken, vol. 12 (see n. 17), p. 156, 'My, my is dit aanzijn straf,/ En ik reikhals naar het graf.', translation by Gwynne van Zonneveld.

19 Cf. Thomas Vaessens, *Geschiedenis van de moderne Nederlandse literatuur*, Nijmegen 2013, p. 87.

20 Cf. Rick Honings, 'De mythe van de dichter. Willem Bilderdijks beroemdheidscultus', in: *Nederlandse Letterkunde* 19 (2014), pp. 1–32.

21 On psychiatric diseases in history: Herman F.J. Horstmanshoff, *Over phrenitis. Dissertatio medica inauguralis De Phrenitide; Utrecht, 30 augustus 1757*, by Michaëlis Jacobus de Vries, Delft 2011. On depression: Jan Godderis, *Kan men een hemel klaren, even zwart als drek? Historische, psychiatrische en fenomenologisch-antropologische beschouwingen over depressie en melancholie*, Leuven 2000.

on illness in the early nineteenth century. Isaäc da Costa, for example, a student of Bilderdijk's, was of the opinion that physical and mental illnesses are imperative. They are given by God to punish man; one ought not to resist them. Coming from that same perspective in 1823, Abraham Capadose wrote his Bilderdijkian pamphlet *Bestrijding der Vaccine* (*Against Vaccination*), in which he takes exception to the cowpox vaccination, which he considered reprehensible. Bilderdijk's own symptoms, as well as his views on the body and soul, sickness and health, and physical and existential pain, have already been exhaustively expounded upon by Joris van Eijnatten.[22] In this article we choose to take a retrospective approach, constantly, however, mindful of the dangers that entails.[23] This type of research has already been conducted on other artists, such as Vincent van Gogh, Robert Schumann and the Dutch nineteenth-century writer Multatuli.[24] The psychological make-up of Goethe, to whom Bilderdijk was often compared in his time, has likewise been the focus of a study using a retrospective approach: 'Goethe's self-assessments in his works and letters as well as the description of him by others are analysed by phenomenological and hermeneutic methods from the perspective of current psychiatric classification and psychotherapeutic knowledge.'[25] A comparable methodology will be utilised here for Bilderdijk: his symptoms will be interpreted in the light of present-day psychiatric theory.

With regard to source material, however, there is an important difference between studying Bilderdijk and studying Goethe. Whereas hundreds of first-

22 Van Eijnatten, Hypochondrische ziel (see n. 12).

23 Karl-Heinz Leven, "At times these ancient facts seem to lie before me like a patient on a hospital bed' – Retrospective Diagnosis and Ancient Medical History', in: Herman F.J. Horstmanshoff and Marten Stol (eds.), *Magic and Rationality in Ancient Near Eastern and Graeco-Roman Medicine*, Leiden 2004, pp. 369–386; M. Stolberg, 'Möglichkeiten und Grenzen einer retrospektiven Diagnose', in: Waltraud Pulz (ed.), *Zwischen Himmel und Erde. Körperliche Zeichen der Heiligkeit*, Stuttgart 2012, pp. 209–227.

24 There have been multiple publications on the psychiatric state of Vincent van Gogh. Cf. J. Bos, 'Vijftig manieren om met Van Gogh af te rekenen', in: *Tijdschrift voor biografie* 2 (2013) 3, pp. 22–29. Much has been published on the mental state of Robert Schumann. Cf. Eliot Slater and Alfred Meyer, 'Contributions to a pathography of the musicians: Robert Schumann', in: *Confinia Psychiatrica* 2 (1959), pp. 65–94. On the relation between biography and psychology in general: cf. Jacques Dane and Hans Renders (eds.), *Biografie & psychologie*, Amsterdam 2007. There also have been publications on the mental state of famous characters from Dutch literature: Cf. (on Hedwig de la Fontayne) H.C. Rümke, *Over Frederik van Eeden's Van de koele meren des doods. Een essay*, Amsterdam 1964; Rene Marres, 'Waarom vermoordde Willem Termeer zijn vrouw? Het interpreteren van motivatie in 'Een nagelaten bekentenis' van Emants', in: *Tirade* 29 (1985), pp. 181–197; Frans de Jonghe, *Eline Vere bij de psychiater*, Bloemendaal 1994.

25 R. Holm-Hadulla, M. Roussel and F. Hagen-Hofmann, 'Depression and creativity. The case of the German poet, scientist and statesman J.W. v. Goethe', *Journal of Affective Disorders* 127 (2010), p. 2.

hand accounts of the German author have been preserved, in Bilderdijk's case we are limited to his own writing. This renders it impossible to check the extent to which his ailments were authentic or fabricated. It would obviously lend more credence to our study were we to possess such sources. That is unfortunately not the case. A critical stance is therefore essential, as Bilderdijk can by no means be deemed a reliable source. Even so, the fact that no one to this day has ever studied Bilderdijk as a patient, is nothing short of an act of injustice, for if ever a poet were a case for psychiatrists, then it is he.

3 A Child Prodigy with Headaches

To get to the beginning, we must go back to Bilderdijk's childhood. The relatively scanty information available to us is what he himself later chose to reveal. From this emerges the image of a child prodigy.[26] Looking back as a fifty-year-old, he claimed he had been able to read at the age of one, though he was not yet able to pronounce all the letters correctly. At the age of one and a half, he was pouring over the work of the seventeenth-century Dutch poet Jacob Cats, and was already reading books in French. He said to have mastered Latin by the age of five, and that he independently went about learning Greek from Sophocles, Italian from Boccaccio, German from Mendelssohn and English from Shakespeare. He reported acquiring Hebrew as well, and he studied the Heidelberg Catechism. The Bible and mythology also fell within his domain, and writing soon became one of his many talents. He said to have recounted history to his grandmother, seated on her lap. Yet whenever he found himself unable to explain a print, he felt deeply depressed.

All that studying had negative consequences for Bilderdijk's health. Early on, he is said to have been tormented by a ringing head and 'buzzings'. These afflictions made his life hellish, as he later claimed. He was not able to sleep because of them, and began to long for death. Because of his wounded foot, Bilderdijk stayed largely indoors. He no longer went to school, but was taught by his father. In between lessons, he inevitably sat with his nose in a book.

While still a child, Bilderdijk suffered from insomnia. Periods of activity, excitement and restlessness alternated with intervals of depression. Gloomy thoughts drifted through his mind, he later reported. The young Bilderdijk was irritable, felt lonely and was given to melancholy ruminations.[27] He was often

26 On Bilderdijk as a child prodigy: Honings and Van Zonneveld, De gefnuikte arend (see n. 2), p. 22 et sqq.

27 Isaäc da Costa, *De mensch en de dichter Willem Bilderdijk. Eene bijdrage tot de kennis van zijn leven, karakter en schriften*, Haarlem 1859, p. 11.

tired and listless. He would later claim to have entertained thoughts of suicide during this period. He said more than once to have toyed with the idea of bringing his life to a violent end.[28]

Thanks to awards he received from literary societies around the age of twenty, Bilderdijk's name as a writer became established, and yet this did not content him. It seems as though he was practically incapable of experiencing pleasure from his accomplishments. Regularly, he fell prey to bouts of melancholy and gloom. In 1780, he lamented his weakness of mind, which he felt limited his possibilities. It kept him from 'doing at least enough useful things to make having gone to the trouble of being born, worth the while.'[29]

By exaggerating his youthful accomplishments, Bilderdijk placed himself in a classical tradition. The childhood of numerous great men from history have given rise to the most curious of tales. Hugo de Groot, the Dutch attorney and writer, was, for example, a recognised child prodigy. At the age of eight he wrote his first elegies. At eleven he went to university at Leiden, where some three years later he received his doctorate. Constantijn Huygens, the Dutch writer and scholar, was able to reproduce songs at the tender age of two. At the age of five, he spoke French as though it were his first language. As a seven-year-old he gained proficiency in Latin, Greek, drawing and the writing of verse. Frans Blom has shown that Huygens consciously created this image of himself, employing a topos from antiquity that goes back as far as Ovid: the child attracted to the Muses.[30]

How would a psychiatrist have looked upon Bilderdijk? To begin with, it is evident that Bilderdijk's childhood years differ from most people's. The injury to his foot isolated him from his peers while growing up. Other than the contact he had with his close relatives, he lacked interaction with other children. This type of association is, however, a prerequisite for normal development of the personality – that complex whole of psychological characteristics which determine how one deals with emotions, thoughts and behaviour. A disturbance in personality development during childhood can lead to later problems. The social isolation in which Bilderdijk found himself, may have had a negative influence on the further course of his life.

Constrained by his foot disability, Bilderdijk threw himself into literature at an early age. However, few children are capable of this. The way in which the young Willem Bilderdijk was able to read classical authors as a toddler, conjures up the image of a child prodigy. The ability to read at a young age is termed

28 Willem Bilderdijk, *Brieven*, 5 vols., Amsterdam 1836–1837, vol. 4, p. 340.
29 Bilderdijk, Brieven, vol. 1 (see n. 28), p. 76.
30 Constantijn Huygens, *Mijn leven verteld aan mijn kinderen*, Frans Blom (ed.), vol. 1. Amsterdam 2003, p. 30.

hyperlexia. Early on, such children primarily learn to recognise individual words; around the age of three, they are often able to read whole sentences. This leads most parents to conclude that their child is a child genius or prodigy. Hyperlexia is not without problems, however, and there can be difficulties comprehending what has been read.[31]

From the description of Bilderdijk's childhood, it is not possible to determine whether he had a properly comprehended what he read. Looking at his development in light of hyperlexia is nonetheless interesting. Leo Kanner (1968) described boys and girls with autism who possessed exceptional reading abilities.[32] Autism is one of the five syndromes in psychiatry which fall under the category Pervasive Developmental Disorders ('pervasive' used here in the sense of 'permeating'). These disorders are characterised by limitations in reciprocal social contact, verbal and non-verbal communication, and narrow and rigid patterns of interest and behaviour.[33] Later studies have shown hyperlexia to occur in five to ten percent of those with a pervasive developmental disorder.[34]

From Bilderdijk's account of his youth, it is apparent that he was socially underdeveloped. He attributed this to his foot, which kept him housebound. In addition to limitations in social interaction, a pervasive developmental disorder involves limitations in communication. This, too, was true for Bilderdijk. Finally, a pervasive developmental disorder entails repetitive, stereotypical patterns in behaviour and interest. The young Bilderdijk seems to have been almost obsessively occupied with poetry and language. Precisely as we are considering a communicative disorder, it is necessary to consult eyewitness accounts of others to establish a diagnosis. These, unfortunately, have not been left to us.

Bilderdijk further recounts moments of activity alternating with periods of gloom. When an adult reports such symptoms, bipolar disorder is immediately considered. With this, a patient experiences manic episodes in which he is more active than normal, needs less sleep and often has grandiose or delusional ideas. In addition, he goes through depressed episodes during which he is down and unable to enjoy anything. Bipolar disorder usually develops between the ages of fifteen and twenty-five, and rarely presents in early childhood. Bilderdijk as a child does not meet the criteria for diagnosing bipolar disorder. It is, however, possible that he did develop this at a later age, for clinical experience teaches us that patients with this affliction often can retrospectively pinpoint having ex-

---

31 Elena L. Grigorenko, Ami Klin and Fred Volkmar, 'Hyperlexia: disability of superability?', in: *J Child Psycho Psychiatry* 44 (2003), pp. 1079–1091.

32 Leo Kanner, 'Autistic disturbances of affective contact', in: *Acta Paedopsychatrica* 35 (1968), pp. 100–136.

33 Michiel Willem Hengeveld and Antonius Jospehus Leonardus Maria van Balkom (eds.), *Leerboek psychiatrie*, Utrecht 2005, pp. 533–549.

34 Grigorenko [et al.], Hyperlexia: disability or superability? (see n. 31).

hibited mild characteristics of the illness in childhood. Mood problems and sleeplessness may nonetheless be the reaction of a highly intelligent child to the impossibility of having normal interaction with children his own age. Bilderdijk's fervent embrace of literature can, in this light, be seen as a coping mechanism; a way to deal with the unpleasant situation in which he found himself as a result of his foot injury.

4 An Aggression Issue

After completing his law degree, Bilderdijk began practising in The Hague. The work of a lawyer proved more difficult than he had anticipated. Despite his best efforts, he felt unsuited to his job, and to life in general: 'I am not, I find, made for this world.'[35] He had in the meantime fallen in love with Catharina Rebecca Woesthoven, whom he married in 1785. She, too, listened to him complain that he felt sad, depressed and dejected, particularly on days when he did not see her.[36] The marriage was not a success.[37] Bilderdijk was increasingly prone to fits of rage. After his wife gave birth in 1789, he charged the housemaid to give her nothing except milk and rusks. Seeing that Catharina was not regaining her strength, the maid went ahead and served her some bread. When Bilderdijk discovered this, he flew into a rage. He ran upstairs to his wife, hit her on the head and in the face, and proceeded to drag her by her hair out into the corridor. The maid began screaming, whereupon Bilderdijk, beside himself with anger, cast the plate with the bread out the window.

The housemaid declared that not a day went by without tirades and physical mistreatment. Back in 1786, during one of Catharina's pregnancies, he had also exhibited similar behaviour. Bilderdijk had demanded she wait up for him whenever he came home late, and make him tea. On one occasion, she went ahead and turned in early. In the middle of the night she awoke to find him at her bedside with a dagger, threatening to pierce her heart. She fled to the cellar. It took the manservant to keep the furious husband at bay. Another time, Bilderdijk was sitting working when the fire went out. When Catharina failed to get it relit, Bilderdijk became enraged and barred her entry to the house, forcing her

35 Rhijnvis Feith, *'Zo als men aan gemeenzaame vrienden gewoon is te schrijven'. De correspondentie van Rhijnvis Feith, 1753–1824,* ed. J.C. Streng, Epe 1994, p. 81.

36 *Mr. W. Bilderdijk's eerste huwelijk. Naar zijne briefwisseling met vrouw en dochter (1784–1807),* ed. Johannes Cornelis ten Brummeler Andriesse, Leiden 1873, p. 104.

37 Dini Helmers, 'Leven met Bilderdijk. Echt of onecht; besluiteloos of spelen op zeker? De echtscheiding van Catharina Rebecca Woesthoven en Willem Bilderdijk', *Het Bilderdijkmuseum* 22 (2005), pp. 1–12. The information in this paragraph is to a large extend based on the research conducted by Dini Helmers.

to take refuge at the house of an acquaintance. Not long thereafter, a note arrived there in which Bilderdijk had written 'I'm sitting without light and fire, and find neither wife, nor child, nor housemaid. I am stiff from the cold, and unable to dress. Why am I being avoided? [....] Does not my wife know who I am, and that I love her above all else, and adore her more than God himself?'[38]

So much is evident: Bilderdijk was subject to mood swings. He was capable of dragging his wife through the house by her hair and calling her every name under the sun, while in the same period writing her for example 'yes, my dear one, I love you beyond all that may be given the name of love'.[39] Meanwhile the poet continued to grumble about his health in his letters.He complained repeatedly of mental exhaustion. Rheumatic fevers rendered him mentally absent, as he put it. Once again he yearned for his moment of death – he fervently hoped for a deadly disease.[40]

As here, too, there are no first-hand accounts or observations, it is difficult to draw any definitive conclusions. It is, however, clear that Bilderdijk exhibited aggressive behaviour on multiple occasions. Most people learn to solve conflicts without aggression during their childhood. Aggression in adulthood can indicate a lack of learnt skills for conflict-solving. It is possible that, due to the large measure of isolation he experienced in childhood, Bilderdijk failed to learn how to deal with conflict. Aggression may have been the only means he had at his disposal.

Aggressive behaviour can also appear concurrently with a psychiatric disorder that decreases self-control. Many kinds of psychiatric conditions can lead to aggressive behaviour, including psychotic, mood, personality and developmental disorders. Aggression is quite often present in antisocial personality disorder. This is diagnosed in people with a lack of respect for the rights of others, who also meet at least three out of seven established criteria.[41] Bilderdijk may fit three of the seven: he is impulsive, quickly irritable and aggressive, and he appears to show no guilt or remorse after assaulting his wife. Naturally, such a diagnosis must remain a matter of conjecture.

Bilderdijk's behaviour may also point to character traits fitting borderline personality disorder. There is for example evidence of an intense yet unstable relationship with his wife, in which he continually switches between idealising her and belittling her. His impulsiveness, extreme mood swings and difficulty controlling rage also match with this diagnosis.

Finally, Bilderdijk's continually reiterating the fact that he was not made for

38 Mr. W. Bilderdijk's eerste huwelijk (see n. 36), p. 264.
39 Mr. W. Bilderdijk's eerste huwelijk (see n. 36), p. 161.
40 Bilderdijk, Brieven, vol. 1 (see n. 28), pp. 192–193.
41 *Diagnostic and Statistical Manual of Mental Disorders* (1994).

this world, may indicate a narcissistic personality disorder. This is characterised by the person seeing himself as more important and special than others, and he expects excessive admiration for his achievements. He may also be preoccupied with his own genius. Based on the known facts, it is not possible to come to a definitive conclusion regarding Bilderdijk's personality. His aggression, however, does seem to stem largely from his personality issues.

5 Lifelong Suffering

Throughout his life, Bilderdijk complained of an endless series of physical and mental agonies, but was never so morose as during his exile (1795–1806). He could not tolerate the air, for instance, and took to despising all things German, like heating stoves and duvets. Embittered, he wrote in 1798:

> Meanwhile my body and mind waste away and decay; illnesses come one after another, I'm losing my memory, my capacity for thought, and all disposition for study or science.[42]

While in London, he fell in love with Katharina Wilhelmina Schweickhardt, twenty years his younger. She followed him to Germany, but, as they were unmarried, living together, or even in the same city, was out of the question. As often as he could, Bilderdijk travelled from his residence in Brunswick to see Wilhelmina in Hildesheim, and later in Peine. The long journeys on horseback through marshlands were trying. Again and again, he bemoaned the many inconveniences. On 10 November 1799, he wrote to her in English, as had been their custom since meeting in London: 'I was somewhat hungry and exhausted without finding any thingh to eat but bread, my headach returned on a sudden, and I was obliged to take opium.'[43] This is quite probably the first time this drug appeared in his correspondence. This tranquillising, addictive medicine would come to play a significant role in Bilderdijk's life in the years that followed.[44] He was often in a bad way, he claimed. He would feel sick, suffer from itching, use a laxative and take opium in order to be able to sleep a few hours. 'My head is so embarassed, my dearest, that I can n't write,' he wrote in his broken English to

42 Willem Bilderdijk, *Mr. W. Bilderdijk's briefwisseling 1798–1806*, ed. M. van Hattum, Utrecht 2007, p. 157.

43 Bilderdijk, Mr. W. Bilderdijk's briefwisseling 1798–1806 (see n. 42), p. 398.

44 Much has been published on opium in the 19th century. Cf. A.J. Dunning, 'Opium. Een oude geschiedenis', in: *Nederlands tijdschrift voor geneeskunde* 139 (1995), pp. 2629–2632. On Bilderdijk's use: M. van Hattum, 'Een 'Bilderdijk-voor-beginners' (met onzin over opium)', *Het Bilderdijk-museum* 24 (2007), pp. 17–22; B. Büch, 'De geopiaceerde wereld van Willem Bilderdijk', in: *Jaarboek van de Maatschappij der Nederlandse Letterkunde 1981*, Leiden 1982, pp. 27–36.

Wilhelmina. Another time he wrote, 'I can n't tell you how unhappy I feel my-self. Lowspirited as I am, (and so it is every time) every thingh goes contrary to my wishes, and the whole world conspires to my ill-luck [...] I can n't describe the weakness of my head, and how I suffer with giddiness, headache &c.'[45]

In 1805, he subjected himself to bloodletting seven times in the space of three weeks in the hope of its helping calm him down. He had been unable to sleep for some time. Sleep he considered to be an unnatural stupor at the root of chronic headaches.

> It used to be that I rarely slept more than once in three nights; now I spend 7, 8, yea 10 nights without slumber coming to my eyes, yet finally I succumb and fall into that sleep that is typical for me; and if not, I have to bring it to pass with opium.[46]

At this same time Bilderdijk experienced fits of 'verse mania'. For no apparent reason he would lapse into a kind of delirium, as he himself described it. He became more productive than was good for him, and, by his own account, spoke in verse for nights on end, as though swept away in some kind of whirlwind.[47] At other times he was capable of nothing, and referred to himself as old and listless.

The end of Bilderdijk's exile in early 1806 did not bring much improvement in his condition. He was finally able to return to the Netherlands, yet even the journey back proved a trial. He became feverish and ill, and used 'Spanish fly plasters'(canthariden) to treat himself. Such plasters were employed to cause blisters or irritate the skin. He shuddered to think that he might not be able to secure enough opium en route.[48] He reported having cramps in his legs and feet at night. The tops of his fingers were cracked open and full of painful abscesses, so that he lamented,

> Heaven may assist me, for I am in the most deplorable and despairfull state, one can imagine [...] No, no body suffered what I am deemed to! I can n't hold the pen, nor withhold my-self from crying aloud! – Heaven, see down, see down, and at least make an end of such an ill-fate![49]

Once back, Bilderdijk was constantly sick and depressed. To aid him in his recovery, Louis Napoleon, King of Holland, invited Bilderdijk to his palace Soestdijk in the summer of 1808. He did not remain there for long, fleeing on the third day as he could not tolerate the air.[50] That seems exaggerated, but years later his wife remembered: 'We were hardly two days at Soestdyk [...] but that he took miserably ill, and fell into a deep melancholy, with bouts of complete

---

45 Bilderdijk, Mr. W. Bilderdijk's briefwisseling 1798–1806 (see n. 42), p. 539.
46 Bilderdijk, Mr. W. Bilderdijk's briefwisseling 1798–1806 (see n. 42), p. 775.
47 Bilderdijk, Mr. W. Bilderdijk's briefwisseling 1798–1806 (see n. 42), p. 789.
48 Bilderdijk, Mr. W. Bilderdijk's briefwisseling 1798–1806 (see n. 42), pp. 819–821.
49 Bilderdijk, Mr. W. Bilderdijk's briefwisseling 1798–1806 (see n. 42), pp. 833–837.
50 Letter of W. Bilderdijk to J. Valckenaer, 18 July 1808, Leiden University Library, BPL 1039.

unconsciousness such that the doctors, who I had summoned against his wishes, thought it prudent to return with haste once more to Leyden.'[51] In the years that followed, Bilderdijk continued to complain about his health. He rarely experienced joy. His constitution made it no easier. He reported not even being able to walk along a green hedgerow without his body reacting to it, with fever and harmful effects to his nervous system as a result. As he had had to remain indoors during his childhood, he believed himself to have become allergic to the whole of nature. He claimed that, when he felt a draught, rheumatic pains and other ailments ensued.[52]

In 1815, things once again took a turn for the worse. That this was not a ploy to call attention to himself is once more apparent from a letter written by his wife Wilhelmina. Her husband reportedly suffered from 'bouts of absence of mind'. She did not dare go on a country outing for fear that things might again go awry, given his greatly agitated state of mind. 'While I'm writing, he's dozing in a chair, but I cannot look upon his countenance without coming to the saddest of realisations: he feels so very unhappy and all his features tell of it!'[53] And still the poetry kept flowing. Dark days of depression and despondency – primarily spent in bed daydreaming and moaning according to Bilderdijk – alternated with manic intervals of intense activity. It was in this period that he wrote to a friend about another recent attack that had caused him to spew verse for twenty-four hours non-stop.[54]

Bilderdijk suffered from a wide variety of ailments in the course of his life. It is a recognised phenomenon that patients with depression often experience physical problems for which no cause can be found. This is termed *somatisation.* The symptoms can be very diverse, ranging from assorted pains, nausea and dizziness, to memory loss and other neurological phenomena. From the letters Bilderdijk wrote, we can ascertain that he in all probability suffered from depression. The core symptoms (a gloomy mood, and a loss of interest and pleasure in practically all activities) are after all quite pronounced in his case. His wife recounted, moreover, that he had 'bouts of absence of mind'. Perhaps she was referring here to a decrease in his attention and concentration, likewise symptoms of depression. His recurring thoughts of death, his sleeplessness and fatigue fit with this diagnosis as well.

Patients with depression are usually capable of very little. Given the thousands

51 Letter of K.W. Schweickhardt to J. Valckenaer, 21/28 April 1815, Leiden University Library, BPL 1039.

52 *Briefwisseling met de hoogleeraren en mrs. M. en H. W. Tydeman, gedurende de jaren 1807 tot 1831,* 2 vol., ed. H.W.T. Tydeman, Sneek 1866–1867, vol. 1, p. 94.

53 Letter of K.W. Schweickhardt to J. Valckenaer, 21/28 April 1815, Leiden University Library, BPL 1039.

54 Briefwisseling met de hoogleeraren en mrs. M. en H. W. Tydeman (see n. 52), vol. 2, p. 165.

of lines of verse Bilderdijk wrote, there must also have been periods during which he was not depressed. With a bipolar disorder, both depressed and manic periods occur. A manic episode is currently seen to have occurred when there is an elevated mood for at least seven days, accompanied by delusions of grandeur, a decreased need for sleep, a rise in talkativeness and an increase in goal-oriented activity. Manic symptoms lasting at least four but fewer than seven days, indicate a hypomanic episode. These occur in patients suffering from what is called bipolar II disorder. Here depressed episodes alternate with hypomanic ones.

This condition has been diagnosed in the German composer Robert Schumann (1810–1856). On the basis of his letters, research has convincingly shown a connection to have existed between his mental state and his productivity. During depressed periods he achieved significantly less than during hypomanic episodes.[55] Recent research also claims that Johann Wolfgang von Goethe may have had this same bipolar disorder.[56] The descriptions of Bilderdijk's 'verse mania' in which he spewed verse like water from a fountain, would certainly fit with a hypomanic episode. That would mean that Bilderdijk had a bipolar II disorder, but of this we cannot be certain.

6 Old and Confused

In his sixties, between 1817 and 1827, Bilderdijk privately tutored a small number of students in Dutch history in Leiden. Once, when a friend came to look him up there, the door remained closed, which Bilderdijk later explained thus: 'I lay abed mad with headaches and intoxicated with opium'.[57] He still sat up without sleeping night after night, and took more opium than could have been good for him. Repeatedly, he complained of headaches, insomnia, dizziness and memory loss. He often wore a damp cloth around his head to alleviate the pain somewhat. On 11 May 1818, after yet another headache attack, an irritable Bilderdijk wrote that he could no longer endure living.[58]

At times, things appeared to go better with him. Yet invariably a backlash ensued. Early in 1820 he experienced a particularly bad stretch. He reportedly did not utter a word for eight days straight. This event heralded in a new phase. Bilderdijk began to complain of old age. He claimed that his memory failed him more and more frequently, and he was no longer able to work. He could not

55 Slater and Meyer, Contributions to a pathography of the musicians (see n. 24).
56 Holm-Hadulla, Roussel and Hofmann, Depression and creativity (see n. 25). On Bilderdijk and Goethe: cf. Rick Honings, 'Levenslijden versus levensgenot. Bilderdijk en Goethe: verwant en verschillend', in: *Nieuw Letterkundig Magazijn* 30 (2012), 2, pp. 42–46.
57 Letter of W. Bilderdijk to J. Valckenaer, 3 June 1817, Leiden University Library, BPL 1039.
58 Letter of W. Bilderdijk to J. Valckenaer, 11 May 1818, Leiden University Library, BPL 1039.

concentrate on his galley proofs because, as he himself put it, he could no longer understand what he had written.[59] He felt dull and vacant. Be that as it may, the need to write verse still returned unexpectedly from time to time.

His opium consumption only caused his confusion to worsen. To his student Da Costa he wrote in 1826: 'The dullness which is mine to complain about these few days, is the consequence of several days use of Opium.' He found he needed to increase his intake to achieve the same effect.[60] This process only worsened after Bilderdijk moved to Haarlem in 1827. More and more often he sat staring vacantly into space. He no longer knew what day of the week it was, nor the month, and writing letters grew increasingly difficult. He had all but stopped reading. It was as though puppets were dancing in his brain, he claimed, and he compared the sensation to drunkenness.[61]

From about 1799 to the end of his life, Bilderdijk took opium pills as a tranquilliser. That in and of itself is nothing special; this remedy was readily available from the apothecary in the nineteenth century. His wife took it as well. A great number of writers, such as Coleridge, Keats, Poe and Baudelaire, used it,[62] as did the Dutch author Multatuli. The Englishman Thomas de Quincey even wrote a book on the subject: *Confessions of an English Opium-Eater* (1821). In it he discusses the 'pleasures' and 'pains' of using the drug, and describes the 'horrors of opium', such as insomnia, and terrifying nightmares and visions. Withdrawal symptoms, even when De Quincey attempted to break his habit gradually, proved formidable as well. After four months, he was still 'agitated, writhing, throbbing, palpitating, shattered; and much, perhaps, in the situation of him who has been racked'.[63] One conspicuous point in Bilderdijk's case is that he considered himself to be a doctor of medicine and wrote his own opium prescriptions, more than one hundred of which have been preserved.[64]

Opium is a juice extracted from the plant *Papaver somniferum*. It contains various substances, including morphine and codeine, both of which are still being used as painkillers today. Opium, like heroine which can also be obtained from it, is a highly addictive substance. Within several hours to days after discontinuing use, withdrawal symptoms appear. An overdose, on the other hand, produces symptoms of intoxication.

In addition to employing opium to combat his many ailments (itching, agitation, headaches and many other types of complaints), Bilderdijk used it to get to sleep. Sleep disturbances can occur in both hypomanic and depressed epi-

59 Bilderdijk, Brieven (see n. 28), vol. 4, p. 231.
60 Bilderdijk, Brieven (see n. 28), vol. 4, p. 277.
61 Briefwisseling met de hoogleeraren en mrs. M. en H. W. Tydeman (see n. 52), vol. 2, p. 265.
62 Cf. Alethea Hayter, *Opium and the Romantic imagination*, London 1968.
63 Thomas de Quincey, *Confessions of an English opium-eater*, Boston 1851, p. 102, 126.
64 Van Hattum, Een 'Bilderdijk-voor-beginners' (see n. 44), pp. 20–21.

sodes. Insomnia can also be a symptom of opium withdrawal. This can have induced Bilderdijk to reach repeatedly for opium in order to be able to get to asleep again. In fact, many of the symptoms he describes can be the result of opium withdrawal. Bilderdijk said himself that he used opium for his headaches. Yet headaches are known to arise when opium use is temporarily ceased.[65] Memory loss, but also 'idleness of the intestines' can have resulted from his drug use; opium brings about constipation. Sleepiness is likewise a side effect, as is a 'disorderly pulse'. Fever can also occur during opium withdrawal.

With regard to Bilderdijk's opium use, we have one important witness: the Haarlem poet Jan van Walré. He experienced Bilderdijk first-hand during the last years of his life, and commented later: 'I for my part would dare to claim that the excessive use of opium, to which he had accustomed himself, often contributed much to the causticity of his style. I have seen him not once, but on multiple occasions, in a particular kind of delirium which I could attribute to nothing else. He would then imagine seeing, in the vicinity of the Great Church, of which he had a view from his dwelling, lights, ghosts, and all manner of curiosities.'[66] This is a clear indication that Bilderdijk's opium use had a negative effect on his memory and mental well-being.

7 Conclusion

The notion that a true artist ought to be melancholy by nature was widespread by the end of the eighteenth century. Glorifying mental afflictions was the fashion of the day, and Bilderdijk kept in step with that fashion. He fell within the centuries-old discourse on melancholy, and spent his whole life an ardent exponent of the romantic image of the suffering poet. Eyewitness accounts, however, reveal that he quite often was truly sick. Anyone venturing to state anything about Bilderdijk's psychiatric condition is therefore treading on thin ice.

In this article, we looked at Bilderdijk as a psychiatric patient. This approach entails one significant danger: any present-day pronouncement on Bilderdijk's state is anachronistic from the outset. Bilderdijk lived in a different age with different views on illness. We have determined that we may be looking at a case of *somatisation* with respect to Bilderdijk: his physical symptoms were possibly related to his mental condition. The poet's own interpretation of his illness was

65 Marco de Marinis, Luigi Janiri and A. Agnoli, 'Headache in the use and withdrawal of opiates and other associated substances of abuse', in: *Headache* 31 (1991), pp. 159–163.

66 Nicolaas Beets, *Het dagboek van de student Nicolaas Beets, 1833–1836*, ed. Peter van Zonneveld, Den Haag 1983, p. 136. Translation: Gwynne van Zonneveld.

naturally different. He offered a religious explanation for it: sicknesses are sent by God and are therefore imperative; man must above all accept them.

That afflictions were viewed differently in the early nineteenth century does not imply that a modern diagnosis cannot offer us interesting insights. Operating on this premise, we have in this article attempted to shed some light on Bilderdijk's physical and mental ailments. It is not easy to attach a label to the poet. Biographers are not psychiatrists after all, nor are psychiatrists biographers. From the available sources, an image emerges of a man with a complex mind. His childhood was disrupted by the injury he received to his foot, which hampered him in his association with peers. This may have interfered with his personality development, leading to problems, most notably in adulthood. His aggression toward his wife would seem to stem from such a personality developmental disorder. It's striking moreover that Bilderdijk shows the characteristics of a bipolar II disorder; periods in which he was incapable of anything alternated with hypomanic episodes during which he was extremely active and wrote much. In this regard he resembles both Goethe and Robert Schumann. For the latter, the relationship between depressive and manic periods and his productivity have been captured in statistics. Such a study cannot reasonably be conducted for Bilderdijk, as it is not clear from his letters exactly when he wrote what. Bilderdijk's use of opium had an unintentional effect: he resorted to this remedy as a tranquilliser, but it produced yet other complaints, including memory loss in his later years. These are but a few aspects of Bilderdijk's complicated and fascinating character. Biographers and psychiatrists joining forces more often than is now the case, may well be worthwhile for both.

What has a retrospective psychiatric approach added to our knowledge of the person Bilderdijk and his writing? Bilderdijk was an author who consciously applied himself to cultivating his eccentric image. Yet his authorship is more complex than this would suggest. Even those convinced that Bilderdijk practised self-fashioning, must assume that this was only partially self-directed. Like every human being, the poet was also affected by factors over which he had no control, such as his mental constitution, formed in childhood. In this article we set out to draw attention to this second aspect, which up until now has received insufficient attention in the literature. Naturally we do not presume to have made the definitive diagnosis here. What we do hope to have achieved, is to have shown that Bilderdijk is a clear candidate for the psychiatrist's couch, and shall remain so for some time to come.

Arnold Lubbers

Oddities, or Illness and Health as Topics in the Early 19th-Century Dutch Readers' Digest

In the long nineteenth century, institutional reading culture flourished in Western Europe.[1] Several different types of institutions of reading catered to a growing reading audience. People could become members of subscription libraries – in general large scale societies that formed book collections and had reading rooms – or visit circulating libraries – commercial ventures, often of bookseller-publishers, that provided the cheapest access to thousands of books and magazines – long before the introduction of public libraries. On a smaller scale there were book clubs: usually consisting of no more than a few dozen men who met once or a handful of times a year to democratically choose between 20 and 30 books in a national language and magazines which would circulate amongst their ranks. In the Netherlands the number of book clubs seems to have been plentiful, more so than in any other country.[2]

Even though we are not able to examine the minds of the Dutch men and women of the nineteenth century, a study of institutional reading culture allows us to gauge their interests, the ideas they were fascinated by and the thoughts they were keen on. By analysing the books and magazines that contemporary readers purchased or borrowed, institutions of reading provide unprecedented insight into their minds. In the Netherlands, subscription libraries developed mainly in the second half of the nineteenth century and typically served the upper middle and upper classes; the subscription fees were generally too high for people from the lower classes to afford. Circulating libraries catered to all classes: for only small fees, books and magazines could be borrowed. These enterprises often presented their customers with holdings containing thousands of titles, which makes the analysis time consuming using conventional historical

1 Many thanks to Mark Towsey for reading an earlier version of this paper and providing me with useful and necessary suggestions.

2 Arnold Lubbers, *'Een republiek in het klein'. Noord-Nederlandse leesgezelschappen en hun lectuurkeuze in het Verenigd Koninkrijk der Nederlanden, 1815–1830*, dissertation University of Amsterdam 2014, p. 140.

research methods. For this reason book clubs were chosen as points of access to the minds of people from the past.

In this paper, I have analysed the choice in reading material made by the members of book clubs in the Northern provinces of the Netherlands between 1815 and 1830, the period of the United Kingdom of the Netherlands. The question that I intend to answer is to what extent illness and health were popular topics in the books and magazines that those members purchased. In order to draw conclusions, what follows first is an introduction on Dutch book clubs and their general purchasing habits.

Book clubs recruited their members amongst the Dutch middle classes. They contributed to the emancipation of those classes by providing an environment in which people could practice basic democratic principles. For example: books and magazines were chosen by majority vote and rules and regulations streamlined the interaction of the members during their meetings. By doing so, book clubs were key to the spread of the democratic ideals that stimulated societal consensus in order to avoid conflict and debate. Consensus was favoured in the period of the United Kingdom of the Netherlands, 1815–1830, after decades of revolutionary upheaval and foreign occupation.[3]

In order to try to look into the minds of some of the Dutch in the early nineteenth century, I have analysed the remaining archives of twenty book clubs in the period of the United Kingdom of the Netherlands, in which information can be found about the books and magazines that their members purchased. These are the following:

- *Leeslust Baart Kunde* (*The Desire to Read Gives Birth to Knowledge*) – Alkmaar
- Unnamed book club – Barneveld
- *Daar Vrede Bloeid Ook Vriendschap Groeid* (*Where Peace Blossoms Friendship Grows*) – Cadzand
- *Legendo Discimus* (*Reading to Learn*) – Den Bosch
- *Eerste leesgezelschap* (*The First book club*) – Dordrecht
- Book club of Classis Dordrecht, Ring Dordrecht – Dordrecht
- *Utile et Jucundum* (*Useful and Pleasant*) – Dordrecht
- *Oefening baart Verlichting* (*Practice gives birth to Enlightenment*) – Gorinchem
- Unnamed book club – Grijpskerk
- *Tot Meerder Oeffening* (*For More Practice*) – Hoorn
- *Liefde voor Waarheid en Deugd* (*Love for Truth and Virtue*) – IJzendijke
- Unnamed book club – Leens

3 Lubbers, Een republiek in het klein (see n. 2), pp. 291–294.

- *Amica Veritas* (*Friends of Truth*) – Leeuwarden[4]
- *Leest, Leert en Betracht* (*Read, Learn and Practise*) – Leeuwarden
- *Leesgezelschap van godsdienstige geschriften* (*Book club of religious works*) – Leeuwarden
- *Onderlinge Vriendschap* (*Mutual Friendship*) – Sommelsdijk
- *Voor Wetenschap en Deugd* (*For Science and Virtue*) – Steenbergen
- *De Eendragt* (*The Unity*) – The Hague
- *Oefening* (*Practice*) – unknown place
- Unnamed book club – Waddinxveen
- Book club of Classis Rhenen, Ring Wijk – Utrecht

This source base is limited in the sense that remaining archives are all of book clubs that existed in the Northern provinces (encompassing what is currently the Netherlands). In the Southern provinces (currently Belgium and Luxembourg) institutionalised reading culture had developed differently: commercial circulating libraries and literary societies catered to the needs of the reading audiences, and book clubs were much less common. The remaining archives provide information on about 10 % of the book clubs that existed between 1815 and 1830.[5]

1 Reading in book clubs

In the early nineteenth century book clubs in the Netherlands were criticised for supposedly buying only 'that what appears new on a daily base'.[6] The content was supposedly of no importance, the members of book clubs were just out to get their hands on whatever they could find, as long as it was recently published. A phrase from a review in the magazine *De Vriend des Vaderlands* (*The friend of the fatherland*) illustrates this idea. In the review, a historical novel was lambasted by a reviewer. He also made a snide remark to another magazine, which had previously reviewed the same novel. About his competitor's magazine, the reviewer comments:

4 Due to the size of the corpus of texts this book club purchased, their titles were not analysed for the information in Graphs 1 and 2.

5 Lubbers, Een republiek in het klein (see n. 2), pp. 55–58, 231–232.

6 Han Brouwer, *Lezen en schrijven in de provincie. De boeken van Zwolse boekverkopers 1777–1849*, dissertation Utrecht University 1995, p. 191 [hetgeen dagelijks nieuw uitkomt]. The criticism levelled at book clubs was penned down by a group of well-off gentlemen, who founded a library in Zwolle in 1827 in order to stimulate the circulation of useful knowledge and results of scientific research which they deemed necessary for general prosperity and national wealth.

> [...] because you, since long having the luck of owning better magazines, having banned this from your Book club; or at least, in your capacity, only having read the last part, like the rest of us have to, for the news of the day, take a look through so many a miserable Journal.[7]

Even though the phrase mainly demonstrates the reviewer's opinion of a rival magazine, it also shows the conventional assumption that in book clubs, people were only interested in 'the news of the day'.

Those who received their reading matter through book clubs were viewed as readers who were primarily concerned with quantity, instead of quality:

> That, which they call the general reading audience, is the crowd, that usually gets served the food for the mind by book clubs, circulating libraries and similar large tablespoons, because there it comes down more to the quantity, than the quality.[8]

Although critical contemporaries negatively classified the members of book clubs as the large reading audience; that in itself offers starting points for investigation. The question remains what it was that this general reading audience read. It is still unclear what was meant with that so-called 'news of the day'. It furthermore remains to be seen whether or not illness and health were part of their reading digest and if so, to what extent.

2 Categories

The reading matter that book clubs bought between 1815 and 1830 were above all novels and collections of stories, followed by books on geography and travelogues.[9] Historical reading matter and biographies come third. In the Groningen town of Leens these categories totalled over 40 %, as shown below in graph 1. The travelogues and books on geography made up 17 % in the *Eerste leesgezelschap*, 14 % in *Utile et Jucundum* (both in Dordrecht in South Holland) and 13 % in

7 *De vriend des vaderlands; een tijdschrift toegewijd aan den roem en de welvaart van Nederland en in het byzonder aan de hulpbehoeftigen in hetzelve* 1 (1834), p. 27, [[...] dewijl gij, sinds lang het geluk naar waarde schattende, van betere Tijdschriften te bezitten, dit uit uw Leesgezelschap geweerd hebt, of ten minste, alleen uit hoofde uwer betrekkingen, het laatste gedeelte ervan laast, even als wij allen, om het nieuws van den dag, zoo menige ellendige Courant inzien].

8 *De Gids. Nieuwe Vaderlandsche Letteroefeningen. Boekbeoordelingen. Eerste Deel* (1831), p. 502, [Datgene, hetwelk men het groote lezend publiek noemt, is die menigte, aan welke gewoonlijk de spijzen voor den geest wordt voorgediend en opgeschept door leesgezelschappen, leesbibliotheken en soortgelijke groote soeplepels, dewijl het hier meer op de hoeveelheid, dan wel op de hoedanigheid neerkomt].

9 All information on the percentages of purchased categories and languages of literature in the following paragraphs is based on: LUBBERS, 'Een republiek in het klein' (see n. 2), pp. 231–287.

Cadzand in Zeeland. A clearly different percentage can be found in the book club of the Ring Dordrecht – part of a church community of the Dutch Reformed Church. The members of that book club spent their money evidently on other categories of reading matter, because novels, collections of stories, travelogues and books on geography made up less than 5 % of all the books they had circulating. The percentages in Cadzand, two of the three book clubs in Dordrecht and in The Hague show a high degree of similarity with previously established percentages of book clubs' interests in and around the Zeeland city of Middelburg.[10] The reason the book club of the Ring in Dordrecht spent less on novels and travelogues was because their primary goal was to have religious reading matter circulate amongst the members.

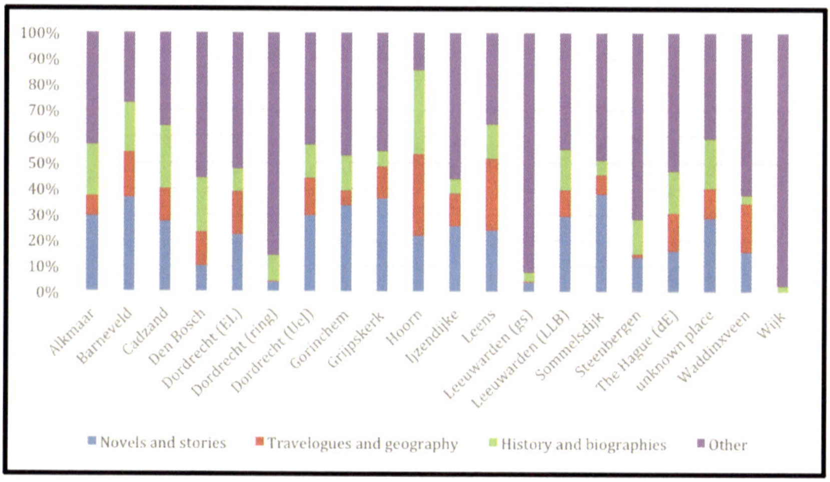

Graph 1: Categories of reading matter bought by book clubs

3 Novels

Around 25 % of all reading matter purchased by book clubs consisted of novels. The majority of these was translated. In the book clubs of Leens, the novels made up 27 % of all books they bought. In Cadzand, the *Eerste leesgezelschap* and *Utile et Jucundum*, they numbered up to 27 %, 22 % and 30 %. The members of *De Eendragt* chose to make 15 % of their purchases to be novels, but, since nearly 50 % of all books and magazines they bought was in French – and those numbers

10 Joost Kloek and Wijnand Mijnhardt, *Leescultuur in Middelburg aan het begin van de negentiende eeuw*, Middelburg 1988, p. 63.

are not included in graph 1 – it is well conceivable that to a certain extent their interest in novels was already satisfied by French novels.[11]

To quench their reading thirst, to a large extent, book clubs bought translated reading matter which is no surprise when we take a look at the original Dutch novel production in the early nineteenth century. In this period, the book market underwent professionalisation and the reading public became emancipated and demanded a more diverse choice of books. Translated publications became formidable competition for original Dutch publications.[12] Countries such as France and England needed less translations from foreign works: 'these two countries *produce* a lot of novels (and good novels, too), so they don't need to buy them abroad.'[13] This raises the question: where did the books that the Dutch read in their book clubs originate from?

4 Original language

Graph 2 shows that even though the majority of the combined reading matter by the investigated book clubs was originally Dutch, a sizeable portion consisted of translated work. The translations were most of all originally German, and to a lesser extent French and English. In Leens this percentage was 49 %, in Cadzand 39 % and in *Utile et Jucundum* no less than 53 %, just to name a few. In two book clubs the numbers were substantially lower: the book club of the Ring Dordrecht only read 12 % of their books and magazines in translation and for *De Eendragt* this number was 27 %. The low percentage for the Ring Dordrecht can be explained again by pointing out their principal intentions: the book club was part of a church community and their choice in reading matter primarily featured religious, Protestant, works. It could be that, because the topics they read about were largely focussed on the religious situation in the Netherlands, original Dutch work offered them more of what they were interested in. The relatively low number in *De Eendragt* can likely be explained by the fact that about half of all their purchases was original French work. A potential demand for French translations would have been curbed that way and it is even possible that potential interest in translations of original German or English works was already met by French translations of those works. Original German and English works

11 Dutch book clubs read almost exclusively original Dutch publications in Dutch. Only a small percentage of book clubs read books in other languages. For this study, only the publications in Dutch – both original Dutch work and translations – were analysed.

12 Gert-Jan Johannes, *De lof der aalbessen. Over (Noord-)Nederlandse literatuurtheorie, literatuur en de consequenties van kleinschaligheid 1770–1830*, The Hague 1997, p. 63.

13 Franco Moretti, *Atlas of the European Novel 1800–1900*, London/New York 1999, p. 151.

were only read in book clubs specifically founded for the purpose of reading books and magazines in those languages.

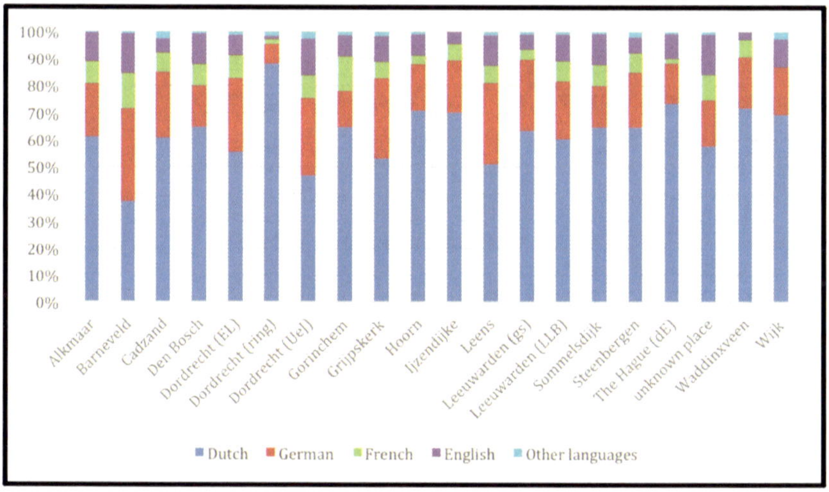

Graph 2: Original language of reading matter bought by book clubs

5 French, German and English

Some of the numbers stand out and give an idea of the amount of translated reading matter that was purchased by Dutch book clubs:

- 29.9 % of the books read in the Groningen town of Grijpskerk was translated from German, just like 28.8 % in *Utile et Jucundum* and 30,2 % in Leens. In Barneveld it is 33.8 %
- 12.7 % of the books read by book club *Oefening baart Verlichting* from the Zuid-Holland town of Gorinchem was translated from French as well as 12.4 % in Barneveld
- 14.7 % of the reading matter that circulated at the book club in Barneveld was translated from English, just as 13.6 % in *Utile et Jucundum* and 14,8 % in the book club named *Oefening*

As mentioned before, the Dutch book clubs in general read original Dutch reading matter. The percentages of translated works range from 53.3 % (in *Utile et Jucundum*) to 11.9 % (in the book club of the Ring Dordrecht). If the religious book club is ignored, however, the book club with the least translations still read 29.9 % in translation (in the Zeeland town of IJzendijke). This means that around

30 % to 50 % of all books and magazines read in Dutch book clubs was translated, which is an impressive number of titles.

In contemporary magazines, a sizeable collection of translations received criticism. Author, lector in German language and literature and professor in Dutch language, literature and history, N.G. van Kampen labelled the practice of translating French literature 'the dead sleep of the eighteenth century'.[14] People spoke about a translating frenzy. According to critics in magazines, Dutch authors themselves were too lazy to write books and Dutch readers, because of a limited relationship with their national culture, lacked a preference for decent, patriotic reading matter.[15] A choice for translations supposedly meant cultural subservience and a misguided lack of self-esteem.[16] The critique on translations after 1800 clearly had a nationalistic hue.[17] During his inaugural speech as professor of Dutch language and rhetoric in Groningen in 1815, B.H. Lulofs remarked:

> A civilized People feels the need for Poetry, for Rhetoric, and other fine arts and sciences […]. When this need of a People cannot be met by the National production, or the National language and fine arts are neglected, or, even though they do not want to make use of their fruits, it will come forth from this, that such a Nation will try to satisfy its need through the Foreigner, that which in their own country they cannot or they do not want to satisfy.[18]

---

14 Luc Korpel, *Over het nut en de wijze der vertalingen. Nederlandse vertaalreflectie (1750–1820) in een Westeuropees kader*, Amsterdam/Atlanta 1992, p. 16; N.G. van Kampen, *Beknopte geschiedenis der letteren en wetenschappen in de Nederlanden*, vol. 3, Delft 1826, p. 219, [de doodslaap der achttiende Eeuw].

15 Johannes, De lof der aalbessen (see n. 12), p. 64.

16 Johan Heilbron, 'Nederlandse vertalingen wereldwijd. Kleine landen en culturele mondialisering', in: Johan Heilbron, Wouter de Nooy and Wilma Tichelaar (eds.), *Waarin een klein land. Nederlandse cultuur in internationaal verband*, Amsterdam 1995, p. 217.

17 Luc Korpel, *In Nederduitsch gewaad. Nederlandse beschouwingen over vertalen 1760–1820*, The Hague 1993, p. 8.

18 Korpel, Over het nut en de wijze der vertalingen (see n. 14), p. 56; B.H. Lulofs, *Over de noodzakelykheid van de beoefening der eigene taal en letterkunde voor de zelfstandigheid en den roem van eene natie, gehouden bij het aanvaarden van dezelfs waardigheid op den vijftienden van slagtmaand 1815*, Groningen 1815, pp. 48–50, [Een beschaafd Volk gevoelt behoefte aan Dichtkunst, aan Welsprekendheid, en andere fraaije kunsten en wetenschappen […]. Indien nu aan deze behoefte bij een Volk door Vaderlandsche voortbrengselen niet voldaan kan worden, wijl, of de Vaderlandsche taal en fraaije Letteren verwaarloosd zijn, of, wijl men van derzelver vruchten geen gebruik wil maken, zoo zal hieruit natuurlijk volgen, dat zulk eene Natie bij den Vreemdeling den honger zoekt te stillen, dien zij in haar eigen land niet verzadigen kan, of niet verzadigen wil].

6 Recreational reading

The dependency on foreign production of reading matter is significant for book clubs in which the members – at least according to the aforementioned contemporary critique – read randomly chosen recently published reading matter. This could mean that rather than a well-considered choice in reading matter, book club members cared principally about the activity of reading. The content of what was read, for them, could have been of secondary importance, whereas the democratic environment that book clubs offered had their primary attention. In that case reading could have been a tolerable, pleasurable activity. An analysis of the borrowings from the *Leesmuseum* (subscription library) in the North Holland city of Haarlem in the second half of the nineteenth century is a first indication for an increase in demand for recreational reading matter during the nineteenth century. Above all, visitors borrowed novels, but in those days mostly original Dutch work, followed by translations.[19]

It is well conceivable that the demand for recreational reading matter was already present during the period from 1815 to 1830, but could not be met by the Dutch novel production. Publishing houses in the early nineteenth century made an effort to get acquainted with the demands of readers and tried to meet those with their production. This could explain the dependency on translations.

It is certainly true that book clubs in the United Kingdom of the Netherlands purchased recently published reading matter. A sample of the reading matter that circulated in book clubs in 1823 revealed that the titles appeared above all in 1822 and 1821, followed by 1823 and 1820.[20] However, this does not immediately imply that book clubs selected their books and magazines randomly. At least one third of the book clubs under consideration subscribed to the monthly *Namelist* of Amsterdam bookseller A.B. Saakes, a bibliographical magazine listing the most recent publications on the book market.[21] In their extensive sets of rules and regulations there were some clear stipulations in regards to the choice of reading matter. In general controversial reading matter was to be avoided, which effectively barred most religious, judicial and medicinal works from the book clubs.[22] In short, the topics that the members of book clubs allowed to be read about were socially acceptable.

This reading matter was not a random choice: the members of book clubs

19 Boudien de Vries, 'Lezende burgers. Cultuuridealen en leespraktijk in burgerlijke kringen in de negentiende eeuw', *Stijlen van burgers. Groniek* 40 (2007) 175bis, p. 59.

20 Lubbers, 'Een republiek in het klein' (see n. 2), pp. 282–283.

21 A.B. Saakes, *Naamlijst van Nederduitsche boeken, als mede van Fransche en Latijnsche werken, oratiën, dissertatiën, konstprenten, pourtraitten, landkaarten, enz. geduurende de jaaren ... in ons vaderland uitgekomen*, Amsterdam etc. 1794-[1855].

22 Lubbers, 'Een republiek in het klein' (see n. 2), pp. 221–231.

purchased recent reading matter, likely because of a wish to stay up to date with recent societal, cultural and literary developments. Now that we know that members of book clubs had a preference for novels, story collections and travelogues, which were originally Dutch, but to a high degree also translated foreign work, the question still remains to what extent illness and health are topics in the books and magazines that circulated.

7 Illness and health

Based on the analysis of the titles of all books and magazines that circulated in Dutch book clubs, some topics that are related to illness and health seem to have been of particular interest. It seems it did not matter where in the Netherlands a book club was located: some book clubs did not purchase any titles related to such themes and others ordered multiple books and magazines. It is however possible that more reading matter which was bought contained the topics, even though the title does not reveal it as such. Based on this information, the subjects could not count on any interest in the book club in Grijpskerk, the *Book club for religious works* and *Leest, Leert en Betracht* both from the Friesland city of Leeuwarden, the book club of the Ring Dordrecht, *Oefening baart Verlichting* from Gorinchem, *Onderlinge Vriendschap* from the South Holland town of Sommelsdijk and a book club in Zeeland: *Liefde voor Waarheid en Deugd* from IJzendijke.

The book clubs read about various illness and health related themes. The three themes that received the most attention were animal magnetism, sea baths, and the discussion surrounding the cowpox vaccine. In the following paragraphs these themes and the associated titles will be discussed as well as some books and magazines that were not related to either of those topics.

8 Animal magnetism

Animal magnetism was the idea, much in vogue in the late eighteenth and early nineteenth century, that all living beings exerted a free stream of invisible energy that could provide healing. Illnesses were considered blockades in that stream that could be healed by inducing static energy through rubbing and stroking. Five book clubs had nine books circulating on animal magnetism; some of the titles were purchased by multiple book clubs.

At *Legendo Discimus* a book by A. Beeler was bought,[23] which received a

23 A. Beeler, *Het Dierlijk Magnetismus, beknopt in deszelfs verschijnselen en manier van*

mixed review in *Vaderlandsche Letteroefeningen* (*Letter exercises from the Fatherland*). The author, a pharmacist and 'chimist' from Amsterdam, felt compelled to publish the book, because animal magnetism was one of the most spoken about topics in France and Germany, but was judged unfavourably in the Netherlands. He discusses the most notable works on animal magnetism and added some of his own experiences. The history of the discovery of animal magnetism he writes about contains the basic principles: heavenly bodies, Earth and living bodies influence each other; there is a 'flow' that permeates everything; the flow functions according to natural laws, much like the regularity of high and low tide; the flow works on the nerves and is comparable with the effects of a magnet on living bodies; mirrors reflect the flow; sound enhances the flow; there are opposing magnetic forces in living bodies that conflict with the flow running freely; by regulating the flow, nerve diseases can be treated.[24] The book was intended for laymen in the field of magnetism, but according to the reviewer it did not add any additional information on the topic. The author was praised for his observations of treatments of nerve diseases, but also because of his reluctance to apply magnetism as a general treatment. The reviewer said he found it difficult not to denounce the book completely, because even though the treatment seemed so simple and so insignificant, the results were so extremely effective and so complicated, that it should never be trusted in the hands of the public.[25]

The same book club bought *The secrets of magnetisers and sleepwalkers debunked for sane and virtuous people.*[26] It also circulated in *Voor Wetenschap en Deugd* in the town of Steenbergen in North Brabant and in *Amica Veritas*. The anonymous author was much opposed to the growing interest in animal magnetism that he had noted in magazines. According to the author people who believe in the positive effects of animal magnetism were 'gullible disciples'.[27] Animal magnetism, he wrote, could be a new invention by Satan.[28]

This harsh rejection elicited a response from Jan Hoogendorp, pastor of the

---

aanwending voorgesteld, volgens de ervaring van vele verdienstelijke Mannen, met derzelver eigene waarnemingen vermeerderd, The Hague 1814.

24 Beeler, Het Dierlijk Magnetismus (see n. 23), pp. 6–8.

25 *Vaderlandsche letteroefeningen*, Boekbeschouwing (1814), pp. 383–384, [Wij durven de lezing van dit boekje […] niet geheel veroordelen[…]. Het middel schijnt zoo eenvoudig en zoo onbeduidend; het is echter inderdaad zoo hevig werkend en zoo ingewikkeld, dat het nimmer in de handen van het publiek te vertrouwen is].

26 *De geheimen der magnétiseurs en somnambules ontmaskerd voor weldenkende en deugdgezinde menschen*, 1816. [Translated from an unknown French title by Jan Hoogendorp].

27 De geheimen der magnétiseurs ontmaskerd (see n. 26), p. 2, [ligtgeloovige aanhangers].

28 De geheimen der magnétiseurs ontmaskerd (see n. 26), p. 4.

Dutch Reformed Church in St. Maartensdijk.[29] Hoogendorp denied the influence of Satan in the so-called animal magnetism. According to the pastor, physicians who did practise magnetism did so with nothing but good intentions, trying to further health and happiness.[30] Hoogendorp went even further: 'Why would a Deist refute the Hidden secrets that appear in the Bible? Why the Wonders, that confirm the Doctrine in it?'[31] This response was purchased for the *Eerste leesgezelschap.*

The members of *Amica Veritas* also bought *Test of an idea of animal Magnetism as Medicine* by C.A.F. Kluge.[32] According to a reviewer, upon release the book must have received enormous attention from physicians, because the original German print had received lots of praise.[33] Kluge hails three discoveries in the previous century as the most important advancements in medicine: electricity, galvanism and animal magnetism. The latter was the discovery of the greatest importance, because of the lasting effects it has.[34] Kluge lists some of the practical aspects involved in treatments using animal magnetism: the effect of wearing gloves, whether the physician or the patient is a stronger or weaker magnet, sleepwalking, feelings of ecstasy and many more.[35]

In Steenbergen the members purchased two more books.[36] In Leeuwarden at *Amica Veritas,* another book was purchased the title of which I could not identify. At *De Eendragt* three more books were bought,[37] one of which was a book written by Hufeland which was also read by the *Eerste leesgezelschap.*[38] In the introduction to this book the editors mentioned that by publishing a

29 Jan Hoogendorp, *De ontmaskeraar van De geheimen der magnetiseurs en somnambules voor weldenkende en deugdgezinde menschen ontmaskerd*, Dordrecht 1816.

30 Hoogendorp, De ontmaskeraar (see n. 29), pp. 4–5.

31 Hoogendorp, De ontmaskeraar (see n. 29), p. 10.

32 C.A.F. Kluge, *Proeve eener voorstelling van het dierlijk Magnetismus*, Amsterdam 1812. [Translated by F. van der Breggen Cornz. from German: C.A.F. Kluge, *Versuch einer Darstellung des animalischen Magnetismus als Heilmittel*, Berlin 1811].

33 *Vaderlandsche letteroefeningen*, Boekbeschouwing (1813), p. 299.

34 Kluge, Proeve eener voorstelling (see n. 32), p. 6.

35 Kluge, Proeve eener voorstelling (see n. 32), pp. 91–240.

36 G. Bakken, *Bijdragen tot den tegenwoordigen staat van animalisch Magnetismus in ons Vaderland*, Groningen 1818; J. Crans, *Het werkdadig magnetismus, of Dagverhaal van drie zieken, waaraan de magnetische behandeling met het gelukkigst gevolg is toegepast: met eene vooraanstaande inleiding ter beknopte verklaring van den aard en de uitoefening van het magnetismus*, Dordrecht 1815.

37 Pieter Gabriël van Ghert, *Mnemosyne of aantekeningen van merkwaardige verschijnsels van het animalisch magnetismus*, Amsterdam 1815; A. Numan, *Verhandeling over het dierlijk magnetismus, als den grondslag ter verklaring der physische levensbetrekkingen of sympathie tusschen de dierlijke ligchamen*, Groningen 1815.

38 Cristoph Wilhelm Hufeland, *Belangrijke waarnemingen omtrent het slaapwandelen, of het droomleven, zonder den invloed van het magnetismus*, Dordrecht 1817. [Translated by an unknown translator from German: C.W. Hufeland and J.C.F. Harles, *Journal der practischen Heilkunde* (1796–1836)].

translation of Hufeland's work they hoped to take away some falsehoods about animal magnetism.[39] In his book the German physician had collected observations of colleagues, who noticed incredible spams amongst their patients or who had patients who sleepwalked, which were not caused by animal magnetism.[40] Hufeland presents three cases of sleepwalkers in detail in order to convince the reader that sleepwalking can be triggered by several physical and mental causes, instead of using the popular diagnosis of animal magnetism.

It seems Beeler was correct in writing that animal magnetism was a popular topic in the early nineteenth century, as the theme was read about in plenty of book clubs. The books that their members purchased were mostly introductions to the topic, but critical responses to the popularity of animal magnetism were chosen as well. Book clubs seem to have been interested in the topic mainly because it was a new development in healthcare in the early nineteenth century and was much talked about in the Netherlands.

9 Sea baths

As mentioned before, the so-called sea baths were a theme that received a considerable amount of attention in book clubs. The sea baths were popular around 1800, when physicians started pointing out the health effects of bathing in the sea. Resorts became popular for people seeking curative and therapeutic treatments. For the well-off guests of sea bath facilities, there were special closed off carriages, bathing machines, that allowed people to enter the sea in privacy.

The members of the *Eerste leesgezelschap* bought *The sea-bath*, in which the sea is described as 'without a doubt one of the most natural and effective of resources'.[41] Bathing in the sea is recommended to further general hygiene:

> This goal, the purity and affluence of the skin, namely, can now only be achieved, through functional washing, bathing, rubbing and other things like those, which exerts an immediate effect on the skin.[42]

---

39 Hufeland, Belangrijke waarnemingen (see n. 38), pp. iii–iv.

40 Hufeland, Belangrijke waarnemingen (see n. 38), p. 8.

41 Gijsbert Swartendijk Stierling and Anthonij Moll, *Het zee-bad, of Overzigt over den oorsprong en de nuttigheid der baden in het algemeen: benevens eene meer opzettelijke beschouwing van den invloed der zeebaden in het bijzonder, of de bevordering of herstelling der gezondheid, door geneeskundige waarnemingen gestaafd: met een aanhangsel nopens de nieuwe zeebad-inrigting te Scheveningen*, Dordrecht 1819, pp. iv, [ontegenzeggelijk een der natuurlijkste en werkzaamste hulpmiddelen].

42 Stierling and Moll, *Het zee-bad* (see n. 41), p. v, [Dit oogmerk, de zuiverheid en welgesteldheid der huid, namelijk, nu kan door geen middel beter bereikt worden, dan door doelmatige wasschingen, baden, wrijvingen en wat dies meer zij, als op de huid eenen onmiddellijken invloed uitoefende].

The authors provide instructions on the length of bathing, the consumption of drinks and food before and after bathing, sleeping and resting after bathing, the use of bathing as a way to cleanse, to stimulate rest and to heal. The book further contains explanations of healthcare, specific illnesses and the effect of sea bathing on the body and these illnesses. The authors Swartendijk Stierling and Moll note that agitation, irregularities in bowel movements, acid reflux, burning sensations, congestions, haemorrhoids and gassiness could all be cured by taking a sea bath.[43]

From one of the authors, the physician Moll, a previous book was published on sea bathing, which was read in *De Eendragt.*[44] According to Moll, he wrote the book 'for the well-being of our Countrymen in general'.[45] Moll stayed in the sea bath facilities in Scheveningen for several weeks. Bathing in the sea had a long history dating back to the practise in Ancient Greece, but only since the second half of the eighteenth century, had a London-based physician rediscovered the curative effects, writes Moll. The first Dutch facility was opened in Scheveningen, where visitors could bathe in the sea using bathing machines and special carts. After suffering from typhoid in 1815, Moll was looking for a way to cure various afflictions. The facilities in Scheveningen offered comfortable rooms with several means of bathing using different temperatures of water.

Another book on sea bathing in Scheveningen circulated amongst the members of *Amica Veritas.*[46] The author wanted the general public, as well as other physicians, to become familiar with sea baths in various places, which often had to close down because of low numbers of visitors.[47] During the bathing season of 1828, 6,699 people took a sea bath in Scheveningen.[48] As an example, the author presents several success stories, such as the one of the 28 year old D.J., a Roman Catholic priest, who suffered from a skin disease and a slimy tongue due to intense studying, but after a couple of sea baths, paired with internal use of sea water, he was healed.[49]

As the first sea bathing facility was opened in Scheveningen in 1818, the topic likely caught the attention of anyone interested in current developments in general, but perhaps also because of the general appeal of health benefits. The members of the book clubs were mainly from the middle classes and they often

43 Stierling and Moll, *Het zee-bad* (see n. 41), pp. 226–227.

44 Anthonij Moll, *Gemeenzame brieven over het Scheveninger-zeebad, ten nutte van lijders, half-lijders en niet-lijders*, Arnhem 1814.

45 Moll, Gemeenzame brieven (see n. 44), p. 1, [tot de welvaart onzer Landgenooten in het algemeen].

46 L.F. d'Aumerie, *Zeebad-inrigting te Scheveningen en het badsaisoen van 1828*, The Hague 1829.

47 d'Aumerie, Zeebad-inrigting (see n. 46), unnumbered page in introduction.

48 d'Aumerie, Zeebad-inrigting (see n. 46), p. 45.

49 d'Aumerie, Zeebad-inrigting (see n. 46), pp. 49–50.

viewed the activities of the upper classes as something worth emulating. The sea bath in Scheveningen was frequented by royalty, nobility and other wealthy folk. Combined with the fact it was an intriguing new development in physical healthcare, this could have been the reason for the interest of the Dutch book clubs.

10 The cowpox vaccine

After the British physician Edward Jenner discovered in the second half of the eighteenth century that people who had been in contact with cowpox were resistant to the dangerous and deadly smallpox, he professed the idea to inoculate people with cowpox. The Rotterdam physician Levie Salomon Davids tested the idea in 1800 and saw favourable results. He was one of the co-founders of the Society for Cowpox vaccination. In 1818, king Willem I of the United Kingdom of the Netherlands handed out golden medals to physicians who had inoculated at least 50 people. The vaccination was first only mandatory for the poor, but over time general vaccination was pushed for. In 1823 the cowpox vaccine became mandatory for children who went to school for the first time.

Even though it also featured elsewhere (for instance at the *Health-magazine*), two book clubs (*Amica Veritas* and *De Eendragt*) seem to have had a more than average interest in this topic, with members reading several works on the cowpox vaccine. The Portuguese Jewish physician Abraham Capadose, who was part of the Dutch Réveil – the Christian revival between about 1815 and 1865 fathered by Willem Bilderdijk – wrote a critique in which he delivered medical and philosophical considerations.[50] Capadose takes a stance against preventive vaccinations and made a connection between the vaccinations and animal magnetism. According to Capadose the vaccination of children is a form of heathen medical practice and he feels it is a criminal act if practised.[51] Capadose writes it goes against the will of God to treat healthy people. Medical practitioners should only deal with the ill.[52] At the same time he protests animal magnetism being taught 'ex professo' at Dutch academies.[53]

The work of Capadose evoked multiple responses, of which only some were published. The members of *De Eendragt* read four of those, amongst which an anonymous pamphlet, the author of which placed Capadose in the circle of

50 Abraham Capadose, *Bestrijding der vaccine, of De vaccine aan de beginselen der godsdienst, der rede en der ware geneeskunst getoetst*, Amsterdam 1823.
51 David Kalmijn, *Abraham Capadose*, dissertation Utrecht University 1955, p. 106.
52 Kalmijn, Capadose (see n. 51), p. 106.
53 Capadose, Bestrijding der vaccine (see n. 50), p. ix.

Bilderdijk and said Capadose only wrote the work to be counted as a pious man.[54] To support the general health of the public, he felt it was necessary to speak out against Capadose.[55] In The Hague the response of F. van der Breggen Cornz. was also read.[56] This Amsterdam professor of Medicine showed that the appeal of Capadose actually had an opposite effect to the one he intended: parents had their children vaccinated *en masse.*[57] C.G. Ontijd, a doctor from The Hague, also wrote a response that was read by *De Eendragt.*[58] Ontijd counts Capadose amongst the 'Bilderdijkian sect', accusing them of thinking that everyone who does not agree with them is influenced by the Devil. He further says that animal magnetism, even though he has his doubts, could have a positive outcome when treating certain nerve diseases. Together with some experienced physicians he remarks that the work of Capadose is lacking in accurate observations or reliable argumentation. He even casts doubt on Capadose's Christian love.[59] Another work that was read in response was written by Johan Samuel Swaan, which was not only a critique on Capadose, but also on Isaäc da Costa's *Bezwaren Tegen den Geest der Eeuw (Objections to the spirit of the century)*, a pamphlet containing critique on enlightened thought, calling for a return to Christian values.[60]

In *Amica Veritas,* the members did not read critiques of the original work of Capadose, but were interested in Capadose's replies to critical reviews and publications. His first response was specifically to take on Van der Breggen's arguments.[61] This response by Capadose was also read by the members of *De Eendragt.* A second response by Capadose, in which he replied to several reviews and publications, was only read in *Amica Veritas.*[62] A reviewer of *Vaderlandsche*

54 *Voorlopige aanmerkingen op dr. Capadoses Bestrijding der vaccine*, Amsterdam 1823.

55 Arend Kagchelland and Michiel Kagchelland, *Van dompers en verlichten. Een onderzoek naar de confrontatie tussen het vroege protestantse Réveil en de Verlichting in Nederland (1815–1826)*, Delft 2009, pp. 516–517.

56 Frans van der Breggen Cornz., *Voorloopige brief aan den schrijver van de Bestrijding der vaccine, of De vaccine aan de beginselen der godsdienst, der rede en der ware geneeskunst getoetst, aan Abraham Capadose, med. doct.*, Amsterdam 1823.

57 Kagchelland and Kagchelland, *Van dompers en verlichten* (see n. 55), p. 510.

58 Conrad Gerard Ontijd, *De waarde der koepok-inënting gehandhaafd, en op nieuw aanbevolen aan ouders en kunstgenooten, tegen de bestrijding derzelve van den med. doct. Abraham Capadose, of De vaccine aan de beginselen der godsdienst, der rede en der ware geneeskunst getoetst*, The Hague 1824.

59 Kagchelland and Kagchelland, *Van dompers en verlichten* (see n. 55), pp. 519–520, [de Bilderdijksche secte].

60 Johannes Samuel Swaan, *Bedenkingen, op de Bezwaren tegen den geest der eeuw van mr. I. da Costa, toegelicht door mr. W. Bilderdijk, gelijk ook tegen de toetsing der vaccine van godsdienst en rede, door Mr. Capadosa*, Amsterdam 1824.

61 Abraham Capadose, *Bijdrage tot de bestrijding der vaccine: antwoord op den Voorloopigen brief van F. van der Breggen Cz., med. doctor en hoogleeraar enz.*, Amsterdam 1823.

62 Abraham Capadose, *Nieuwe bijdrage tot de bestrijding der vaccine behelzende de ont-*

Letteroefeningen (*Letter exercises from the Fatherland*) decided to stop reviewing Capadose's responses, because according to him the potentially dangerous ideas of Capadose had already received enough attention.[63]

Once the cowpox vaccine became mandatory for schoolchildren in 1823, the topic immediately became a societal issue. In several religious circles the mandatory vaccination was heavily criticised and several notable physicians and authors, such as Capadose, set to writing. Various authors, both in favour of and against preventive vaccinations, had their responses published, which made for an interesting corpus of texts for book clubs to choose from. Even though book clubs generally refrained from reading about religion, in order to avoid controversy and possible debate amongst the members, it seems that arguments in the cowpox vaccine debate – in part driven by religion – made them overlook this common practice. Clearly, this topic was deemed to be of high societal importance.

11 Miscellaneous work on health and well being

In the Leens' book club the only health and illness related reading matter was a book by A.F.M. Willich, the *Healthbook*.[64] In this work, doctor Willich states that too many people live unhealthily in the first half of their lives. For him, that was the reason to write a book with tips for a healthy lifestyle with the intention to extend the duration people could live. According to a reviewer that was the reason his colleagues looked down on him.[65] In his book, Willich tackles the influence of air in different regions, how to prevent illness in children, hygienic tips to prevent skin diseases, the workings of senses, liquors, spices, electricity and also the previously mentioned sea baths, animal magnetism and cowpox vaccine.[66] According to a reviewer the *Healthbook* is more complete than com-

---

wikkeling van sommige voorname punten en derzelver bevestiging door feiten: vervat in de wederlegging van onderscheide recensien en tegenschriften, Amsterdam 1824.

63 *Vaderlandsche letteroefeningen*, Boekbeschouwing (1824), pp. 337–338.

64 Anthony Willich, *Gezondheidsboek: behelzende wat er al, tot behoud van ligchaamswelvaart en sterkte, reeds bij de opvoeding en verder tot op den ouden dag, ten aanzien van lucht en weder, reinheid, kleeding, spijs en drank, oefening, rust, slaap, gemoedsgesteldheid, zintuigen, vooral oogen, tanden, enz. moet worden in acht genomen: onder vergelijking van menigerlei waarnemingen van in- en uitlandsche geleerden*, Rotterdam 1818. [Translated by an unknown translator from English and possibly an adaptation of (a part of): A.F.M. Willich, *Lectures on diet and regimen: being a systematic inquiry into the most rational means of preserving health and prolonging life: together with physiological and chemical explanations*, second edition, London 1799].

65 *De Recensent, ook der Recensenten* 2 (1819), p. 86.

66 *De Recensent, ook der Recensenten* 2 (1819), p. 87.

parable works of J.F. Martinet and C.W. Hufeland.[67] 'In short, it contains everything that one desires to find in such a Reference work'.[68]

In the book club of Barneveld in Gelderland, the diary of a physically disabled man was read, written by Henry Matthews and translated into Dutch.[69] For the main character his disability was the reason to start travelling. This supposedly was healthy and indeed, at the end of the diary, his disability caused him less problems. A reviewer of *Vaderlandsche Letteroefeningen* (*Letter exercises from the Fatherland*) felt the book was perfectly suitable for book clubs: 'We dare safely recommend the diary, as pleasant and entertaining reading matter, for every book club'.[70] However, the book itself contains little information on his disability; it is primarily a travelogue, taking the readers through Portugal, Italy, Switzerland and Spain and consists of descriptions of natural landmarks, inhabitants, buildings, cultural artefacts, literature, art, food and much more.

The members of *Utile et Jucundum* had a book circulating on people with mental disabilities. In the introduction, the author recommends the book for anyone interested in knowledge of human nature, not just for those who are professionally involved with psychology or anthropology.[71] Mental disabilities are described as a state 'beneath the most despicable animal'.[72] The book features short biographies of inhabitants of a hospital in London, amongst whom are Patrick Walsh, a 'savage madman' with 'bloodthirsty cruelty', who, as a mutineer, killed his captain and part of his crew.[73] Thomas English, a born Greek, is a 'criminal fool'.[74] He tried to mutilate a baker with a razor blade.

67 *De Recensent, ook der Recensenten* 2 (1819), p. 88.

68 *De Recensent, ook der Recensenten* 2 (1819), p. 88, [Kortom, het bevat alles, wat men in zulk Huisboek verlangt aan te treffen].

69 Henry Matthews, *Dagboek van een' invalide, gehouden op eene reis naar Portugal, Italie, Zwitserland en Frankrijk, gedurende de jaren 1817, 1818 en 1819*, Haarlem 1821–1822. [Translated by an unknown translator from English: Henry Matthews, *Diary of an Invalid: being the Journal of a Tour in Pursuit of Health; in Portugal, Italy, Switzerland and France, in the Years 1817, 1818 and 1819*, London 1820].

70 *Vaderlandsche letteroefeningen*, Boekbeschouwing (1824), pp. 171 and 174, [Wij durven zijn dagboek gerustelijk, als eene aangename en onderhoudende lecture, ieder leesgezelschap aanprijzen].

71 *Tafereelen der broosheid van het menschelijk verstand, of Karaktertrekken, anecdoten en bijzonderheden der krankzinnigen, die zich tegenwoordig bevinden in het Bethlehems hospitaal te Londen*, Amsterdam 1824, pp. iii. [Translated by an unknown translator from English and possibly an adaptation of (a part of): A constant observer, *Sketches in Bedlam; or characteristic traits of insanity: as displayed in the cases of one hundred and forty patients of both sexes, now, or recently, confined in New Bethlem, including Margaret Nicholson, James Hatfield, Patrick Walsh, Bannister Truelock, and many other extraordinary maniacs, who have been transferred from Old Bethlem. To the above are added, a succinct history of the establishment, its rules, regulations, forms of admissions, treatment of patients, &c. &c.*, London 1823].

72 Tafereelen (see n. 71), p. iv, [beneden het verachtste dier].

73 Tafereelen (see n. 71), p. 1, ['woeste uitzinnige' and 'bloeddorstige wreedheid'].

A book by H.D. Hermes on Christian, spiritual support for the ill was read by the members of the *Eerste leesgezelschap*.[75] In Leeuwarden in Friesland, the members of book club *Amica Veritas* read multiple titles that are related to illness and health. One of the books contains tips to extend the duration of life,[76] of which a reviewer for *Vaderlandsche Letteroefeningen* (*Letter exercises from the Fatherland*) said it contained false intentions and had a 'quack-like title'.[77] According to the author, professor G.J. Wenzel, one of the ways people could live a long life would be to have a lot of body mass, since large animals like elephants and whales live long lives.[78]

In *Amica Veritas*, as well as in *Daar Vrede Bloeid Ook Vriendschap Groeid* from the Zeeland town of Cadzand, the members also read volumes of the *Health-magazine*, in which a wide range of subjects on illness and health were covered, such as the indecency of maternity visits, the usefulness of investigating urine, the disadvantages of liquor for young people, how to behave in extremely warm weather, the consumption of ice as a dessert, but also the previously mentioned sea baths and cowpox vaccine.[79] The book club members of *Amica Veritas* also read the reply by A. Frölich on a prize contest by the prominent German physician C.W. Hufeland, in which Frölich describes the treatment of various types of fever by the external use of cold water.[80] The author provides guidelines on the use of the thermometer and explains which body temperature warrants a particular temperature of water.[81] A reviewer praised the work because the application of water is such an easy treatment.[82]

The titles presented in this section differ widely from each other. A reference work and a magazine on various health and illness related topics, a travelogue of

74 Tafereelen (see n. 71), p. 10, [misdadige zinnelooze].

75 Hermann Daniel Hermes, *Betrachtingen bij het ziekbedde*, Haarlem 1820, [Translated and adapted by Willem Bilderdijk from German: H.D. Hermes, *Herr, siehe, den du lieb hast, der ist krank! Eine kurze Anweisung zu einem Gott wohlgefälligen Verhalten auf dem Krankenbette*, 1820].

76 G.J. Wenzel, *Kunst, om gezondheid, jeugdige kracht en schoonheid, in al de tijdperken des menschelijken levens, te behouden*, Amsterdam 1817. [Translated by an unknown translator from German: G.J. Wenzel, *Die Kunst gesund, jugendlich, stark und schön auch im Alter zu bleiben*, Vienna 1800].

77 *Vaderlandsche letteroefeningen*, Boekbeschouwing (1817), pp. 592–593, [kwakzalverachtigen titel].

78 *Vaderlandsche letteroefeningen*, Boekbeschouwing (1817), p. 593.

79 *Gezondheids-blad ter onderrigting en waarschuwing voor allen die prijs stellen op leven en gezondheid*, I–XII, Amsterdam 1822–1825.

80 A. Frölich, *Over het uitwendig gebruik van koud water ter matiging der koorts, eene bekroonde Prijsverhandeling*, Gorinchem 1823. [Translated by C. van Eldik from German: A. Frölich, *Abhandlung über die Übergiessungen oder Bäder von kaltem oder lauwarmem Wasser in Krankheiten*, Vienna 1820].

81 *Vaderlandsche letteroefeningen*, Boekbeschouwing (1824), p. 335.

82 *Vaderlandsche letteroefeningen*, Boekbeschouwing (1824), p. 336.

a disabled man, a description of people with different mental disabilities, a book with information on how to prolong life and a text explaining how to treat fever with cold water. Ostensibly these works had nothing in common. When viewed within the context of book club purchasing habits however, it becomes clear these were the topics that were of interest to contemporary readers. Especially the reference work, the magazine and the books on fever treatment and prolonging life show that in the early nineteenth century people were keen to learn to enhance their well being and take care of their health.

12 Conclusion

The members of book clubs in the Northern provinces of the United Kingdom of the Netherlands read dozens of books and magazines every year. They chose their reading matter in a democratic way and had up to date information on the most recent publications on the Dutch book market. Around 50 % of all books they bought consisted of substantial portions of novels, story collections, travelogues and books on geography. Between 30 % and 50 % of everything they read was originally German, French or English work and was read in translation. The content of the reading matter that the members chose was probably not their primary interest; the act of reading and the democratic surroundings that book clubs offered were likely their leading motives.

Those who were active in book clubs showed no unusual or explicit interest in the themes of illness and health. The interest that the members of the book clubs did demonstrate in subjects that are related to illness and health, primarily focussed on three themes: sea baths, animal magnetism and the cowpox vaccine. If the critics of the book clubs were right in saying the members only read 'the news of the day', this would mean that their choice in reading matter reflected certain contemporary trends. And indeed, when we take a look at the three aforementioned themes, we can conclude those were *en vogue*. Around 1800, sea baths were a popular way to treat skin diseases and the first facility opening in the Netherlands in Scheveningen in 1818, animal magnetism was a topic that attracted attention in both professional and laymen circles and the cowpox vaccine became mandatory in 1823 and received immediate criticism. The 'news of the day' consisted, at least in part, of the contemporary issues that society was dealing with and illness and health were – albeit modestly – part of those.

Mary Kemperink

'Am I not Punished Enough?' Confessions of Homosexuals in Medical Studies Around 1900

1 Introduction

In the Netherlands nowadays a refugee is not send back to his homeland, if he or she is homosexual and if in the homeland homosexuality is considered to be criminal. It is upon the authorities, then, to judge whether the refugee standing before them is a homosexual. But how does one recognize a homosexual? Nowadays this question causes serious problems to the Dutch Raad van State (the Dutch Council of State). In this context it is interesting to realize that more than hundred years ago it was physicians who for the very first time asked themselves this same question. As an answer they constructed a brand-new concept: 'homosexuality'.

In his *Histoire de la sexualité* (1976–1984) Foucault departs from the idea that the concept of homosexuality was imposed by medical professionals, as means of power and suppression. In his opinion their definition of homosexuality as a disease served to maintain the 'natural' societal order. This however, seems a somewhat over-simplified view of the matter. The construction of the concept of homosexuality is not to be considered as an exclusively suppressive act by scientific authorities, but can be seen rather as the result of a cooperation between physicians and patients.[1]

In this article I will focus on this cooperation. I would like to demonstrate how literature, in the sense of literary genres and literary rhetorical techniques, played a considerable part in this process. Herewith I will concentrate on confessions published in medical studies on homosexuality. My central question focuses on the relationship between these confessions and (the remaining part of) the medical assessment with regard to vision and especially rhetoric. To what an extent were confessions and medical texts conceived in mutual relation to each other and what rhetorical means were used in this behalf?

1 Philippe Weber, *Der Trieb zum Erzählen. Sexualpathalogie und Homosexualität, 1852–1914*, Bielefeld 2008, p. 206.

I will start with a short overview of the historical development of the concept of 'homosexuality'. For the record, it was only in the course of the twentieth century that the term homosexuality became common. Around 1900 preferably other designations were used, like 'Urning', 'Uranier' and 'invert'.[2] When I speak here of 'homosexual' or 'homosexuality', I use this designation as a meta-term, meaning: 'with a sexual preference for members of the same sex'.

2 The medical discourse[3]

In the second half of the nineteenth century the discussion on homosexuality and on sexuality in general became standard practice in medical science, under the denominator of 'sexuology'. The suffix '-ology' indicates that a real science was here at stake. Before, in light of the current penal code, homosexuality, had rather been a matter for the judge than for the doctor. Only in England anal sexual intercourse was legally forbidden, whereas in 1885 there came a law into force that attached a penalty to so-called 'excessive obscenity' between men. In France after the revolution, from 1791 on, sodomy (in the general sense of 'sexually abuse') in the new penal code was abolished as a punishable crime. The same happened in the Netherlands under French government (in 1809 and 1811). In Italy there existed no legal law whatsoever against homosexuality. In Germany, after the establishment of the German empire in 1871, article 175 was implemented in the penal code, which stated that unnatural obscenity between men of the same sex, or between men and beasts, was to be punished with confinement and loss of all civil rights. At the end of the nineteenth century

2 The term 'Urning' is coined in 1869 by the Hungarian Károly Mária Kertbeny. Anna Katharina Schaffner, *Modernism and Perversion. Sexual Deviance in Sexology and Literature, 1850–1930*, London 2012, p. 13. The term 'Uranier' comes from Karl Heinrich Ulrichs. Herewith he referred to the divine Urania, one of the nine Muses.

3 For this article I made use in particular of following secondary studies: Heike Bauer, *English Literary Sexuology. Translations of inversion, 1860–1930*, London 2009; G. Hekma, *Homoseksualiteit, een medische reputatie. De uitdoktering van de homoseksueel in negentiende-eeuws Nederland*, Amsterdam 1987; Elena Mancini, *Magnus Hirschfeld and the Quest for Sexual Freedom. A History of The First International Sexual Freedom Movement*, New York 2010; Klaus Müller, *Aber in meinem Herzen sprach eine Stimme so laut. Homosexuelle Autobiographien und medizinische Pathographien im neunzehnten Jahrhundert*, Berlin 1990; H. Oosterhuis, *Stepchildren of nature. Krafft-Ebbing, Psychiatry, and The Making of Sexual Identity*, Chicago/London 2000; G. Robb, *Strangers. Homosexual Love in the 19th Century*, London 2004; Schaffer, Modernism and Perversion (see n. 2); Weber, Der Trieb zum Erzählen (see n. 1).

protest was made against this article, also by physicians. It was only in 1994 that it was officially abolished.[4]

Initially the doctor just played an advisory part in the legal procedure. He was the one who had to determine whether there was a physical injury and later on whether there was congenital homosexuality at stake. In the last decennia of the nineteenth century the importance of the physician in matters of homosexuality increased dramatically. This development was caused by a growing interest in medical circles for sexuality and especially for sexual disturbances. This interest can be seen in the light of a growing moral pressure on sexuality and medical interest in human intimate life and in pathology in general. Whole series of even in our time still prevailing 'perversions', as *sadism*, *masochism*, *fetishism*, *voyeurism* and *exhibitionism* were only developed during the second half of the nineteenth century. Towards the end of the century homosexuality was standing in the centre of medical attention and it became more or less detached from a pathological context.

Medical interest also increased because scientists became almost obsessed by the burning question of the nature of abnormal sexuality.[5] How could it be that nature produced something that as a matter of fact was considered unnatural? Medical doctors especially focused on homosexuality between men. This primary interest was related not only to the law, which exclusively pointed towards homosexuality between men, but also to the general idea that the sexual drive was far more violent in men than in women.

Towards the end of the nineteenth century a flood of medical studies dedicated to homosexuality came on the market, first in Germany and a little later also in France and Italy.

In those studies a number of crucial questions were repeatedly discussed time and again. An important one was the question whether homosexuality was acquired of congenital. In the former the person involved was considered to be morally guilty, in the latter he was not. The opinion evolved more and more towards the idea of a congenital predisposition. Possible answers raised new questions. If homosexuality was congenital, was it then pathological? Was it a form of degeneration? Or was it simply a non-pathological, healthy variation of 'normal' sexuality? Those physicians who were more enlightened slowly and with some hesitation leaned towards the concept of the healthy homosexual. In the same line less physicians around 1900 considered homosexuality to be a danger to society. The view that homosexuality implied anal penetration (sodomy) retreated into the background as well. Anal penetration was still

4 In practice, however, all these rather severe laws were often not executed. Robb, *Strangers* (see n. 3), p. 23

5 Weber, Der Trieb zum Erzählen (see n. 1), p. 101.

considered as pathological and blameworthy, but it was not seen any more as a practice inherent to homosexuality.

Medical science happened to be highly descriptive and it tended towards schematizing and categorizing. Krafft-Ebing's aim was to develop a finely-woven classification of the subtypes of homosexuality. He was not the only one. Other physicians shared the view that knowledge had to be based on observation. Hirschfeld began his study 'Ursachen und Wesen des Uranismus' (Causes and nature of uranism) remarking: "Observe, gentlemen, observe!' with these words my honored master, Freiherr von Recklinghausen of the university of Strasbourg, began and concluded almost every class."[6]

Relevant in this respect is that towards the end of the century next to a physiological approach a psychological approach to the patient gained a more prominent place in psychiatry. For Krafft-Ebing, and physicians after him, diagnosis was not entirely based on physical characteristics and external behavior, but on the entire personality, one's perceptions and emotions included.[7] Physicians started searching for cases as an empirical basis for their theories and as illustrations and convincing evidence in their studies. In general a medical case had a fixed format with its causes (etiology), its symptoms and its therapy as recurring components.[8] This meant that in the elaboration of a homosexual case if possible the following points were to be included: heredity (father, mother, grandparents, aunts, uncles), physiologic characteristics of the patient (skull, face, body, genitals, etcetera), psychological characteristics of the patient on the basis of his (or her) own information and of information from relatives and acquaintances and finally the therapy suggested by the doctor and its results.

The problem was that homosexuality was a morally tricky subject and even forbidden by law in some countries. The so-called patients would not easily present themselves in the consultation room of a doctor. Hirschfeld recounts an anecdote of a professional physician in the field, who confessed to him that in real life he had never met one single homosexual. Would Hirschfeld perhaps be so kind to introduce him to one?[9] Thus, at first medical practice did not generate much empiric material, except for some extreme cases of detention or cases of

6 "Beobachten, meine Herren, beobachten!' mit diesen Worten begann und schloss mein verehrter Leher, Freiherr von Recklinghausen, von der Universität Strassburg, fas jede seiner Unterrichtsstunden.' Magnus Hirschfeld, 'Ursachen und Wesen des Uranismus', in: *Jahrbuch für sexuelle Zwischenstufen mit besonderer Berücksichtigung der Homosexualiteit* V (1903), vol. 1, p. 3. Von Recklinghausen was a specialist in the field of genetic diseases.

7 Müller, Aber in meinem Herzen sprach eine Stimme (see n. 3), p. 61.

8 The format of the medic case comes from Philippe Pinel (1745–1826) and from his student Jean-Étienne Esquirol (1772–1840).

9 Hirschfeld, Ursachen und Wesen des Uranismus (see n. 6), p. 4.

mental illness and admission in psychiatric institutions. Where could a doctor then obtain information on the homosexual practice?

One could base one's theory on existing historical sources: memoires and chronicals, and especially on literature (novels, plays) which sketched the perceptions and feelings of homosexuals themselves from the inside. Medical studies on homosexuality richly focused then on literary sources. In the preface to his study *Uranisme et unisexualité* Raffalovitch asks his readers to send him historical as well as literary documents to confirm or contradict his theory.[10] And the physician A. Moll mentions in the introduction to his *Die konträre Sexualempfindung* literature as his most important source. In his book he uses numerous literary examples. Another leading physician, I. Bloch, considered the French novelist De Sade to have been maybe the first sexologist.[11]

3 The confession

The most convincing material for a physician was the personal confession of a patient, written or told to him face to face in the consultation room. The author of a confession (or an autobiography) by definition remolds his own life up to the moment of his writing, into a rounded story. He transforms it into a coherent whole that has a development, a beginning and an end. One great example here is *Les Confessions* (1780) by Rousseau in which the author in search of his own personality, claims to give the reader an unembellished self-portrait.

In self-portraits of homosexuals similar questions rise: who am I? how do I come to be as I am? am I morally guilty? By means of exclamations like: 'When shall I ever find true love again?' and 'Am I not punished enough?', the reader seems to get direct insight into the inner life of the patient with all his fears and despairs.[12]

Although an autobiography may provoke the illusion of authenticity and sincerity, its narrative form implies a strategic coloring.[13] The reader is led, not only by the doctor who selected the confession, but also by the patient himself, in the direction of the desired plot. Therefore, confessions can and should be read and analyzed like literary texts, with the help of a customary set of instruments.[14]

10 Marc Andre Raffalovich, *Uranisme et unisexualité. Étude sur differantes manifestations de l'instinct sexuel*, Lyon/Paris 1896, p. 3.
11 Schaffner, Modernism and Perversion (see n. 2), p. 21.
12 Richard von Krafft-Ebing, *Psychopathia Sexualis. A medico-forensic study*, New York 1939, p. 301.
13 See on the subject: Lut Missine, *Oprecht gelogen. Autobiografische romans en autofictie in de Nederlandse literatuur na 1985*, Nijmegen 2013.
14 Smith and Watson provide in their chapter 'A tool kit: twenty strategies for reading Life

Confessions are often modeled after current literary genres and subgenres like for instance, the adventure novel, the naturalist novel, the romantic love story, and the so-called *Bildungsroman*.

As more doctors began to write on homosexuality in understanding and non-condemnatory terms, homosexuals sought to tell their stories. A confession caused relief: the understanding of a doctor functioned as a kind of forgiveness. Moreover, the confessing patient often hoped that by publishing his life story the outside world would get some comprehension for his nature. For the physician on the other hand, the confession was needed material. In a sense the patient was the expert in the matter. Sometimes he even happened to be a doctor or medical student himself.

So, actually, the confessing homosexual had a lot to gain. He gained a willing ear, he could be set free from guilt and suddenly found himself to be an authority instead of a criminal pervert or a poor wretch. Moreover he could defend his case and be recognized. In turn such documents contributed to an increasing understanding on the side of the doctor. The relationship between doctor and patient was clearly a matter of mutual interplay.[15] More and more medical studies contained cases of homosexuality, written confessions included.[16] Confessions often came from educated people, mostly men, from the upper-middle and higher classes. Their authors often show to have the pen of a ready writer.

The confessions come in two different forms. The first is the dialogue, presented in the third person. Questions and answers are noted by the physician who acts as the unique narrator. The conversation is highly initiated by him. The doctor knows what he wants to ask and uses the case format as a guideline. The second form is the written, usually anonymous confession, which was send to the physician, sometimes even after the death of its writer.[17] Here the homosexual himself is directly speaking and in general he addresses the doctor as a discussion partner. Sometimes those confessions are quiet elaborate. They leave the

Narratives' from their book *Reading autobiography. A guide for interpreting life narratives* (2001) applicable instruments for analyzing self-confessions that fruitfully can be combined with traditional instruments from literary narratology. Cf. SIDONIE SMITH and JULIA WATSON, 'A tool kit: twenty-four strategies for reading life narrative', in: Idem, *Reading Autobiography. A Guide for Interpreting Life Narratives*, Minnesota 2001, pp. 235–251. Here I made use of their 'tool kit' next to traditional narratological concepts.

15 PHILIPPE LEJEUNE, 'L'Autobiographie et l'aveu sexuel', in: *Revue de littérature comparée* 325 (2008), p. 45.

16 The twelfth edition of Krafft-Ebing's *Psychopatia sexualis* from 1903 includes 238 more cases than the first edition from 1886. MÜLLER, Aber in meinem Herzen sprach eine Stimme (see n. 3), p. 206.

17 One of Hirschfeld's first studies, *Sappho und Sokrates oder wie erklärt sich die Liebe der Männer und Frauen zu Personen des eigenen Geschlechts* (1896), was written after the suicide of an officer. He carried in his pocket a letter addressed to Hirschfeld. MANCINI, Magnus Hirschfeld and the Quest for Sexual Freedom (see n. 3), p. 47.

patient full play to present himself in accordance with his own view, choosing freely the style and design of his life story.

On the whole, medical studies contain two kinds of texts: theoretical discussions on the part of the physician and confessions from his patients. This situation evokes a series of questions concerning the relationship between these two categories. Let me mention the following: did the patient tell the doctor what he wanted to hear, in confirmation to his theories (characteristics of the homosexual, classification in subtypes) and was the case perhaps partly selected to meet this aim? Was it perhaps even invented or adapted by the doctor himself?[18] Did the patient give different or new information that proved or contradicted the medical theory? Are there rhetorical similarities between the confessions and the surrounding text? Which rhetoric techniques are used in the confessions? Is there an affinity with specific literary genres? What is the function of the plot, the description of the inner self, space, time and style (metaphors, symbols)? Do the confessions resemble the standard format of the medical case?

Within the frame of this article I will concentrate on the rhetoric of the confessions and the relation to the medical theory.[19] I will focus here on confessions written in the first person. In this form the patient has in principle the opportunity to present himself freely. In my selection of confessions I have further aimed at confessions in studies by physicians who were of different, sometimes even contradictory opinions. It may be presumed that each of them selected and used the confessions in a different way. My expectation is that the chosen confessions will show mutual rhetorical variations as well as a varying relationship with the surrounding text.

In the following paragraphs three leading German and French physicians and their studies are introduced: Richard von Krafft-Ebing, Georges Saint-Paul (writing under the pseudonym 'Dr. Laupts') and Magnus Hirschfeld.

4 Krafft-Ebing, *Psychopathia sexualis* (edition 1903)[20]

Richard von Krafft-Ebing (1840–1902) was a German psychiatrist. His study *Psychopathia sexualis* (1903, twelfth and last edition by the hand of the author himself) shows a vigorous urge to classification. First he makes a general distinction between acquired and congenital homosexuality. Within those two large categories he divides acquired homosexuality in men and women into four

18 Lejeune, 'l'Autobiographie et l'aveu sexuel' (see n. 15), p. 47, suggests that this frequently was the case.

19 Other questions will be addressed in my current research on this theme.

20 The quotes come from the English translation from 1939. Krafft-Ebing, Psychopathia Sexualis. A medico-forensic study (see n. 12).

subcategories, or 'phases', suggesting a possible growth of homosexuality within one person or within one family. In each subcategory the sexual preference for members of the same sex is stronger. Then he cathegorizes congenetical homosexuality among men in four cathegories of growing homosexuality. Congenital homosexuality among women is discussed in a separate chapter and here he also distinguishes four different subcategories in an increasing form on virility. Thus Krafft-Ebing in sum comes to eight different types of homosexual men and women.

The confessions Krafft-Ebing selected for his book serve as illustrations and foundations of the categories in question. He translated scabrous passages into Latin to make them inaccessible to laymen and especially to women. It is remarkable that Krafft-Ebing hardly doubts the reliability of the confessions he uses. In his opinion, people in crisis tell the truth. Only confessions of effeminate homosexuals do awake his doubts. This kind of homosexuals only want to catch your attention, he says.[21] From his book two long cases have been chosen: a man's and a woman's confession. In *Psychopatia sexualis* they are numbered case nr.146 and case nr.166.

Case nr.146 serves as an illustration and affirmation of Krafft-Ebing's second category, the 'Homosexuale oder Urninge' [homosexuals or urnings]. This is the group of congenital, non-effeminate healthy homosexuals. The case is based on two sources. The first, the shortest part of the text, seems to be a resumé by Krafft-Ebing of a summons. The text shortly sums up the facts of what looks like an indecency offence. Two men, having oral sex in the open field, were caught by a watchman. Being no question of anal penetration, no charges were brought to execution:

> On a summer evening, at twilight, X.Y., a physician of a city in North Germany, was detected by a watchman while committing a misdemeanour with a countryman in the field. He was practicing masturbation on him, and then *mentulum alius in os suum immisit [he put his member in his mouth]*.[22]

Only the time of the day is mentioned, not the date nor the exact place in the north of Germany. Together with the passage in Latin these are indications that the text has at least been reformulated by Krafft-Ebing himself.

Then there follows a long letter written by X. and addressed to Krafft-Ebing personally. The aim of this letter is twofold. X. wants to provide Krafft-Ebing with information that will give him more insight into the phenomenon of homosexuality. He presumes to be the obvious person to do so, being an experienced homosexual himself and moreover a physician with a practice, often

21 KRAFFT-EBING, Psychopathia sexualis. A medico-forensic study (see n. 12), p. 309.
22 KRAFFT-EBING, Psychopathia sexualis. A medico-forensic study (see n. 12), p. 374.

visited by a lot of homosexuals. His second, less explicit aim is to present himself as a healthy, virile homosexual, to whom the homosexual nature is congenital and whose life story demonstrates the necessity to abolish article 175 from the penal code.

Krafft-Ebing quotes large parts from this letter. First, however, he compresses it in the format of a medical case (etiology, symptoms), quoting bits and pieces from the letter. The letter offered Krafft-Ebing only partly the possibilities for such a format because the patient refused to be observed and did not want any therapy. He considered his homosexual nature to be healthy and satisfying.

The resumé clearly shows X.'s hereditary defect. Numerous members of his family suffered from nervous diseases (madness, suicide, spinal disease), sexual perversions, hermaphrodism and masturbation. As a child X. was sensitive and nervous. He preferred to comb the maid's hair instead of taking part in boyish games. At the early stage of seven years of age his sexual nature was revealed. At thirteen, he seduced his comrades to mutual masturbation. During adolescence he was in the company of what Krafft-Ebing mentions as 'men of doubtful character' from an artistic background.[23]

During his later life he had several sexual contacts with men. His desire for sex was irrepressibly strong. He got addicted to morphine and later to cocaine. Under the influence of these drugs his sexual passion decreased, but as soon as he gave up drugs, his sexual desire returned in all its vehemence. It was not possible to suppress it in any way. Other homosexuals, he noted, have that same experience. He considers homosexuality as a congenital trait, as an intrinsic part of his personality. At one single glance he can notice whether someone is a homosexual or not.

He describes himself physically as virile in shape: he is tall, possesses a full beard and well developed genitals. Explicitly he informs Krafft-Ebing also on his sexual preferences. Politely he excuses himself for the candor of this description.[24] Krafft-Ebing translated this passage into Latin. In short X. usually satisfies his partner orally, whereas he himself comes between his thighs. At present he leads a very regular life. He smokes and drinks moderately.

X.'s confession offers the overall confirmation of Krafft-Ebing's subcategory of the congenital, non-effeminate healthy homosexual. The for this type important characteristics of 'healthy' and 'non effeminate' are brought out even more clearly when X. supplies information behind the scene of other kinds of homosexuals. He offers Krafft-Ebing so to say the ammunition for subcategories that will follow in his study. He professes to know homosexuals who behave in an extremely effeminate way; they tart themselves up and use girls names. In those

23 Krafft-Ebing, Psychopathia sexualis. A medico-forensic study (see n. 12), p. 376.
24 Krafft-Ebing, Psychopathia sexualis. A medico-forensic study (see n. 12), p. 379.

circles cross-dressing is no exception. Against this group of sissies X. positively stands out as a healthy and virile homosexual.

So far this confession only seems to offer an instructive but rather neutral enumeration of facts. At the same time, however, this information is rhetorically loaded by means of the direct insight the reader gets in the personal perception of the I-narrator. Whereas Krafft-Ebing mentions X's seducing ('seduces his comrades'), X. himself speaks of love ('I loved him wildly'). And when Krafft-Ebing describes X's young friends as 'men of doubtful character', X. himself tells how he met his first real love in this circle ('he was my first love').[25] In his letter X. himself brings up the incident that Krafft-Ebing mentions at the start of the case, but now perceived through his own eyes. He tells that two years ago he settled in the German countryside, in order to overcome his addiction to cocaine. He succeeded, but from the moment he abstained from the drug his sexual hunger returned. And then it happened: 'one evening, while out in the fields near the city amusing myself with a man, I noticed that I had been detected by the authorities and advertised.'[26] In this context the sexual incident receives a different over-tone. Here we see a man who succeeded to overcome his drug addiction, and so evidently possesses willpower. What he is doing in the fields is nothing immoral or illegal, but something innocent that takes place without any force ('amusing myself'). Furthermore, the discovery by the watchman does not happen by accident: it is the result of a determined effort to catch homosexuals. X. here fashions himself as the hunted quarry. The end of the letter coincides with the end of case nr 146 (as a whole). X. concludes his letter with a plea for the abolition of article 175 from the German penal code. Apparently Krafft-Ebing agrees with his patient's opinion: he allows him the last word.

The story of X.'s life presents the reader with a loving, virile, healthy and culturally instructed homosexual, who does not practice anal penetration. Nevertheless, sadly enough, the world does not allow him to live in accordance with his own nature. In fact, Krafft-Ebing borrows X's own rhetoric, not only to confirm his type of the healthy 'Urning', but also to ask for tolerance towards this group of homosexual men.[27] The virile and healthy character of this type shows so much the better, when after this confession Krafft-Ebing moves on to the subtype of the 'Effeminatio', the effeminate homosexual. He stresses the ab-

25 Krafft-Ebing, Psychopathia sexualis. A medico-forensic study (see n. 12), pp. 375, 376, 376, 377.

26 Krafft-Ebing, Psychopathia sexualis. A medico-forensic study (see n. 12), p. 378.

27 Only on one single point Krafft-Ebbing does not agree with his patient. X.'s statement that homosexuals recognize each other from the first second is a myth, he states further in his book. Cf. R. von Krafft-Ebing, *Psychopathia Sexualis. Mit besonderer Berücksichtigung der conträren Sexualempfindung. Eine medicinisch-gerichtliche Studie für Ärzte und Juristen*, Stuttgart 1903 (12th edition; first edition 1886), p. 312.

normal, feminine emotional life of this type that is totally colored by the sexual preference for its own sex. Jealousy, vanity, weakness, cross-dressing and passive anal sex are frequent here. All the features labeled as 'feminine' have a negative overtone, with the exception of some semi-artistic talent. This type does not have Krafft-Ebbing's sympathy and neither the sympathy of X. himself.

Whereas effeminacy in men is judged negatively by Krafft-Ebing, virility in women ('Gynandry') stands in a positive light. This is strikingly demonstrated in case nr 166. It deals with the notorious life story of the Hungarian count Sandor who in fact turns out to be countess Sarolta. This gender transgression comes to light when in 1889 Sarolta is arrested and put in prison on a charge of having swindled her father-in-law. Physicians, among whom probably Krafft-Ebing himself took part, examined this extraordinary case.[28]

The presentation of the case in *Psychopatha sexualis* has more or less the same structure as the previous case 144. It starts summing up the judicial facts. Then follows a description of the life of Sarolta, written in the third person. The required facts are collected from her autobiography and from some of her love letters. She sent this material herself to the judicial and medical authorities in charge with her case. This case description is interlarded with quotations from her letters and her autobiography.

Sarolta descends from a noble Hungarian family that on her father's side shows serious hereditary defects. In her ancestry hysteria, eccentricity, delusions and nervousness are frequent. Nevertheless Krafft-Ebing underlines the intelligence and the kindness of this family and he calls her eccentric father 'foolish' instead of 'insane'. This father brings up his daughter Sarolta like a boy; and that is how she sees herself. She has many relationships with women, pretending to be a man. She even becomes an esteemed literary author. Then she meets Marie, her great love. She succeeds to marry her with the help of a fake priest and a false marriage contract. Marie has no suspicions what so ever: she beliefs herself to be married to a man she deeply loves and she would like to have children with him. In a letter to Sarolta she writes: 'I don't like children any more, but if I had a little Bezerl or Patscherl by my Sandi – ah, what happiness, Sandi mine!'[29]

Krafft-Ebing explains Marie's extreme naïveté by her innocence and by the convincing masculinity that Sarolta by nature possesses. Her love letters to Marie, written after her arrest, speak of her great and sincere love. Krafft-Ebing notes: '[…] she expressed emotions which were such as only could be felt – not

28 P. Pognant, 'Le comte qui était comtesse: un cas de gyandrie au tribunal de Vienne (1890)', in: *Droit et Cultures. Revue internationale interdisciplinaire* 20 (2010), pp. 113–127.

29 Krafft-Ebing, Psychopathia sexualis. A medico-forensic study (see n. 12), p. 432.

simulated.'[30] She keeps on writing desperate letters, though she knows they will never reach Marie. Krafft-Ebing quotes parts of those letters, full of poetic phrasings like: 'Thy dear sweet voice; the voice whose tone perchance would raise me from the dead; that has been for me like the warm breath of Paradise!'.[31] The confession ends with Sarolta's plea to the authorities to do her justice. She acted purely out of love and what 's more, God has created her the way she is:

> Gentlemen, learned in the law, psychologists and pathologists, do me justice! Love led me to take the step I took; all my deeds were conditioned by it. God put it in my heart. If he created me so, and no otherwise, am I then guilty; or is it the eternal, incomprehensible way of fate?[32]

In fact, the vision Sarolta has of herself is completely shared by the medical authorities, Krafft-Ebing first of all: she is not immoral but driven by sincere love. Her emotional life, her physical shape and her behavior are natural and convincing. Her letters and her confession prove her to be an intellectual, religious and highly-minded person, who fell victim to her inner loving nature. Her plea for understanding and mercy to her judges is a plea to us readers as well. In this respect her case is a match to the previous case of the German physician.

What strikes in those two cases is the difference in Krafft-Ebing's vision as well as the opinion of the patients themselves on effeminate men and on virile women. An effeminate man is considered to be highly objectionable: he is clearly debased. 'Effeminate' by definition means 'false', 'vain' and 'weak'. This is the opinion of the homosexual X. A virile woman, on the contrary, enhances her status. Sarolta is proud of her own virility and she hates to show weakness. In this respect Krafft-Ebing mentions her acknowledged literary talent with admiration. Exactly by her masculine force this woman, in contrast to normal women, has proved able to develop into a real artist. The confession of Sarolta is the most literary of the two. It is the story of a tragic life that, due to predisposition and circumstances had to end unhappily, just like in a naturalistic novel. The heroine in the story is not to be blamed: she simply is who she is.

5 Laupts, *Tares et poisons* (1896)

Dr. Laupts was the pseudonym of the French general physician Georges Saint-Paul (1870–1937). He wrote several medical studies, of which *Tares et poisons* (Defects and poisons) deals with homosexuality. Although Laupts in his study claims to be impressed and influenced by Krafft-Ebing's *Psychopathia sexualis*,

30 Krafft-Ebing, Psychopathia sexualis. A medico-forensic study (see n. 12), p. 433.
31 Krafft-Ebing, Psychopathia sexualis. A medico-forensic study (see n. 12), p. 433.
32 Krafft-Ebing, Psychopathia sexualis. A medico-forensic study (see n. 12), p. 433.

his own vision on the matter is far less enlightened. In Laupts' eyes homosexuality is chiefly infectious: slowly but surely it undermines a nation. Often homosexuality is acquired, although Laupts also recognizes some cases of congenital homosexuality. For him homosexuality is not only a psychological but also a social affair.

Laupts' study, published under pseudonym, is greatly influenced by Émile Zola.[33] The preface on the book is written by Zola and the long confession it contains, is passed on to Laupts by the novelist himself. Zola was sent this anonymous confession by the author with the request to use it as material for a novel. Zola considered the theme far too delicate; he preferred to give it in the hands of a professional. Laupts publishes this text here in full under the literary title *Le roman d'un inverti* (The novel of an invert).[34]

'Le roman d'un inverti' serves as the colorful illustration of Laupts' subtype of 'l'inverti-né féminiforme', that is to say the effeminate congenital homosexual. This type shows feminine features, physically as well as psychologically. The invert is the male pendant of Krafft-Ebing's Sarolta. His genitals are male, but his secondary sexual characteristics are for a large part feminine. The readers is given the whole confession, without interventions by Laupts, who has saved his comments for the end. He only translates the daring passages into Latin, just as Krafft-Ebing does.

The confession consists of two long letters and a postcard that was posted shortly after the letters. The present from which the confession is written, is far more specified than in the former confessions. The given letters are said to have been written in an Italian hotel during three successive days. The 'I' reports whom he meets in the hotel and what he is doing there. His interlocutor is no doctor, but the famous author Zola. From time to time the 'I' addresses Zola in flattering words: Zola with his eagle eyes will see his own sensitive and artist soul and he will discover the sorrow that lies behind his words.[35] The document is divided into paragraphs, apparently by the author himself. It follows the format of a medical case, starting from his ancestry, completed with an elaborated physical and psychological self examination.

The 'I' recounts that he is a progeny of an old noble Italian family. He offers detailed pictures of his parents. Apparently there is a degenerative element in his ancestry on the mother's side. At thirteen his sexual feelings awake; from the start he prefers men to women. He feels irresistibly attracted to strong, older men. When he is masturbating he dreams of them. Sexual intercourse with

33 Saint-Paul had literary aspirations himself. Under the pseudonym Espé de Metz he wrote theatre pieces, poetry and novels.

34 Earlier Laupts had published this confession in the *Archives d'anthologie criminelle*. LAUPTS, *Tares et poisons. Perversion et perversité sexuelle*, Paris 1896, p. 46.

35 LAUPTS, Tares et poisons (see n. 34), p. 48.

women disgusts him. He wants to change, but he does not succeed. In his own opinion he is nature's mistake.

For Zola, as he puts it, he sketches a detailed portrait of himself. He is a ravishing beauty (revealingly he compares himself with the lover of the roman emperor Hadrianus). He definitely has female secondary sexual characteristics: large hips, a large pelvis, small feet, gorgeous hands, a childish face, a soft female chin, very light growth of beard and a sweet melodious voice. His skull shape is characterized by a receding forehead, dented temples and a protruding occiput. He does not say so himself, but for contemporary readers his skull definitely shows degenerative characteristics.

When he is nineteen years old and in military service he seduces a sergeant of humble origin. This seduction scene is sketched in detail. When deep kisses and mutual masturbation are at stake, Laupts translated the text into Latin. Later, however, he regrets his seduction as a result of a cursed, poisonous passion.[36] It was lust, not love. When he hears, half a year later, that his sergeant has by accident been killed, he feels no grief whatsoever.

At present he lives like a virgin, he declares. 'Am I not punished enough?', he asks.[37] It is here that the first part of the confession ends. The narrator presents himself so far as an unhappy human being, driven by a natural but forbidden lust to which he will not give way anymore. The following part of the letter shows that he lied.

This second part is written the day after. He wants to make a confession, although it is 'a filthy history'.[38] He tells now how at sixteen he was seduced by an elder man, heterosexual by nature, who during his life acquired homosexuality. This seduction is sketched in full color, just like the previous one with the sergeant. In this relation the 'I' plays the female part: he sits on the captain's knee, is carried by him to bed and when they have sex he lies under. He experiences lust and cruelty. Afterwards he feels no shame, but pride and happiness. From this moment on his life began, he declares.[39] As their relation continues the captain turns out to be a real satyr. He demands anal penetration. The 'I' doesn't think to refuse, for to him it seems a very natural desire. In practice however it appears to be a painful affair. Disappointed they leave it at this first attempt. For the rest the 'I' executes obediently all other sexual favors the captain asks from him, having apparently a sadomasochist character.

So far the confession, he says. He feels deeply unhappy; only sexual passion can brighten him up. 'Why would I be ashamed of what I have done? Is it not

36 Laupts, Tares et poisons (see n. 34), p. 69.

37 'Ne suis je donc pas assez puni?'; Laupts, Tares et poisons (see n. 34), p. 71.

38 'un récit assez sale'; Laupts, Tares et poisons (see n. 34), p. 71.

39 'Je n'avait jamais eu de jours plus brillants et plus heureux, et il me semblait que je ne commençais à vivre que depuis ce jour-lá.' Laupts, Tares et poisons (see n. 34), p. 75.

Nature that made the first mistake condemning me to eternal sterility?', he asks.[40] Besides self-pity he also feels some horror and disgust with his sexual desires, although they feel natural to him. He trusts to find comfort in religion at the end. Here the second part of the confession ends in the tragic tone of a victim seeking understanding.

In a postscript in a few lines the 'I' tells that he has conceived a burning passion for a young man who is staying in the same hotel. He has only seen him from afar. He would rather prefer him dead than being the lover of someone else. This is a different tune then in the lines above. The 'I' obviously plays a game with fact and fiction in his letters. Rhetorically the postscript also functions as a so-called 'cliff hanger'. What will happen next?

Presently a next letter arrives. The 'I' has supposedly written his last letter on a rainy day and during the following rainy morning. At that time he was pessimistic. At present he writes Zola in a different mood, after a copious diner in cheerful company. Thus he shows to be extremely moody. All of a sudden he judges the whim of nature that put him on earth in a far more favorable way. In fact he is a very special person, he states, gifted with a female spirit and a divine beauty, to be compared with Ganymedes en Hyacinthus. He stands not beneath but above common people. He considers himself the degenerated product of the end of the century, and exactly this gives him his special character.[41] He is hooked to his hard and cruel captain. He calls him 'mon maitre' (my master).[42] He would like to flee from him but he doesn't. For both sides it is more sex than love. He himself wishes the penetration by the captain to succeed. So far they have tried it three or four times, without success.

He continues by giving some more information about his inner self. He has never had a job and he takes it for granted to live at his father's expense. He is an aesthetic with an exclusive preference for artificial beauty. He is not a religious person although he loves the catholic pomp. He is mad about sumptuously decorated rooms with antiquities and chinoiseries. He considers himself to be the spitting image of Madame Dubarry in cross-dressing. Explicitly and without any hesitation he calls himself 'effeminate'.[43] Only people of the highest classes and artists are subjects of his interest. The remaining humanity doesn't count for him. He prefers a beautiful pedigree dog to a workman. He has sadist traits: it arouses him to hurt. He likes anything that is special and extraordinary and he dislikes ordinary things. He loves novels that show the inevitable development of

40 'Pourquoi aurais-je donc honte de ce que j'ai fait? N'est-ce pas la Nature qui a fait la première faute et me condamne à une stérilité éternelle?' Laupts, Tares et poisons (see n. 34), p. 77.

41 '[...] je me console en pensant que je suis le produit vicieux et gracieux d'une civilisation raffinée et délicate.' Laupts, Tares et poisons (see n. 34), p. 84.

42 Laupts, Tares et poisons (see n. 34), p. 84.

43 'efféme'. Laupts, Tares et poisons (see n. 34), p. 87.

the inner life of a character. In fact that is the kind of novel he wants Zola to write about himself.

The information he supplies Zola with, concerning his aesthetics, his emotional life and his lifestyle matches in detail the fin de siècle decadent heroes of writers as J.-K. Huysmans and Gabriele d'Annunzio. In this kind of decadent literature short shrift is given to moral and social scruples in favor of an aesthetic against the grain.[44] In the same line, this homosexual Italian allows himself anything that is considered to be immoral. He ends his letter encouraging Zola to describe not only the psyche but also the appearance of his characters. He trusts to have given Zola ample information for such a description. He is delighted with Théophile Gauthier's *Mademoiselle de Maupin* (1835), a novel he has just read, in which lesbian love and cross-dressing are central themes. It follows that Zola should write a similar novel but now with the 'I' himself as the protagonist. This letter ends with a postscript: he has just met a man in the hotel with whom he plans to start a sexual relation.

The very last document is a post card. It recounts how he has been with the man from the hotel and to his greatest joy anal penetration has succeeded this time: 'all of them failed, where he succeeded!'[45] he exclaims triumphantly.

In this case Laupts presents his readers from within an example of the 'inverti-né féminiforme'. He can be followed in his decadent preferences, not only sexually but also aesthetically and morally. It becomes clear that this patient cannot do anything about his abnormal behavior: he is born this way. In this life things went as they necessarily had to go.[46] Nevertheless there is disapproval of his life and lifestyle, at erratic moments even by the 'I' himself: 'a cursed passion had bitten and poisoned me'.[47] Predominantly, however, he is condemned implicitly by his own immoral actions and thoughts. He seduces an innocent poor heterosexual sergeant and he maintains a sadomasochist relation with a pervert heterosexual. He knows no compassion whatsoever. He is vain, egocentric and unreliable. Consequently he evokes no sympathy. He may be a lamentable figure, but above all he is a pernicious and dangerous element in society. His antagonist, the captain, is an example of an even more despicable type, that of the pervert heterosexual sadist seducing young men. Laupts two types of the 'pervert' and of 'l'inverti-né féminiforme' are the central protagonists in this confession. Together they sap the vitality of the human race, that is the leading idea.[48]

---

44 J. Goedegebuure, *Decadentie en literatuur*, Amsterdam 1987; M. Praz, *The romantic agony*. Translated from the Italian by Angus Davidson, 2th edition, London/New York 1970.

45 'Là où tous avaient *échoué, il a réussi*.' Laupts, Tares et poisons (see n. 34), p. 95.

46 'Mais ce qui devait arriver arriva.' Laupts, Tares et poisons (see n. 34), p. 65.

47 '[...] une maudite passion avait mordu et empoisonné.' Laupts, Tares et poisons (see n. 34), p. 69.

48 Raffalovitch as well uses in his study a part of this confession to underpin his own

6 Magnus Hirschfeld, 'Ursachen und Wesen des Uranismus' (1903)

In his medical publications and practice the German physician Magnus Hirschfeld (1868–1935) set himself up as an emancipator in the discourse on homosexuality. In his study 'Ursachen und Wesen des Uranismus' (Causes and nature of uranism) Hirschfeld provides a profile of the homosexual. He based it, he says, on his own observation of 1500 homosexuals. Furthermore he states that every human being, the homosexual as well as the heterosexual, possesses to some degree features of the opposite sex. Hirschfeld designs two opposite series of masculine and female characteristics. The homosexual man, who plays the leading part in his book, shows an outspoken mixture of those female and masculine features; he is a specimen of the so-called 'third sex'.[49] In Hirschfeld's opinion homosexuality is always congenital. One is and stays a homosexual, even if one does not practice his homosexuality.[50]

Hirschfeld ends his book with a long confession under the title 'Lebensgeschichte des urnischen Arbeiters Franz S.' (Life story of the urning worker Franz S.) This story counts 34 pages and follows immediately after Hirschfeld's following statement: 'I for my part will never stop to battle for the right of these repressed persons, not for want of glory, but because I could not bear to be a passive initiate in this enormous injustice.'[51] Hirschfeld does not note the origin of this confession, nor does he deal with the question of its authenticity.

This confession appears to be a romantic love story with as its tragic hero the worker Franz S. Just before the start of the confession Hirschfeld notes that homosexuality can be found in all social classes. In other words, it is not a phenomenon belonging exclusively to the (degenerated) upper classes. The confession itself makes clear that the lower working classes are depicted in idealized (biedermeier) colors. The fourth estate is natural, innocent and hardworking. So is our Franz. His life story develops from light (a sunny youth) to dark (the lonely present), with in between some lightening sparks caused by love. Like a protagonist in an adventure novel Franz has many changes of fortune. His story bears also features of the coming-of-age novel, as far as Franz slowly acquires a clear insight in his own homosexual nature. Moreover his story

abhorrence of effeminate homosexuals. Raffalovich, Uranisme et unisexualité (see n. 10), pp. 109–113.

49 Hirschfeld, Ursachen und Wesen des Uranismus (see n. 6), p. 68.

50 Hirschfeld, Ursachen und Wesen des Uranismus (see n. 6), p. 15.

51 'Ich für mein Teil werde nicht aufhören, für das Recht dieser Unterdrückten zu kämpfen, nicht aus Ruhmbegier, sondern weil ich es nicht ertragen könnte, untätig Mitwisser eines so gewaltigen Unrechts zu sein.' Hirschfeld, Ursachen und Wesen des Uranismus (see n. 6), p. 159.

has a didactic tone: it should also lead to an understanding of homosexuality by the intended reader.

The story is told by Franz from a vague dark present. The focus lays on the life behind him. Franz had a happy childhood, although born in a poor family. Already as a young boy he had to roll up his sleeves. At the age of five he shows a girlish mind and girlish behavior. This is exact the age at which, according to Hirschfeld, homosexual predisposition appears. He easily blushes and weeps and he has a preference for girls games and household tasks. He is peaceful and sacrificing, with a predominant interest for aesthetics. Here we get one by one all the (positive) female characteristics that according to Hirschfeld are applicable to the male homosexual. They are the congenital features of his nature.

Franz's first great love is Willy. He is thirteen years old then. At first sexuality stays out of his feelings: he has only a strong desire for friendship. Keywords in his description of his relationship with Willy are: 'pure', 'innocent' and 'natural'. 'Which rosy haze of sweet innocence was spread over these naïve children's games!' he exclaims.[52]

The natural innocence of their friendship also speaks from its setting in the pureness of nature instead of in the immoral city. The scenes in which Franz evokes their friendship are depicted alive with dialogue and local color. He sketches Arcadian meetings in which Willy's head rests in his lap, while he himself twains garlands. Even the classic rhetorical motive of the so-called *locus amoenus* (an idyllic spot in nature as a setting for love or friendship) is present: 'Then we often lay hidden at the foot of a hill or in the bushes and listened to the singing of the larks above our heads and we followed their movements when those little singers jubilantly took off into the blue ether.'[53] The use of the German word 'lauschten' here instead of the more average 'hörten' gives an even more literary touch to this passage. The pastoral setting of the scene does not only stress its innocence, but also gives it an almost metaphysical dimension. Traditionally the lark is to be the singer of God flying up into the sky in His honor. Moreover the use of 'Äther' (the atmosphere of the gods) points in the direction of a higher world. In this way their impressions of nature resemble a prayer.

Nevertheless, already the first symptoms appear of the irresistible homosexual passion that will determine his further life. Franz compares it to a tremendous subterranean fire.[54] It is a force of nature. This passion is stopped by

52 'Welch rosiger Hauch holder Unschuld lag über diesen naiven Jugendspielen ausgebreitet!' Hirschfeld, Ursachen und Wesen des Uranismus (see n. 6), p. 160.

53 'Dann lagen wir oft an einem kleinen Abhang oder im Gebüsch versteckt und lauschten dem Gesange der Lerchen über unseren Häuptern und folgten ihren Bewegungen, wenn die kleine Sänger jubelnd in den blauen Äther aufstiegen.' Hirschfeld, Ursachen und Wesen des Uranismus (see n. 6), pp. 163–164.

54 Hirschfeld, Ursachen und Wesen des Uranismus (see n. 6), p. 164.

Willy's abundantly clear heterosexual nature. In vain Franz tries to keep him with him. Through interior monologues the reader gains direct insight in his feelings and desperate romantic plans: 'I traced out all: to travel on foot through the world, cities and villages, yes perhaps to see foreign countries, and to be always together! Did we not have to spend the night in hostelries during our travelling?'[55]

Franz's use of the Latin 'per pedes' instead of the more common 'zu Fuss' (on foot) shows the intellectual education (*Bildung*) Franz has acquired by now. Willy, however, does not share these dreams. He flirts with women all the time right and left. At the end, although infected with venereal disease, he marries a girl only for her money. In other words: this so-called normal and tolerated heterosexual love is in fact immoral. In contrast to this dirty opportunism Franz's pure and sincere homosexual feelings stand out favorably.

When Franz is nineteenth years old he enters into a sexual relationship with a fifteen year old boy. He feels a deep and self-denying love for him. He sees their relationship as morally correct: 'O no, I could not see something immoral in this [relationship], I even didn't think of the possibility, that someone could come and say: 'Your feelings are criminal!'[56] In other words: the world is evil, not him. One day Franz and his minor friend are caught together. Hand in hand they stand in front of the judge and Franz is sentenced to a half year's imprisonment.

After his release his relatives try to keep him on the right path. They do not succeed: his craving for a homosexual relationship cannot be stopped. Lonely he wanders around the world. Among other jobs he signs up as a fireman on a boat to America. Meanwhile he continues to work on his intellectual development by reading a lot. Finally he returns to Europe and arrives in 'ein kleines idyllischen Nestchen' (a little idyllic nest) in Germany.[57] There, against his better judgement, he marries the kind daughter of a friendly family. He loves her like a sister, not like a beloved. He begets children by her, while dreaming of men during the sexual act. His marriage is no success: he keeps on craving for men. Then he falls in love with Ludwig, a young worker. Together they read poetry and make music. They study and philosophize. Although they have no sexual relationship, Ludwig being heterosexual, he is Franz's great love. As their friendship continues,

55 'Alles hatte ich mir bereits ausgemalt: Per pedes die Welt durcheilen, Städte und Dörfer, ja vielleicht fremde Länder sehen und immer beieinander sein können! Mussten wir nicht auf unsern Reisen in Herbergen übernachten?' Hirschfeld, Ursachen und Wesen des Uranismus (see n. 6), p. 174.

56 'O, nein, ich konnte nichts Unmoralisches darin finden, dachte gar nicht daran, dass wohl irgend Jemand kommen könnte und sagen: "Deine Gefühle sind verbrecherisch!"' Hirschfeld, Ursachen und Wesen des Uranismus (see n. 6), p. 175.

57 Hirschfeld, Ursachen und Wesen des Uranismus (see n. 6), p. 187.

Ludwig realizes that he has alienated Franz from his family. They part in tears. Poor Franz finds himself lonely again.

His confession ends with following plea, formulated as well in name of his fellow-sufferers: 'Release us from our chains: it won't harm society and will do credit to the honor of mankind.'[58] Franz substantiates his plea not only by moral but also by cultural values. He implies that culture is represented *par excellence* by the homosexual part of the nation, as he demonstrates himself by all his reading, writing, philosophizing and music making.

The life of this worker is one great defense of homosexuality and a plea for the abolition of article 175. His story is rhetorically arranged so as to make the intended reader sympathize with this lonely, loving and virtuous homosexual. The protagonist utters his sincere feelings by evoking pity for his cruel fate and by sketching his high-minded character, his sense of responsibility and his spirit of sacrifice. Additional self-evident ideologies that support this vision on Franz are the pureness of nature and the high value of *Bildung*. Significant for this chaste homosexual is the fact that he gives no scabrous information on his sexual practices. No need here for Latin translations.

7 Concluding

In the studies of Krafft-Ebing, Laupts and Hirschfeld – all medical specialists – confessions provide insight in homosexual personalities and serve to confirm and to illustrate the often finely-woven medical classifications stipulated in their studies. The reader gets to know the high-minded Franz (Hirschfeld), the healthy virile physician X. (Krafft-Ebing), the noble virile countess Sarolta (Krafft-Ebing) and the degenerated effeminate Italian from the highest classes (Laupts). The cases depict the homosexual from within, in the first person and by means of interior monologues. The I-narrators rely on suggestive rhetorical questions, metaphors, symbols and rhetorical *topoi*. They employ sharp contrasts: the dark present versus the happy past, the innocent youth versus the guilty adult, the pure love versus the denunciating world. The confessions bear close resemblance to current literary subgenres: the adventure novel, the idealised (Biedermeier) love story, the naturalistic novel, the decadent fin de siècle novel and the coming-of-age novel. As is the case in 'real' literature, they often show a symbiosis of subgenres.

In each study the reader is acquainted with different types of homosexuals,

58 'Erlöst uns, nehmt uns die Fesseln ab: der Kultur wird es nicht zum Schaden, der Menschheit aber wird es zur Ehre gereichen.' Hirschfeld, Ursachen und Wesen des Uranismus (see n. 6), p. 193.

according to the theories and the taxonomy of the physician in question. The confessions also show differences concerning their narrative function. The German doctor X. as well as the countess Sarolta of Krafft-Ebing are complete confirmations of the two homosexual (masculine and female) types under which they are classified. Not only the inner and external features fit, but also the vision both have on their own nature as congenital, degenerated but not perverted. In terms of Krafft-Ebing himself: they show 'Perversion', but no 'Perversität'. He agrees with them one hundred per cent. The Italian in Laupts' book is the perfect illustration of the 'l'inverti-né féminiforme', with the type of the 'pervert' as his antagonist. Otherwise than in Krafft-Ebings' study Laupts' I-narrator supports Laupts' views on the type of the effeminate homosexual by means of his own unreliability. Exactly by presenting himself in all his vanity, effeminacy, immorality and self-satisfied pride, he deservedly evokes not only Laupts' disapproval but also the disapproval of Laupts' intended reader. In the case of Hirschfeld, worker Franz is the striking illustration of Hirschfeld's universal type of the male homosexual (a man with idealized female traits), and is also the spokesman of Hirschfeld himself.

The question arises whether these confessions are untrue or false, in the sense of manipulated or even written by the physicians themselves; in case of Laupts perhaps in close collaboration with Zola. An ultimate answer to this question can only be given on the basis of examination of the subsequent medical archives. In the case of Krafft-Ebing such a research has been carried out by Oosterhuis.[59] Without having checked all confessions from *Psychopathia sexualis*, he shows that Krafft-Ebing indeed possessed hundreds of confessions. The case of countess Sarolta was even notorious in its time.[60] Research on the Laupts' archives has not been done as far as I know; the archives and library of Hirschfeld have been destroyed by the Nazis.[61]

The texts themselves do raise doubts as to their authenticity. Let me mention the following possible clues. Nowhere does Hirschfeld give any information on the provenance of Franz S.'s confession, or its authenticity. It comes out of the blue. In fact it doesn't seem very probable that a poor worker wandering all over the word would be able to transform his own life story into a literary novel of this kind. Moreover, all parts of his life that do not concern his love affairs, like his relatives, his work, his wife and his children, are kept in the vague. Those aspects are not only considered to be unimportant for the story Franz wants to tell, they hardly ever seem to exist. His love affairs on the contrary are elaborately de-

59 Oosterhuis, Stepchildren of nature (see n. 3).
60 Pognant, Le comte qui était comtesse (see n. 28).
61 The Bundesstiftung Magnus Hirschfeld affirmed me that there were no traces of any case documents within the remains of the Hirschfeld archives.

picted. Nonetheless they appear clichéd. Franz's innocent games, his romantic walks in the German forests, his excessive reading, philosophizing and music making, his standing hand in hand with his lover before the court and his sailing as a fireman on a ship to America; that all seems exaggerated. The scenes seem to have stepped right out of a mixture of adventure novel, didactic novel, romantic story and the coming-of-age novel.[62]

The Italian in Laupts' book possesses not only the stereotype effeminacy of Italian men, moreover he renders the fin de siècle decadent after the style of French and Italian contemporary literature. Zola himself abominated decadentism and effeminacy. Judging by his preface in Laupts' book he completely shared Laupts' points of view, and in his own literary work of that time he advocated a strong and healthy society, with virile men and feminine women and lots of childbirths. Did he perhaps together with Laupts fabricate this decadent confession? And did they then deliberately situate this excessive example of immorality and effeminacy beyond the French border in order to spare their own nation a little? The southern effeminate Italy that functioned as a refuge for homosexuals was an obvious location. The title 'roman' points in the direction of literature as well. Moreover, this supposed Italian writes amazingly good French, in spite of his own excuses for his poor use of this foreign language.

Remarkably enough all four confessors follow the format of the medical case. They all show familiarity with medical studies and especially with studies on homosexuality. The question whether these confessions are manufactured, intentionally or unintentionally, in close connection with the medical studies their writers were familiar with, can be answered positively. The question whether these confessions were manipulated or completely invented by the physicians themselves can be answered less univocally, unless material from their archives would offer clear evidence. A rhetorical and literary analysis, however, of the two cases in Laupts' and in Hirschfeld's studies definitely reveals them both as highly suspicious.

62 It should be mentioned that Hirschfeld himself in his younger years was active in the literary field and had aspirations to become a writer. MANCINI, Magnus Hirschfeld and the Quest for Sexual Freedom (see n. 3), p. 18.

Frans-Willem Korsten[1]

Poet-Judge-Physician: Literature as Cicatrix. The Case of Maria Dermoût

1 From scar to cicatrix

Dutch author Maria Dermoût (1888–1962) came from a family that had lived for generations in the so-called Dutch Indies during the 19th and early 20th century. She started to publish only later in life, in the fifties of the 20th century, when, due to the weak health of her husband, the family had already moved back to the Netherlands some decades beforehand. The setting and themes of her work nevertheless deal exclusively with the colonial situation in the Dutch Indies. With this in mind, I want to consider one story and one novel as synecdoche for both Dermoût's work at large, and as a specific paradigm for literature's diagnostic and healing powers. Or, more specifically, I want to consider two of Dermoût's texts as paradigmatic cases in relation to literature's ability to both show and heal societal wounds. As will become clear, literature is doing the basic work of healing, here, just as prescriptions, medical actions and acts of care would do in the case of illnesses. It does not do so by *describing* the process of healing, although this is a possibility. A stronger possibility, performative in nature, is that literature, or art in general, captures and engenders a healing process by embodying what I will come to call a *cicatrix*.

A good example of both a constative description of a healing process and the performative enactment of one, can be found in one of Dermoût's stories, never officially published during her lifetime as part of a volume but taken up in her *Collected Works*, entitled 'The Kenari Woman'.[2] The story ends with a dialogue that is paradigmatic for the situation in the Dutch Indies when the colonial system was still firmly in place, although its impending collapse was palpable. A Dutch colonial family is about to leave for the Netherlands, and their house in the Indies will be sold. The lady of the house has gone back to see that the furniture

1 This article profited immensely from the response that I got from Sara Polak, Joost Haan, and the editors and I thank them for it.

2 Maria Dermoût, 'De kenari-vrouw', *Verzameld werk*, Amsterdam 1990, pp. 655–667.

in the house is auctioned properly. She meets her former Indonesian gardener and asks him whether an indigenous woman whom she has known still comes to collect kenari nuts on the square in front of the house. The gardener answers as follows:

> The gardener looked at her in astonishment. 'No,' he then said, 'the kenari woman doesn't come anymore, she is dead, doesn't my lady know? Long dead – let see! – almost a year. When the little boy was so sick, here – let see! – on that day, on that night, when my lord doctor had been sleeping here – surely this my lady remembers – then she passed away. Didn't my lady know?'[3]

The gardener informs his mistress, astonished, that the indigenous woman who had befriended the youngest son of his mistress, is dead. The reader, meanwhile, knows that this so-called kenari woman may mysteriously have saved the life of the mistress' delicate son when he was on the point of dying.

Clearly, the story is about someone who was severely ill: the young boy who caught typhoid and came close to dying. He recovered, though severely weakened, and was taken to a healthy place in the mountains to strengthen. This is the description of a disease and a healing process. Yet in a more complicated, performative way, the story also provokes another process of healing. The very question with which this passage ends – 'Didn't my lady know?' – may illustrate the point. The question is open to an answer, in that it invites one. At the same time it is closed in that the answer is apparent on the level of the diegesis: the lady did not know. However, this implicit answer of not-knowing in turn painfully opens up unfinished business, not so much on the level of the diegesis but on the level of Dutch society, whether in the fifties and sixties of the previous century or now.

The gardener's question implies a polite diagnosis concerning *two* diseases. This is captured by a difference between two tenses of the verb as he asks the question twice: …'doesn't my lady know' and 'didn't my lady know?' The question hurts with regard to both the present and the past. This happens in first instance with respect to the disease that is the story's theme. Here, the question opens up a gap that relates to the past of a negligible death, namely of the old and poor woman, and a fortunate recovery, of the young and wealthy boy. As this opposition suggests, the question also pointedly implies a diagnosis of the present in relation to a symbolic dis-ease, a societal one, more specifically: the colonial one in the Dutch Indies. The diagnosis is not a judgment in the sense of a verdict. Whether it concerns the 'does not' or 'did not', the gardener will not give a verdict but poses a question that *implies* a judgment and calls upon one, appealing to all the parties involved, who will all have to give their own answers.

---

3 Dermoût, De kenari-vrouw (see n. 2), p. 667; my translation, FWK.

Here the story performatively provokes a process that both opens and thereby shows a wound and may close it. The readers will have to ask themselves whether they belong to the knowing or not-knowing part, and this has decisive implications for their ability to both accept and close the colonial wound.

With respect to the societal or colonial dis-ease, a form of healing is hinted at, in the story, by an equality of names, or non-names. Throughout the story, the young boy is called 'the little boy', who is 'barely six years old'. It is telling that the little boy's name is just mentioned once, when his father forbids him to see the kenari woman any longer, by means of which he installs the colonial divide. Then the son is called 'Jantje' – Little John. The narrator even explains: 'this was the little boy'.[4] The explanation suggests that the proper name places the boy out of context, or better that it places him within a context that he rejects, as becomes evident when he attacks his father because of the latter's verdict. Throughout the story, then, the societal wound, or the gap between the world of colonial rulers and subjects, is closed by means of the fact that both the kenari woman and the little boy are, in a sense, nameless. Their equal status in this respect connects to the story's major theme: the impossible and yet possible friendship between the old, poor, Indonesian woman and the precious, well to do, Dutch boy.

The two meet one another for the first time when the woman comes to gather kenari nuts. The young boy begins to collect them with her and for her. In the process they start to talk and befriend one another, much to the concern of the mother who distrusts both the nature and the depth of this friendship. The friendship is restricted in terms of space, though, when another structural colonial divide shows itself. Each time they have met, the little boy wants to follow the kenari woman back home to her 'kampong' – the neighborhood of the poor indigenous people. Each time again, she sends him back, knowing well that taking the child of a colonial ruler to her home is impossible under the colonial circumstances. The story now suggests that, when the boy is on the brink of dying because he has been struck with typhoid, she sends him back as well. As the reader can gather from the hallucinatory words that the boy is mumbling, the kenari woman is on her way home again, and he wants to go with her, just as he would have wanted in everyday life. She, however, is leaving for death. This is a home to which she cannot take the boy along either, so she sends him back, to life.

The story deals with literal disease, then, as a theme, with the little boy catching typhoid but recovering. In terms of the metaphorical or symbolical disease, the story does much more than deal with it as a theme. It takes it as its subject, as something that is not frozen in time but that is actively presented to be dealt with. The story painfully shows the open colonial wound *and* closes it, by

4 Dermoût, De kenari-vrouw (see n. 2), pp. 656, 663.

narrative means. If there is healing involved on this level, this is surely not in the sense of a recovery. The image that comes to mind is more that of a scar, or better: a cicatrix.

The scar, etymologically speaking, has two origins, one going back to Greek, Latin and French, *eskhara*, *eschara*, *escarre* – indicating the scab covering a wound – and the other to the Norse *skore* – indicating a mark, a cut, an incision. In common usage the word has come to indicate what can be described more adequately and precisely, scholarly speaking as *cicatrix*. Tellingly, this word has an unknown etymological origin. It appears as if new, which is in concordance with the fact that cicatrix indicates the new tissue that closes the wound and then contracts into a permanent bodily sign. The cicatrix is material in its own right, that is, also in this sense that it is a matter of *specific* tissue. Although it is an index to the former wound, then, it can never be reduced to it. It is, in a distinct sense, something that is *added* and there to stay, whereas the scar, in the basic sense of the word as the scab that covers a wound, is 'dressing it' to then disappear. The former becomes part of the body, the latter does not (and note that I deviate here from the common usage of this term). The Dutch term 'litteken' actually captures quite nicely what the cicatrix indicates, again etymologically speaking. 'Litteken' consists of 'lic', meaning body or flesh, and 'teken' meaning sign: a body-sign.

Likewise, literature is not something that is applied, or something that is 'dressing' something else, like the scab that is functional in covering up a wound to then disappear. Literature is even not only or simply an index to former societal wounds and presently healed bodies. Literature as cicatrix is a materially real, indexical, iconic and symbolic sign *in its own right* that is part and parcel of what it partakes in. It is indexical in that it is caused by, borders on, and refers to a once open societal wound and its process of closure. It is iconic in that it shares properties with newly formed tissue, a tissue that exists in its own right. It is symbolic in its cultural action, taking upon itself the task of showing a wound, diagnosing it, judging it, and partly through judging it, healing it, by closing it. In the latter shift, from healing to closing, there is a painful residue. Real wounds can never be *healed* as if there is no material presence of the wound any more, as would be the case in certain forms of magic. Real wounds can only be closed by means of significant new tissue, leaving the element of healing in permanent doubt.

My considerations in these matters were helped and provoked by Maria Dermoût's work, of which Pamela Pattynama stated that it is exceptional in the colonial context because it makes all subjects speak on an equal level.[5] As will

5 The story of the kenari woman proves Pattynama's point the more, that, within the Dutch context: 'Dermoût is one of the few colonial authors who systematically give indigenous

become clear, in acting as both a cultural physician and a judge, Dermoût's work operates in a specific way, here, that is distinctly different from the well-known and one could even say dominant image of the cultural physician as it was proposed by thinkers of the philosophical avant-garde such as Friedrich Nietzsche and Gilles Deleuze. Dermoût's work, in terms of its being a cultural physician, is practical and situational. In contrast, the modernist doctor appears to be of a typical or a general category, one that longs for a general cultural diagnosis and a revolutionary solution defined by the New. Let me deal first with this powerful *Type* of the modern or modernist cultural physician in order to then assess how Dermoût's work is made possible by another, specific kind of poet/judge/physician.

2 'I am modern: I am sick'

The work of healing needs to be instigated and facilitated by some sort of physician. The question then poses itself whether, by analogy, we would have to think of a specific type of writer, author, or storyteller in the case of literature and societal diseases, just as there are many different kinds of physicians – including such physicians as shamans and witch-doctors. Another question that needs to be raised is whether literature, in order to diagnose or to both show and heal a societal wound, could ever take the role of a healer or physician only. Would it not, as was already indicated, also require a diagnosis that implies a *judgment*, since most societal wounds are not just a matter of coincidence or physical affliction but are caused by forms of injustice? To put this differently, the question here is whether we can think of literature's healing powers only in terms of a medical analogy.

When Friedrich Nietzsche and Gilles Deleuze proposed that the modern artist is a 'cultural physician', this was provoked, obviously, by the idea, dominant since Romanticism, that the modern world is ill, not just ill at ease with itself, but ill to the core: addicted, mad, insane, distorted, in pain, and so forth. Although capitalism was not yet the favorite opponent of the Romantics (it could have been, already, or should have been), it would become the major culprit of modern man's illness, propelling him through and even outside of history. The storm from paradise that blew away Paul Klee's, or rather Walter Benjamin's angel, was a metaphor for capitalism's acceleration, for the destruction it caused and left behind. With respect to this Nietzsche and Deleuze considered literature

characters a voice.' [My translation, FWK] See PAMELA PATTYNAMA, 'Totdat Constance kwam: Het inheemse in het werk van Maria Dermoût', in: *Indische Letteren* 24 (2009), pp. 132–144, here p. 135.

and art as the major agents that could diagnose, and by implication, judge, the disease of modernity.

In general, just as newspapers are better at bringing bad news than good, most modern philosophers have been better at defining and diagnosing modernity or capitalism as an illness than at presenting a cure, let alone healing. Or, when some of them presented a cure for the disease of modernity, such as the big ideologues of communism, fascism or neo-liberalism claimed to do, they were dialectically bound to it, in the end worsening the disease. In this context, art acquired a paradigmatic position. Although tapping into millennia old ideas of the powers of poets as legislators and healers of the world, Nietzsche and Deleuze were not alone and clearly modern in their project of defining the task of the poet as a 'cultural physician'. Tellingly, this physician also had to relate to the function of poets as legislator, which is where the element of diagnosis and judgment is implied. A sick world, this is to say, answers to the wrong law, or answers wrongly to an already existing law. In Roland Bogue's *Deleuze on Literature* (2003) the three – poet, legislator, physician – come together as follows:

> As healer the physician creates new possibilities for life, functioning in this regard as an artist affirming metamorphosis and transformation and a legislator fashioning new values.[6]

Bogue, in this case, is bringing the good news first, when he mentions healing upfront as the ability to 'create new possibilities of life'. In line with Deleuze's vitalism, healing gets a distinct quality in that it has to create *new* possibilities of life. This is in accordance, in this quote, with the poet's ability to affirm metamorphosis or a legislator's to make new laws.

With regard to the position of the physician, a shift is taking place in the course of Deleuze's work. Aidan Tynan aptly describes Deleuze's development as a move from symptomatology to schizoanalysis, a term that originates in the cooperation with Félix Guattari. To be sure, for Tynan the literary clinic is 'present from Deleuze's early works and persists throughout his career'.[7] Yet symptomatology relates to the early phase in which Deleuze is dealing with the potential of art 'to explore the intensities of life without being stuck in a moralistic attitude,' capturing instead, and rendering sensible 'the anomalous complexities of life'.[8] Here, we have the compassionate doctor, and the reassuring suggestion is that the cultural physician is, at least, not a moralist, which is to say he is not judging in terms of some sort of verdict. That said, there is more to literature and art than that it renders sensible 'anomalous complex-

6 Roland Bogue, *Deleuze on Literature*, New York 2003, p. 13.
7 Aidan Tynan, *Deleuze's Literary Clinic: Criticism and the Politics of Symptoms*, Edinburgh 2012, p. 2.
8 Anne Sauvagnargues, *Deleuze and Art*, London 2005, p. 26.

ities'. In terms of literature's task as a cultural physician, it is to relate to the modern situation as follows:

> The negative will to power comes to infect all humans with reactivity and *ressentiment*, with a ubiquitous hatred of life. The disease of negativity is the universal disease, and for this reason the philosopher of affirmation must be a physician, both a diagnostician who interprets properly the signs of the disease, and the healer who prescribes a cure.[9]

With respect to the general modern characteristic of this 'hatred of life,' art and literature have to take up the disease of the world, then, heroically, to go through it, to show its extremity and severity, without dying from it. For this they have to diagnose the disease and to prescribe a cure, which connects to the judging part as a medical analogy of a verdict.

This is where the work of Dermoût makes a difference. One reason is that her work shows modernity in a different light, not so much as 'a ubiquitous hatred of life', but instead as a collision of worlds. This becomes evident especially in her novel from 1955 entitled *De Tienduizend Dingen* (*The Ten Thousand Things*). In this novel, that appears at first sight as a set of stories only connected by a theme, murders are central to each of its chapters. These are examples of murders that could happen anywhere. Yet, they are also embedded in the exuberant, complex, and, yes, sick and unjust situation of the colonial Dutch Indies. It is a situation, however, that cannot be characterized by a so-called hatred for life. The murders that take place in fact form the contrast for what is an immense love of life, not just human life but life in general. The novel cannot be reduced to its theme of murder or violent death, that is. One reading of the novel could even take the human conflicts as marginal in relation to the natural environment. As for the human conflicts, the novel testifies of a love of life that is clearly aware of the fact that different forms of world are colliding, and painfully so. The colonial context is not just *couleur locale*. In fact, all stories testify of what is characteristic for the work of any physician, or judge: they have to diagnose and by implication judge specific situations of conflict, with people form very different cultural, ethnic and social backgrounds colliding. To be sure, the position of the judge is slightly more complicated, here, especially in the colonial context, in the sense that he speaks on behalf of a state. Whereas doctors are bound by an oath to help everybody, regardless of whatever kind of socio-cultural difference, judges have to maintain an ideologically invested order. Yet, they are supposed to do so 'blind-folded', in a non-biased way. As will become clear, the character that connects all the stories in *The Ten Thousand Things* and that turns the sum of them into a novel, is precisely such a type of impartial judge and physician, although she clearly belongs to a certain side.

---

9 Bogue, Deleuze on Literature (see n. 6), p. 13.

In terms of its specific situation, Dermoût's work helps us to ask, in relation to literature's diagnostic, judging and healing task, in what way it connects, by analogy or comparison, with the everyday business of physicians and judges. It is Dermoût's pragmatic and situational approach that appears to stand in contrast with the Nietzschean and Deleuzean ideas on the poet/physician's heroic powers. With respect to these, as we have just seen, Deleuze emphasized especially the cultural physician's ability to diagnose and work through the disease of modernity. In the context of capitalism's line of flight Deleuze comes up with the idea of the cultural physician's inability to be outside of modernity, which leaves him with the only possibility to merge with its illness. This is how he formulates it:

> [...] the writer as such is not a patient but rather a physician, the physician of himself and of the world. The world is the set of symptoms whose illness merges with man. Literature then appears as an enterprise of health.[10]

There is also some good news, here: literature deals with health. Yet it is good news with a desperate undertone. Even if literature is an enterprise of health, it can only be so by means of the writer's merging with the illness of the world (much, by the way, as Jesus would merge with its sins). This is partly distinct from Nietzsche's idea of the cultural physician, but it stays well within the parameters of the Nietzschean, or modernist and avant-garde idea of the immense, heroic role the artist has to take upon himself with regard to the world.[11] The poet's task and ability is, in the end, no less than 'to shape the world' in a 'creative deployment of forces in new configurations'.[12]

In one way, here, Dermoût's 'love of life' attitude connects very well to Deleuze's material, sensuous, always situational approach. Yet the Deleuzean physician, almost identical with the Nietzschean one, appears to be concerned more with the present and the future, in the sense of a 'there must be a way out of this'. The past and the present almost get out of focus. As a result, his type of physician appears to miss the pivotal characteristic of any physician's or judge's basic task: to love life so much that the first task is to preserve life, to make life and society live-able, to address illnesses in the light of a cure, to correct wounds that have been produced, or to close wounds. The function of legislators is not only to make new laws but to preserve justice on the basis of existing ones. Likewise, the major task for physicians is not that they morph patients into new beings but that they restore bodies as good or as awkward as the case may be; that they heal wounds, making whole what was split, fragmented, cut, torn, or

10 Gilles Deleuze, 'Literature and Life', in: *Essays Critical and Clinical*, London 1998, pp. 1–7, here p. 3.
11 On this see Daniel Ahern, *Nietzsche as Cultural Physician*, Pennsylvania 1995.
12 Bogue, Deleuze on Literature (see n. 6), p. 2.

damaged, which is not so much a matter of metamorphosis but of preservation or restoration. If we want to use the model of the physician/judge for literature and art in the light of this basic task, the major question becomes not how we can get out of the mess of modernity but how literature relates to the past and present of societal bodies in terms of healing. With respect to this, it is telling that Dermoût's work has been described in terms of past and present not as being nostalgic, but in terms of her 'irrevocably presenting the past in the now'.[13]

In relation to past and present literature has to take upon itself the humble yet so complex task of restoring what was destroyed, healing what was wounded, curing what was ill, correcting painful injustices, instead of bringing us the forever New as a solution for the modern problem, a modern problem, moreover, which can be characterized itself as an obsession with the new. For this purpose, I need to take a closer look at the powers of closure apparent in Dermout's work.

3 Narrative closure and the ability to judge all parties concerned

One of the dominant targets of postmodern criticism with relation to narrative, and by implication history, was the element of narrative closure. More in general one could argue that both postmodernists and poststructuralists took open-ness as their point of departure and arrival. In Hutcheon's influential analysis of postmodernist literature, closure was always related to a power-grab on the level of representation. Or, as Ernst van Alphen described it:

> One aspect of the realist plot, for instance, is its closure: everything comes to an end, an end that somehow satisfies. And more often than not, that end is good. If the very shaping of facts into a narrative, however truthful, is inherently unable to do justice to the facts, then the only mode of representation that might satisfy, however poorly, is the archival mode: the collecting, ordering and labeling of facts, items, pieces of evidence, testimonies.[14]

Apparently, the pivotal point, here, is a narrative representation's inability to do justice to the facts, in the context of which closure is either inadequate or always, somehow, beside the point. The alternative that is presented here, the archival mode, meanwhile, will clearly not work for any cultural physician, if she wants to

13 My translation; PAMELA PATTYNAMA, '27 Pamela Pattynama', YRA VAN DIJK, *'Geloof mij Uw oprechte en dankbare Vriend'. Brieven uit de Nederlandse letteren verzameld en van commentaar voorzien door vrienden van Marita Mathijsen*, 30 oktober 2009, p. 27; <http://www.dbnl.org/tekst/dijk069math01_01/dijk069math01_01_0028.php> [last retrieved on March 2, 2015].

14 ERNST VAN ALPHEN, 'Visual Archives as Preposterous History', DEBORAH CHERRY (ed.), *About Mieke Bal*, London 2008, pp. 64–75, here p. 65.

heal, that is. With respect to history's wounds, or, to use a term that is both more technical and concurrent with contemporary uses of the word in the humanities and social sciences, history's *traumas*, closure is of the essence if one wants a wound to heal, or, in terms of justice, if one wants to close a case. For such healing closure one could even argue that narrative is the most adequate generic form, as Julie Stone Peters argued in the context of her dealing with the South African Truth and Reconciliation Committee. Narrative may heal due to its gradually developing plot aimed at closure.[15]

Closure in the case of wounds can only take shape in the form of a cicatrix that implies a complex dynamic of closure and opening. The body that was whole first, even if it was porous, was in a sense closed. Then, due to a wound, it is opened, which is why it needs to be reclosed. The body will never achieve its former whole-ness, however. There is new tissue that both indicates and closes off access to the former wound. The cicatrix is a sign of a history, one that has come to a certain end and that can be told to have come to an end; the wound became closed. As a sign it may indeed indicate narrative closure but it also provokes a story to open up, to be told from the very beginning. It provokes the question of what caused the wound. Closure here, that is to say, is not the closure of historiography and power in the sense of a covering up (which would define it as a scar), but it is closure in the sense that something is being contracted as new tissue, as a form of healing.

The dynamic of closure and opening through the cicatrix is explored in Dermoût's work, not only in this small story 'The Kenari Woman' but also, perhaps most powerfully so in her novel *The Ten Thousand Things*. In the former case, the story seems to have come to and end, indeed has come to an end, with the boy being cured and the kenari woman being dead. Yet the question of the gardener embodies a cicatrix, in the sense that it both closes the story and demands that we return to its beginning. Likewise, *The Ten Thousand Things* works through the dialectic of narrative opening and closing. As said, the novel does not set out as a novel at all on first sight, but as a collection of stories with a similar theme: murder, or some sort of violent death. Each time anew a story seems to open, to open up a wound also, both literally and figuratively, and close, without the pain being forgotten. Yet the collection ends in such a way that all the previous stories are framed and concluded or closed as a result, including the wounds of trauma. All specific situations, captured in the seemingly independent stories, are brought together when all the souls of the murdered people are remembered by one of the characters who had been introduced in the

15 Julie Stone Peters, "Literature,' the 'Rights of Man,' and Narratives of Atrocity: Historical Backgrounds to the Culture of Testimony', in: *Yale Journal of Law and the Humanities* 17/2, 2005, pp. 253–285.

first story, 'Lady Kleyntjes'. The latter does so, annually, on All Souls Day, a day that she distinctly de-christianizes because it matters not much to her whether the people concerned 'faithfully departed'. Although she clearly belongs to one side, she does not judge from it.[16]

The character that opens the collection of stories and closes them as a novel, Lady Kleyntjes, both embodies and differs from Deleuze's idea of the writer as a cultural physician. Of the latter Deleuze states:

> The writer returns from what he has seen and heard with red eyes and pierced eardrums. What health would be sufficient to liberate life wherever it is imprisoned by and within man, by and within organisms and genera? It is like Spinoza's delicate health, while it lasted, bearing witness until the end to a new vision whose passage it remains open to.[17]

Dermout's character fits this description as for the way in which Lady Kleyntjes has been struck by life, has heard and seen the pains of the world and has remained open to it nevertheless. As for delicate health, the narrator is explicit about her being in pain:

> As much as she had tasted bitterness, more bitter than the most bitter water from the bitter martavan jar, as much she knew now the pain, from inside and from outside – and what is there to ease the pain?[18]

Lady Kleyntjes can be seen as a victim herself here, struck by the violent death of her son, and the repetition of the word 'bitter', four times, is an icon for her being in pain continuously, as if a wound has not been closed. As if to strengthen the iconic dynamic, the image of the martavan jar also captures this eternal opening. At the same time the jar is an icon for closure. So Lady Kleyntjes is wounded, and not beyond pain. This does not mean that the wound has not somehow been closed. It is precisely because of this that she can become a diagnostic cultural physician, weighing cases time and again, diagnosing them, judging them and trying to heal the wounds that have been struck. This is where she becomes distinctly different from Deleuze's 'writer'.

For Deleuze writers have to diagnose critically in the sense that art and

16 I have been using the Dutch original: Maria Dermoût, 'De tienduizend dingen', *Verzameld werk* (see n. 2), pp. 119–298. I have used the Dutch version and my translation of it for reasons of precision. Literary translations for an international audience must be more free than a translation that demands scholarly rigor. For the most recent English translation, see: Maria Dermoût, *The Ten Thousand Things*, New York 2002; an earlier one was published in 1983.

17 Gilles Deleuze, Literature and Life (see n. 10), p. 3.

18 Dermoût, De tienduizend dingen (see n. 16), p. 288. In this case, for instance, the martavan jar, though used consistently in Dermoût's work as the translator of the 1983 version acknowledges, is left out of the translation. In the 1983 version, the translator opts for 'a bitter spring'; p. 232; see also p. 304.

literature cannot simply heal without having *confronted* us with the acknowledgment that we are sick. They diagnose our illness that is, judge it, but not so much to begin a process of healing. Or if a healing is involved, it will consist in creating a new situation. In contrast, Lady Kleyntjes' mode of judging and healing consists in terms of acceptance. Her diagnosis shows itself in the principal distinction she wants to make, even quarreling about it with the ghost of her deceased son, between murder and death, between dying and being murdered. The one is acceptable, even if it happens because of accidents or accidentally used poison. Murder, however, is unacceptable and one can never get 'beyond it' or 'above it' as the text says.[19] It is telling in this respect that the cases dealt with by Lady Kleyntjes have never been brought to court and solved. Their injustice lasts and provokes remembrance. The cases, that is, are not closed. Still, their histories come to a closure in this novel because, for the first time this year and much to her surprise, Lady Kleyntjes meets the ghosts of the murderers as well, remembering and in a sense commemorating them as much as their victims.

The fragile status of closure and of a judgment by means of which murdered and murderers are considered together in their own right, in their connection, is emphasized when Lady Kleyntjes at the very end of the novel is called inside by her servants and she decides to go inside 'to drink her cup of coffee and to again try to live further.'[20] The wound is closed, then, but this does not suggest full healing or an escape towards the new. Life cannot be lived further as if nothing has happened. In fact the very sign that something was a wound and that it has now been closed remains materially real. The cultural physician as it appears in Dermoût's work works distinctly different, here, than the one proposed by Nietzsche and Deleuze, and this demands a redefinition of its status.

4 Societal healing – against mastery

From the classical age onwards, the idea that the poet-artist had magical powers with regard to society as either healer or legislator was a common one, although it came with a dark and a bright side. On the dark side she had poisonous skills that enabled her to disrupt society. On the enlightening side she had equally magical healing skills. This double nature was captured, notoriously, in the double meaning of the *pharmakon*. With respect to the modern era, Gregg Lambert translates this duality adequately when he entitles one of the chapters in *The Non-Philosophy of Gilles Deleuze* (2002) as follows: 'The uses (and abuses) of

19 See n. 18, p. 288.
20 Dermoût, De tienduizend dingen (see n. 16), p. 298.

literature for life'.[21] Literature can help to solve societal issues of life and death, indeed, but it can also easily topple over from performing symptomatology or schizoanalysis to worsening the disease or radicalizing it by turning into a fascist or nazist, or any other totalitarian mode.

So, (even) if with Deleuze art and literature may have lost their magical powers of healing, they have retained the *powerful* stature of the poet-artist. The modern artist is still heroic, whether for better or for worse. Bogue describes how for Deleuze the relationship between critical and clinical, between literature and the medical, 'comes at the height of his preoccupation with psychoanalytic theory'[22], which is when he is closely cooperating with the French psychoanalyst Félix Guattari. The key characteristic here is that analist and analysand work things through together without either one of them being outside of the situation, and without either one of them having an authoritarian position, as in the classical psychoanalytical situation. With schizoanalysis, the disease is countered by complicating things, multiplying them, as a result of which something new can evolve. There is no healing in the sense of recovering, here. Diagnosis has become a limit, and critical and clinical analysis start to merge in a process that will provide us with an *escape.* This is, clearly, something else than a healing, and it will shun judgment as well. It remains a heroic attempt nevertheless.

Multiplication is clearly also elemental in the work of Dermoût, but in a different way and with a different aim. In its dealing with language, the work answers to a realist code in terms of characterizing the characters by their ways of speaking, as Dutch, Indonesian, or Chinese, as man or woman, child or adult. The work is also modernist in that language is the dominant material for a mode of telling, with a mixture or oral and literary modes of telling and an abundant use of free indirect speech. Finally, the work is partly postmodernist also, in its dealing with the fantastic. Or the stories have a postmodern tendency towards fragmentation and they testify of a preference for small narratives as opposed to big ones. Moreover, the work is both colonial and postcolonial. Its mode of narrating is partly western, partly eastern, as Pamela Pattynama noticed:

> Dermoût grew up with the oral art of telling, developed amongst Indonesians and Indo's. Her much acclaimed 'pointilistic' way of telling by and large imitates speech and consists in repetition, pauses, short dialogues, parlando, silences, short words, and constantly interrupted sentences.[23]

Apparently, Dermoût connects both to a tradition of oral storytellers and to a generation of 'writers', or authors, and both in turn relate to different cultures

21 Gregg Lambert, *The Non-Philosophy of Gilles Deleuze*, New York 2002, p. 132.
22 Bogue, Deleuze on Literature (see n. 6), p. 30.
23 Patynama, Totdat Constance kwam (see n. 5, my translation, FWK), p. 142.

and different types of modernity. The question is how this translates to her position as a cultural physician/judge.

In order to answer this question, a conflict between the author Dermoût and the self-appointed patriarch of Dutch-Indonesian literature, Rob Nieuwenhuis, is revealing. The latter had reviewed Dermoût's newly published collection of stories in 1956, entitled *De juwelen haarkam* (*The Jeweled Hair Comb*), unfavorably, and Dermoût wrote him a letter. In it Dermoût speaks about her work as an author:

> Good heavens, I am not a 'stylist' in a certain sense not a writer because I cannot write, this I know, mastering our language insufficiently, the abc of style, rhythm etc. is simply beyond my knowing, which is why I write so difficult, want to tell a story because I see it somewhere, hear it–I don't know, cannot say this properly (which is also how it should be) – and try to put it all in words in sensing my way (in the blind bitter land of the words as Yeats has it)…
> (Letter from Noordwijk aan Zee, December 1956)[24]

As may be evident, Dermoût willfully and consciously refuses mastery. If she admits that she cannot say things properly with regard to the way in which stories come forward, this is, according to her, 'how it should be'. Literature is implicitly and explicitly described, consequently, as something that is served by someone who has to sense her way into the strange land of words, of language.

Dermoût is well aware, then, of the precarious situations she is confronted with, in the shape of the stories that she somehow sees or hears. With regard to these, she shows no mastery. Instead, her personal, conscientious work is much more humble in nature, just as a real doctor is not the magical healer of an inactive object that he conjures from being sick into being healed and healthy. In the real world, doctors may have vast technical possibilities, their work itself is essentially humble in nature in the sense that they have to sense their way into the strange land of bodies and symptoms, to then facilitate healing. The healing itself is done by the interaction between the physician's prescriptions, the acts of care of nurses, and the responses of the body itself. And the process results in something that implies the end of the process while inevitably referring back to the process.

If we translate this attitude to literature's or the poet's ability to heal societal diseases, we find ourselves at the opposite position of a heroic one. Societies may suffer from all kinds of diseases and there is not one heroic cultural physician that may address them all. It is precisely with respect to the disease embodied in

24 My translation, FWK. On the original of this letter and Nieuwenhuys' review, see Barney Agerbeek, 'Een brief van Maria Dermoût aan Rob Nieuwenhuys: Het verhaal en niet de schrijver', in: *Indische Letteren* 16, 2001. Nieuwenhuys' review was published in *Het Parool*, dd. November 30th, 1956.

the Dutch colonial situation that Dermoût is such an adequate cultural physician. With regard to this situation a position of mastery is impossible, as if the physician him- or herself would stand apart from it and could diagnose and judge the case from the outside. Dermoût was very much part of the colonial situation and of the societal illnesses that came with it. She could not heal that very situation as a writer, from the outside. This is not to say, however, that her way of narrating could not have healing powers.

'The Kenari Woman' may prove the point. The title of the story is telling in that the character it calls upon both is and is-not the main character. It is not in terms of the story's span of attention. It is as if the colonial Dutch family and especially the little boy in it, appear centre stage. Yet this may indeed be a matter of appearance. As becomes clear at the end of the story, there is no 'getting round' the kenari woman, or to come back to a phrase from *The Ten Thousand Things*, to get 'beyond' or 'above' her. As for the theme of illness, both the literal and figural disease are captured in the friendship, the coincidental near-death of the little Dutch boy and the conclusive, but to some unknown and unnoticed death of the Indonesian woman. As it seems, life goes on, and so does death. Once the little boy has been taken to another place in the mountains to fully recover, for him the whole affair is forgotten 'as if it was gone from his memory, as if swiped out by a hand'.[25] Yet he is no older than six or seven years. In contrast, the mother remembers, and so does the gardener. In social traffic, between the gardener and the lady, there is the unforgettable reminder that a wound existed literally that now appears closed. It has been done. That leaves them, and any of the story's readers, with the open and closed societal wound of colonialism. With respect to this, the story works like a cicatrix.

5 Conclusion

In contrast with the high demands of Nietzsche and Deleuze, Dermoût's stories work like a cicatrix, as the embodied sign that both points to former wounds, with the pain implied by them, and to the closure of these wounds, not as the scabs of a scar would do, but as newly formed tissue. The wound has been closed in that it is contracted into a sign, becoming something in its own right that testifies to a closure, which does imply a healing but also differs from it. In introducing and using the term cicatrix I would like to emphasize once more that there is this pivotal distinction with the scar, whether literal or symbolical. In general, the body's first having a wound that was necessarily and functionally covered, is captured in the matter and the shape of a scar. In the context of the

25 Dermoût, De kenari-vrouw (see n. 2), p. 666.

dual operation of literature's diagnosing, judging and healing powers, however, which is to say in terms of its opening and closing potential, I want to use the term cicatrix. I suggest to use the term not to make things scholarly more respectable, but to emphasize that the cicatrix is something else than a scar.

Whereas the scar indicates a mark that covers something and that can be 'counted', as a (temporarily) finished thing, the cicatrix is a dynamic sign, in that it opens up and closes, in that it installs a process by bringing us back each time and again to a specific situation. Whereas the scar will disappear, the cicatrix will not. The scar, in my reading of it, functions on a constative level, of description and covering – or of description as covering. The cicatrix functions on a performative level, where the process of opening and closing is only seemingly finished, and needs to be redone again and again. Whereas the scar is etymologically defined, the cicatrix has an unknown etymological origin, which turns it into a culturally more neutral concept. Such neutrality is crucial in relation to literature's ability to heal societal wounds, of whatever cultural make up. This is not to say that each piece of literature will have to be able to deal in some sort of neutral sense with all the parties involved in relation to societal wounds. On the contrary, literature will always takes sides. Yet it will take *all* sides. In total, as a consequence, literature will have the ability to do justice to all parties concerned, or to treat all forms of disease and all sorts of sick subjects. Again, whereas real physicians will have to take care of anyone, whether perpetrator or victim, literature will tend to pick a favorite. Yet the *total* result of this will be that literature favors all sides. Literature in general, that is, will offer the perspective of all parties, in accordance with Jacques Derrida's contention that literature's task is 'to say all'.[26]

Only on a superficial level the work of literature might seem to resemble the workings, here, of so-called Truth and Reconciliation Committees that have been operative in several societies, most famously so in South Africa at the end of the 20th century. The aim of both literature and the TRC committees would seem to be to *restore*, also in terms of restorative justice. Still, the powers of literature are broader, more radical also, and they can be, and tend to be much more painful. Literature could also respond, for instance, to a call for justice that to some was muffled *by* the Truth and Reconciliation Committee, as a matter of 'political expediency', in a desire to move further and beyond societal cleavages. Literature does not care very much for political expediency and it does not move beyond cleavages either. In order to heal something, it might even provoke cleavages, like when a badly healed bone needs to be broken again. Literature might want to open up a wound that seemed to be closed.

26 JAQUES DERRIDA, "This Strange Institution called Literature': An Interview With Jacques Derrida', DEREK ATTRIDGE (ed.), *Acts of Literature*, New York, p. 36.

In defining literature's ability to serve and facilitate societal healing as a cicatrix, something is both opened up and closed, contracted into a sign. That sign remains telling in its own right, constantly provoking stories of wounds, in (re)opening and (re)closing them. Literature as cicatrix is always of the present, although it intrinsically linked to a past. As for the future, it presents us with the certainty that, even when closed or even as closure, the cicatrix will never symbolize complete healing. It will only close by leaving a dynamic, open sign.

Sander Bax

The Legacy of Incomprehensibility: Trauma, Experience and Historiography in Harry Mulisch's Historical Novel *The Stone Bridal Bed*

1 Introduction

At the end of the Second World War, the city of Dresden fell victim to severe allied bombings. The bombings destroyed most of the city's center and many of the inhabitants were killed. During the course of time, there have been many debates on the number of victims, these numbers ranging from 250,000 (as was thought in the years immediately following the war) to 25,000 (the estimation of a recent committee employed by the city council). According to Dutch journalist Antoine Verbij, the bombing of Dresden had acquired mythical proportions in historiography.[1] It was the ongoing debate on the nature, scale and impact of these bombings (could it justifiably be termed a war crime?) that made the play *Das steinerne Brautbett* relevant and topical. This reworking of Harry Mulisch's novel *Het Stenen Bruidsbed* (*The Stone Bridal Bed*) was staged in the city of Dresden in the fall of 2011. Both novel and play present a controversial account of the Dresden bombings with Mulisch posing fundamental questions on guilt, trauma and historiography.[2]

In *Luftkrieg und Literatur* (1999), German writer W. G. Sebald (1944–2001) brought together a series of lectures he had given in Zürich a few years earlier.[3] The book revolves around the trauma resulting from the catastrophe of the Second World War. He focuses on the traumas of the German people in the last part of that war, experienced during and in the aftermath of the bombings of at least 131 German cities by allied forces. Sebald claims that, in spite of the fact that it was experienced by millions, there are only a few literary accounts of this

1 Antoine Verbij, 'Mulisch herleeft in Dresden', in: *Trouw*, 5-10-2011. 'Het bombardement op Dresden van 13 tot 15 februari 1945 kreeg in de geschiedschrijving mythologische proporties'.

2 Susanne Vees-Gulani, *Trauma and Guilt: Literature of Wartime Bombing in Germany*, Berlin/New York 2003, pp. 172–184.

3 Volker Hage, *Zeugen der Zerstörung. Die Literaten und der Luftkrieg*, Frankfurt am Main 2003.

trauma.[4] He concludes that this 'silence on the part of German authors' is the result of 'the establishment of a taboo surrounding the events immediately after the war'.[5] As a consequence, this traumatic experience has not been shared and not been passed on to the younger generations. It was for obvious reasons – the nation had to come to terms with the guilt of its national-socialist past, the nation had been destroyed and divided – that this historical trauma was suppressed by the people who experienced it. Even the 'Trümmerliteratur' ['the literature of the ashes'], dealing expressly with the reality of the bombed cities in Germany, was deeply influenced by the individual and collective amnesia and was restricted by unconscious processes of self-censorship.[6]

One of the conclusions that we can draw from Sebald's argument is that apparently literature has a fundamental role to play in the process of dealing with (collective and individual) historical trauma, and more generally in the formation of national identities.[7] Its value in coming to terms with the past, both in terms of harm done and in terms of harm experienced, is decidedly therapeutic and can hardly be overestimated. From this perspective, it is striking that a young Dutch writer created an early literary representation of the World War Two bombings of German cities. In 1956, Harry Mulisch (1927–2010) decided to write a novel about the destruction of Dresden. In *Het Stenen Bruidsbed* (*The Stone Bridal Bed* 1959), Mulisch tells the story of an American war pilot returning to Dresden, the city he had helped destroy in 1945. Focusing as he was on representations of trauma in German literature, it is not surprising that Mulisch's novel should have escaped Sebald's notice, although it might have been exactly what he was looking for. The book was translated into German in 1960 by Bruno Loets and published by the Hamburg publisher Nannen Verlag.[8] In the years thereafter, the novel found its way into the Norwegian, English, Spanish and Slovakian literary fields. Here we have a Dutch writer, of Austrian-German-Belgian descent, who not only tried to address the historical trauma, but who also wanted to raise philosophical questions on guilt and historiography.

In *Trauma and Guilt*, Susanne Vees-Gulani offers a thorough account of the debate that ensued around Sebald's lecture series. Some critics challenged the

4 Vees-Gulani, Trauma and Guilt (see n. 2), p. 4.
5 Vees-Gulani, Trauma and Guilt (see n. 2), p. 4.
6 Winfried Georg Sebald, *Luftkrieg und Literatur*, München 1999.
7 Cf. Fiona Schouten, 'Literature, Trauma, and Ethics: Reconciling Post-Structuralism and Collective Memory Studies', in: *A diffuse Murmur of History. Literary Memory Narratives of Civil War and Dictatorship in Spanish Novels after 1990*, Nijmegen 2009, pp. 13–48.
8 In 1995, a new translation was published. It was published by Surhkamp Verlag (Frankfurt am Main) and translated by Gregor Seferens. The novel was also translated into Norwegian (1961), English (1962), Slovakian (1968), Hebrew (1983) and French (1985). A short version was published in Spanish (1963). Cf. Marita Mathijsen, 'Een beknopte drukgeschiedenis van zijn romans', in: Harry Mulisch, *De kamer*, Amsterdam 2000, pp. 11–89, pp. 40–41.

supposed silence about the bombings, others agree with Sebald on 'their complete neglect'. She concludes: 'The strong reaction that Sebald's lectures caused both in the press and among the population illustrates that Germans today also feel a need to explore the experiences of the bombings and their effects in more depth.'[9] In her study, Vees-Gulani explores the texts that have been written about the bombings, for she claims that literature about the bombings 'offers a unique opportunity to gain insight in both the nature of the psychological effects of the bombings and also the short- and long-term reactions to these experiences by the people who lived through them.'[10] In her account of the literature about the bombings, Vees-Gulani places Mulisch's novels alongside Kurt Vonnegut's *Slaughterhouse-Five* (1969) and Henri Coulonges *Farewell, Dresden* (1979) as depictions of the bombings by non-German authors. She claims that these authors deal with the topic more freely, because they 'are not subject to the same issues of guilt and shame as their German counterparts'.[11] That, in her opinion, was the reason that Mulisch was able to write about the bombings, whereas for instance Herman Böll and Günter Grass remained silent.

In her interpretation of *The Stone Bridal Bed*, Vees-Gulani focuses mainly on the concept of guilt. In her account, the novel poses the problem of personal guilt against collective guilt. She describes protagonist Norman Corinth as 'a man marked by internal and external destruction'.[12] She points out this characters' psychological development: his inability to establish social relationships, the dissociation he experiences between his mind and his body, and his loss of orientation in time and space. She claims that Corinth returns to Dresden to 'find access to himself', to 'overcome his guilt' and 'to become whole again and reestablish his place in the world', although his hope of returning to wholeness turns out to be an illusion.[13] At the end of the novel, Corinth concludes that his personal guilt cannot be redeemed and will never disappear: 'his self-destructive act and nearly complete repetition of the past events in the final pages of the novel confirm this acknowledgement.'[14] She concludes that Mulisch 'offers a unique angle by which to analyze the various guilt issues involved in the Dresden bombing as well as in the Second World War in general.'[15]

In this article, I will offer a slightly different interpretation of *The Stone Bridal Bed*, focusing more on a reflection on the complex relationship between the psychological concept of trauma (which is experienced primarily on a personal

9 Vees-Gulani, Trauma and Guilt (see n. 2), p. 6.
10 Vees-Gulani, Trauma and Guilt (see n. 2), p. 9.
11 Vees-Gulani, Trauma and Guilt (see n. 2), p. 9.
12 Vees-Gulani, Trauma and Guilt (see n. 2), p. 174.
13 Vees-Gulani, Trauma and Guilt (see n. 2), p. 177.
14 Vees-Gulani, Trauma and Guilt (see n. 2), p. 183.
15 Vees-Gulani, Trauma and Guilt (see n. 2), p. 183.

level), its adaptation to the field of historiography and memory studies (when trauma is experienced on a collective scale we begin to speak of 'traumatic memory'), and the way literary texts can deal with both individual and collective aspects of trauma at the same time.[16] While Vees-Gulani writes about guilt rather than trauma and only analyzes the development of Norman Corinth, I will pay attention to the connection between trauma and historiography in the novel and ask the question which narrative logic Harry Mulisch employed to represent this traumatic historical event. It seems that literature is the genre par excellence that can bring together the personal and the collective in the worlds and the characters it creates. As it turns out, Mulisch's theories about historiography and literature can be understood much more readily if we avail ourselves of the theoretical concept of 'traumatic memory'. In Mulisch's novel, this traumatic memory is constructed using a mythological narrative structure.

In this essay, I want to show how Mulisch portrays the Second World War in his novels, taking his 1959 novel *The Stone Bridal Bed* as a representative example. In writing the novel, Mulisch had to deal with both the 'incomprehensibility' (Caruth) and the 'unrepresentability' (Van Alphen) that are central to the experience of severe war trauma – in this case the experiences of being in a city devastated by bombings. A close reading of this novel will reveal that the concepts of 'traumatic experience' and 'myth' can help us to understand how Mulisch came to terms with these problems of representation. My thesis will be that Mulisch has the ambition to write 'modern myths' that lay bare the traumatic experience of the transition from the pre-historical and incomprehensible past of World War II to the historical present in post-war society. In doing so, he contributed to the development of a 'trauma esthetics' that could provide an answer to the question put forward by Sebald.

2 Representing (historical and psychological) trauma

In his essay 'De neus van Cleopatra' ('Cleopatra's nose'), Harry Mulisch discusses his views on historiography.[17] He reflects on the relation between literature and historiography and states that the historian always describes the past in retrospect. One of the implications of this is that when we read a historical study on the Second World War, for instance, the fact that the Germans lost the war is taken as a given. Mulisch has serious doubts about the adequacy of this

16 Hans Ester van der Merwe and Etty Mulder (eds.), *Woordeloos tot verhaal. Trauma en narratief in Nederlands en Afrikaans*, Hilversum 2012.

17 The essay was written in 1989 and was presented as a lecture in Groningen, 8–11–1989. It was published in the Dutch newspaper *NRC Handelsblad* on 9–11–1989, the day the Berlin Wall fell down.

kind of historical representation. In an approach like this, he claims, the *real* experience of the war can never be represented. After all, during the war people did not know that the Germans would lose the war. A writer who wants to represent the reality of the war has to overcome this problem in some way. His or her story should at least take people's lack of knowledge into consideration.

> That fundamental insecurity, which first and foremost was 'wie es wirklich gewesen', because no one knew how things were going to turn out, not even Hitler. Historiography is confronted with the paradoxical duty of also having to show what things were like in the past when it was still the present, with all its possibilities and unlikely coincidences. When they occurred, historical events were not historical events; the nature of necessity, the truly historical therefore, historiography in a sense has to put in parentheses.[18]

Mulisch concludes that the literary writer has the potential to recreate the past in such a way that the reader can experience it *as if* it were the present. In doing so, he actualizes the past in the experience of the reader. Although the events in a novel are as fixed as they are in history, one reads the novel as if it is a world of coincidence (and not a world of necessity), which develops in the course of the reading process. Reading a historical novel, therefore, entails that at every point in the story everything is still possible.

> Historiography, on the other hand, rarely succeeds in calling to mind the openness of the 'now' in the act of reading. According to historiography, it always happened 'then', while nothing happened 'then': everything that ever happened, happened in a 'now'. [...] But it should be more like what you have in a literary masterpiece, which the reader can return to again and again, and always discover new elements: it is both unchangeable and not unchangeable – that is the adequate representation of history.[19]

Mulisch emphasizes the differences between historiography and literature. Historiography recreates the past as a closed 'then', whereas literature can recreate the past as a 'now'. For the historian, the past is unchangeable, but the novelist can make the past changeable in the course of writing. Although Mulisch seems to imply that there is a contrast between historiography and literature, his final point is more complex. Central to Mulisch's conception of literature is the idea that the finished novel also has a fixed and unchangeable nature. We may read the novel as if it were 'a changeable now', but at the same time we know that everything in it is fixed and structured by the author. To a certain extent, this means that literary writers are faced with the same problems as historians. A writer who recreates the past in a novel therefore has to deal with two conceptions of the past: it is changeable and unchangeable at the same time. To

18 Harry Mulisch, 'De neus van Cleopatra', in: *De zuilen van Hercules*, Amsterdam 1990, p. 139.
19 Mulisch, De neus van Cleopatra (see n. 18), p. 140.

create an appropriate literary representation, the author has to deal with this paradox.

In this essay, I will interpret Harry Mulisch's theories on historiography and literature from the perspective of memory studies. In the field of memory studies, scholars theorize an opposition between official historiography (creating coherent and reliable stories of the past) and memory (the individual experiences of the past of someone who has not managed to turn the past into a coherent story). Ann Rigney has drawn attention to the way literary texts contribute to the formation of cultural memory. She observes that literary expressiveness and narrative skills 'have a role to play in the creation of memories, that is, of stories that are memorable.'[20] She agrees with Geoffrey Hartman that there is a relationship between literature and 'history of the inside'. The genre of the historical novel will flourish in periods when societies need stories about alternative or marginalized events from the past. When official historiography does not succeed in collecting these stories, literature can function as a 'counterforce' which provides an 'alternative forum for recording memories of the past which were left out of the institutionalized discourses of the time.'[21] According to Rigney,

> literary texts may have a role to play in arousing interest in histories which are *not* one's own, in the history of groups with which one has hitherto not identified. This suggests the importance of seeing literary texts not just as channels for perpetuating certain memorial traditions but also as the source of new traditions and the means for broadening the horizons of what one considers one's own heritage.[22]

To get a clearer idea of the way Harry Mulisch uses this counterweight potential of his literary texts, the ideas of Frank Ankersmit on forgetting may prove helpful. In his essay 'The sublime dissociation of the past', Ankersmit follows Nietzsche's claim in *Vom Nutzen und Nachteil der Historie für das Leben (On the Use and Abuse of History, 1874)* that historians should welcome and contribute to a forgetting of the past.[23] To explain this, he distinguishes four types of forgetting, two of which are relevant to my line of argumentation here. These are the two types of 'traumatic forgetting', which in Ankersmit's categorization are discussed as the third and fourth types.

Some memories are too painful to be admitted to our collective or individual consciousness. The most striking example of this kind of forgetting is the

20 Ann Rigney, 'Portable monuments. Literature, cultural memory, and the case of Jeanie Deans', in: *Poetics today* 25 (2004), p. 380.
21 Rigney, Portable monuments (see n. 20), p. 375.
22 Rigney, Portable monuments (see n. 20), p. 389.
23 F.A. Ankersmit, 'The sublime dissociation of the past. Or how to be(come) what one is no longer', in: *History and Theory* 40 (2001), pp. 295–323.

memory of the Holocaust in the first two decades after the Second World War. Paradoxically, these kinds of traumatic historical experiences are remembered and forgotten at the same time: 'forgotten in the sense that it is successfully expelled from conscious memory; remembered in the sense that the subject of a traumatic experience will be seriously handicapped by it.'[24]

The other type of 'traumatic forgetting' that Ankersmit distinguishes concerns 'the most decisive and profound changes that people in the West have undergone in the course of their history.'[25] Here, he wants us to think of moments when people found themselves in a new world order, such as the Renaissance or the French Revolution. It concerns moments when people entered a new world and could only deal with that by forgetting the previous world and abandoning their former identity. This abandoning of the old world inevitably was a painful process. Ankersmit argues that the experiences involved in these historic changes can also be classified as traumatic experiences. The difference between the two types of forgetting is that 'in the third type of forgetting closure of the trauma is possible, whereas it remains a constant and permanent presence in the fourth type.'[26] In the case of a 'normal' traumatic experience, it seems possible to integrate the traumatic event in the new identity by creating a coherent story that incorporates the traumatic experience. This might help to achieve a reconciliation of experience and identity. In the fourth type of traumatic experience, such a reconciliation is no longer possible, because the previous identity no longer exists. In the next paragraph, I will theorize the concept of trauma in more detail.

In applying this concept of traumatic experience, Ankersmit combines notions of memory and historiography with psychological concepts. In doing so, he enters the debate that has been going on for many years now in the field of 'trauma studies', an institutionalized interdisciplinary field within literary studies and historiography. At first sight, it might seem strange that literary scholars and historians should have become involved with the notion of trauma, seeing that it is first of all a psychological and therefore medical concept.[27] Literary theorists and historians started using the notion of trauma in the wake of their attempts to make sense of the history of World War Two, and more particularly in their attempts to write about the Holocaust. Some scholars have concluded that the Holocaust cannot be represented by traditional forms of

24 ANKERSMIT, The sublime dissociation of the past (see n. 23), p. 300.

25 ANKERSMIT, The sublime dissociation of the past (see n. 23), p. 301.

26 ANKERSMIT, The sublime dissociation of the past (see n. 23), p. 301.

27 STEVEN JAY LYNN and JUDITH W. RHUE, *Dissociation. Clinical and Theoretical Perspectives. Clinical and Theoretical Perspectives,* New York 1994; R. LEYS, *Trauma. A Genealogy,* Chicago 2000; CATHY CARUTH, *Unclaimed Experience. Trauma, narrative and history,* London 1996.

historiography and literature.[28] They witness a 'crisis in representation', which calls for what DeKoven Ezrahi formulates as 'a new aesthetics and ethics of representation [...] with Auschwitz as the ultimate point of reference.'[29]

The concept of trauma appears to pave the way for such a 'new aesthetics and ethics of representation'. The building blocks for such forms of representation were found in the testimonies of concentration camp survivors. In these testimonies, Langer sees a tension between 'deep memory' (trying to recall Auschwitz 'as it was then') and 'common memory' (attempting to restore the self to pre- and post-camp routines).[30] The attempt to integrate these two contradictory forms of memory into one personal identity is often disrupted. 'The tension between imposed isolation and the impulse to community, between the revelations of deep memory and the consolations of common memory, remains unresolved.'[31]

This means that the field of 'trauma studies' or 'trauma theory' is one that operates at the boundaries of medical, historical and literary theories. To a certain extent, these testimonies have been regarded as literary texts, containing as they do several narrative devices. However, these texts also function within a medical context (psychology, psychiatry), being as they are expressions of survivor's traumatic experiences. For scholars of trauma studies, experience is first and foremost a linguistic phenomenon and this is how literary theorists became involved.[32] In *Unclaimed experience,* Cathy Caruth describes the psychiatric concept of post-traumatic stress disorder (PTSD) as 'an overwhelming experience of sudden or catastrophic events in which the response to the events occurs in the often uncontrolled, repetitive appearance of hallucinations and other intrusive phenomena.'[33] The mind of the patient is taken over by an event that it cannot control; therefore it is seen as 'the most destructive psychic disorder'.[34] Caruth emphasizes the importance of using these psychological concepts of trauma to gain an understanding of the way we remember catastrophic events:

> I will argue in what follows that trauma is not simply an effect of destruction but also, fundamentally, an enigma of survival. It is only by recognizing traumatic experience as

28 Hayden White, *The Content of Form. Narrative Discourse and Historical Representation,* Baltimore/London 1987; Saul Friedlander, *Memory, History, and the Extermination of the Jews of Europe,* Bloomington/Indianapolis 1993.
29 Schouten, A diffuse Murmur of History (see n. 7), p. 18.
30 Lawrence Langer, *Holocaust Testimonies. The Ruins of Memory,* New Haven 1991, p. 23.
31 Langer, Holocaust Testimonies (see n. 30), p. 23.
32 Ernst van Alphen, *Caught by History. Holocaust Effects in Contemporary Art, Literature and Theory,* California 1997.
33 Caruth, Unclaimed Experience (see n. 27), pp. 57–58.
34 Caruth, Unclaimed Experience (see n. 27), pp. 57–58.

> a paradoxical relation between destructiveness and survival that we can also recognize the legacy of incomprehensibility at the heart of the catastrophic experience.[35]

A final point of discussion keeps popping up. While Langer deals strictly with testimonies of real Holocaust victims, Ernst van Alphen in his monography *Caught by history* uses the concept of trauma to lay bare the narrative structures of specific literary texts or works of art. Although there have been numerous ethical debates about the possibilities of using fiction or imagination in representing the Holocaust, Van Alphen claims that this distinction collapses when we consider experience to be interpretative itself. 'Event and interpretation cannot be disentangled either, because experience of the event is the only access one has to the event.'[36] This has implications for historiography. Van Alphen claims that even the inmates of the camps needed 'narrative, discursive frameworks' to experience their living through the trauma of everyday life there, so historians cannot claim that they can work without a 'framing mechanism'.

> The unrepresentability of Holocaust experiences has a discursive basis and histories of the Holocaust are necessarily the product of emplotment, which implies a framing activity performed by a subject living in the present. Individual experience, as well as the collective endeavor of history writing, happens within the conditions of the discursive or symbolic realm.[37]

It has become clear that a literary representation of trauma has to deal with both the 'incomprehensibility' (Caruth) and the 'unrepresentability' (Van Alphen) of the traumatic past. This naturally constitutes a fundamental and indeed formidable challenge to the literary writer. We may perhaps find an answer in Ankersmit's study to the question as to how to construct a trauma esthetics. In the essay mentioned earlier, Ankersmit adopts the perspective taken by Victor Turner who describes myths as 'liminal phenomena' that 'derive from transitions' and are 'frequently told at a time or in a site that is 'betwixt and between''[38] Every myth tells the story of a transgression of a fundamental boundary. This transgression is often dramatized 'into a dissociation between prehistorical (or a-historical) and historical time'.

> For the story of a move from one phase to another – which is the nature of all stories about transitions – is now dramatized into a story on *the birth of time itself.* With this dramatization all that should be associated with what preceded the transition has been removed outside historical time. It has become part of pre- or a-historical *nature.*[39]

35 Caruth, Unclaimed Experience (see n. 27), p. 58.
36 Van Alphen, Caught by History (see n. 32), p. 59.
37 Van Alphen, Caught by History (see n. 32), p. 64.
38 Ankersmit, The sublime dissociation of the past (see n. 23), p. 319.
39 Ankersmit, The sublime dissociation of the past (see n. 23), p. 319.

Therefore, myths separate 'a pre-historical world of a perennial and quasi-natural stability' from the world of change that we live in. These stories narrate on the loss that occurs with the birth of time, the loss of the 'perfection and stability of the pre-historical world'. Myths can thus be considered to be stories that lay bare the transition from one world to another, and they are characterized by the traumatic experiences of these transitions. Therefore, one might find in mythological texts ruptures that cannot be solved; ruptures portrayed particularly through the heroes of these stories, who are generally torn between two worlds. In this sense, myths 'perform' the loss that takes place in historical transitions.

> It follows that myth and the historical sublime should not be relegated exclusively to a distant past; myth and the historical sublime accompany us like an ever-present shadow on our path towards modernity. Each time humanity or a civilization enters a truly new phase in its history, a new mythical sublime comes into being as this civilization's cold and fossilized heart that will forever be handed on to those living in all its later phases.[40]

Mulisch's account of the Dresden bombings in *The Stone Bridal Bed* is replete with mythological references. Ankersmit's theories might provide us with insights into the way Harry Mulisch performs the memory of World War II in his novel. To understand the way Mulisch evokes the concept of trauma, a close reading of *The Stone Bridal Bed* will prove helpful to regard it from the perspective of Ankersmit's notion of myth as a transitional text that represents the trauma caused by the boundary between a-historical time and historical time.

3 'Vergiss mich nicht'. Reality in *The Stone Bridal Bed*

The novel *The Stone Bridal Bed* by Harry Mulisch is centered around the American war pilot Norman Corinth. He took part in the bombing of the German city of Dresden in 1945. He and his comrades not only set the city ablaze, they also shot a lot of innocent citizens who had fled into the river Elbe. After the war, Corinth returned home to become a dentist in Baltimore. The story begins when he receives an invitation to a dental conference in Dresden. He decides to go there and the plot unfolds as we witness his experiences during his stay for the conference in Dresden. Corinth has suppressed the traumatic experiences from the past, but when he is confronted with a number of people in post-war Dresden some of these experiences come back to him. Several times he feels like he's

40 ANKERSMIT, The sublime dissociation of the past (see n. 23), p. 321.

being captured by the past: he hears voices and finds himself on the brink of fainting.

In *The Stone Bridal Bed*, the representation of the historical moment ('the massacre of Dresden') shows three different characteristics, which can all be considered as emphasizing the traumatic nature of the event. First of all, we notice that the historical moment is only represented in this text in a roundabout way, implicitly. Secondly, Mulisch lets his character reflect explicitly on the connection between historiography and traumatic events. Thirdly, Mulisch represents the historical trauma by creating a character that experiences the past as traumatic. The novel deals with a historical event commonly regarded as a pointless war crime, because the Germans already were as good as beaten at the time. The bombers used an excessive amount of violence, the most reprehensible part of it probably being the shooting of citizens in the Elbe. There are two passages in the novel that describe these events. The first passage relates the events as told by a couple that experienced the bombing on the ground; the second passage is told from the perspective of the war pilots.

Let me begin with the description of the event as experienced by the German couple. At the end of the first day of the conference, a number of guests are having a drink in a German bar. They meet a local couple who start telling them about their experiences on the fateful day. The man tells a horrifying story about the cruelties of the bombing, the burning of the city, the incredible heat and how his wife wandered through the city with their child in her arms. His wife went to the river Elbe, fleeing from the heat, but the people there were attacked by an airplane. Overcome by fear, feeling like something bit her in the leg, the woman let the baby slip out of her arms:

> Everything was on fire, the whole city, the streets had changed into ovens, but you could hardly see the flames for the smoke. In half a minute, her hair and her clothes were scorched off her body and she was almost choked in the smoke, because the fire consumed all the oxygen. She said there was a smell of roast meat everywhere. [...] Everywhere people were standing stock-still up to their necks in the water, without groaning or speaking, just standing in the water. She wetted the child and took it on her shoulder and went as far as possible into the water and then the plane came. At a height of perhaps thirty feet and with it came the screams of the people. All the guns were firing, but if you ask me she didn't understand it any more. She thought something bit her in the leg and the child slipped away from her and she groped about in the water but she couldn't find it [...].[41]

In this scene, Mulisch makes the main character (one of the attackers) face his victims. Corinth himself was one of the pilots who took part in this last attack on

41 Harry Mulisch, *The Stone Bridal Bed*, translated by Adrienne Dixon, London/New York/Toronto 1962, pp. 64–65.

the city. The narrator describes his reaction as follows: 'Corinth screwed up his face and tried to find her in the black water, but the war was here and he was there, and there was nothing in between.'[42] This is one of those moments where Corinth's traumatic experience of the war crime he was a part of become visible: there is a gap between his present identity in American post-war society and his former identity during the war, and he cannot reconcile the two identities to form a coherent story. Whereas the witness provides us with a realistic representation of the experience, Corinth cannot accept this representation as meaningful or true.

It is important to notice that the historical event in this novel is narrated in retrospect. The thoughts of Corinth as well as the dialogues he engages in with other characters are therefore memories of and reflections on the traumatic historical event this novel attempts to represent. There are, however, moments in the novel where the trauma manifests itself as if it were taking place right then and there. This is the case in the passages in which the past takes hold of Norman Corinth. He himself speaks of the 'green whispering':

> The green whisper could roar as well, a deep male voice in a hall: '*…measure about…*', '*…the revolving turret, and who…*', rising and falling in a wall of night; sometimes it was a woman's voice that was born in his head, saying: '*…really? I see…*' or: '*…all the animals and…*'; and also abusing, laughing, whispering, a loud shout in the void, or a single word, drifting on silence; they were very real voices, belonging to people he did not know or see, but who evoked an image: dock-hands, a woman in her kitchen, a boy watching a street fight; a town, it would happen to him just before falling asleep, occasionally during the day; it used to come at school, during the lesson, he did not understand it. It never meant anything, whatever came out of that town.[43]

Throughout the novel, Norman Corinth experiences a gap between the present and the past. In the present, he is a dentist in Baltimore who psychologically does not have access to the trauma of his past. When he is confronted with the city he took part in destroying, this suppressed trauma surfaces in his mind, entirely beyond his control, causing a feeling of crisis.

In the novel, the historical moment is represented in yet another way. The scene I am referring to here is spread out throughout the book. There are three four-to-five page long passages that are printed in italics and that are called 'zang' (meaning 'song' or 'ode'). In these 'songs', the bombing of Dresden is narrated by an extradiegetic narrator who uses a style that can be seen as a pastiche of Homer's epic texts *Iliad* and *Odyssey*. To illustrate this, let me quote the last sentences of the second 'song' – which itself ends with a song from an operetta:

42 Mulisch, The Stone Bridal Bed (see n. 41), p. 66.
43 Mulisch, The Stone Bridal Bed (see n. 41), pp. 14–15.

> In the black water under the trembling glow of the flames the blue-eyed Corinth sees them: heads, chumps, motionless. And then, in his turret, he laughs the laugh of the victorious and shouts: 'Shall I give them a serenade?' And they all laugh, all the airmen, Jim, Alan, Frank, Patrick and Archie, and then he drives the bullets ahead of him into the water, where the heads burst, tumble, collide, jump, shy, sink, and laughs, all the airmen laugh in the night, singing:
>
> Adieu, mein kleiner Gardeoffizier, Adieu,
> Adieu, und vergiss mich nicht,
> Vergiss mich nicht.[44]

It is striking that the actual historical moment around which this novel revolves should be described in such a grotesque way. In these 'songs', the narrator represents the suppressed memories of Norman Corinth that are coming back to him while he is having sex with the East-German woman Hella Viebahn. From his point of view, the Dresden attack exists as a 'pre-historical moment', which has no place in the historical time of 1956. It is an 'eternal' moment that ruptures his experiences in the present.

This makes these three italic passages even more interesting. They tell two stories at once. First of all, they narrate Corinth's experiences in the war. But the war experiences can also be read as a metaphor for the actual sexual intercourse that Corinth and Hella are having at the same moment. From this perspective, the serenade at the end can be considered a metaphorical representation of Corinth's orgasm. We can conclude that the sexual intercourse that takes place in 1956 mirrors the war scene of 1945. Both scenes also mirror the Trojan War, which is central to Homer's texts. Mulisch thus uses the principle of synchronicity: three historical moments mirroring each other, becoming each other's metaphor. In the course of the novel, more intertexts are added to this layer of metaphors, such as the Napoleonic wars and the burning of the city of Rome during the time of the emperor Nero. In *The Stone Bridal Bed,* Mulisch brings together several historical wars in one mythological structure, at one and the same moment in time. In doing so, he changes the metonymical character of *historical* time into a metaphorical timelessness that Ankersmit calls *a-historical time.* The tension that is the driving force in the novel is the result of this ongoing friction between metonymy and metaphor.

As mentioned earlier, the historical moment is only implicitly represented in this text. We encounter victims who narrate their experiences eleven years after they occurred and Mulisch uses an overtly fictionalized narrator who narrates the past in the present tense. Both representations illustrate the impossibility of representing the past in a direct way. Mulisch is clearly looking for a literary form that helps him bridge the temporal and spatial distance between the mo-

44 Mulisch, The Stone Bridal Bed (see n. 41), p. 83.

ment of writing and the historical event. We might say he was in search of an 'esthetics of trauma'. But Mulisch also uses two other literary strategies to represent the Dresden bombings. There are several passages in the novel where Corinth reflects explicitly on the connection between historiography and traumatic events. Here, the notion of trauma refers to a theoretical or philosophical concept that is used by both the character and the author to understand the past. Corinth contrasts the history of meaningful events with the history of meaningless events:

> Corinth closed his eyes even tighter and thought it never did happen. Damn it. It never happened because it might as well not have happened: it was not part of a strategic plan, of the Second World War, like the massacres of other cities. The others had a purpose, and demonstrable results – like the massacre of Carthage, and Hiroshima; these pointed beyond themselves, as the battle of Troy was not about Troy but about Helen. Dresden was not like that. Therefore the history books will go on writing pages and pages about the Battle of Dresden and a few hundred slaughtered nags and grenadiers of Napoleon's army, but the massacre will be mentioned in small letters in a short footnote, because it doesn't belong to the text.[45]

Corinth's theories might strike us as bizarre. How can he claim the massacre of Dresden did not happen at all? He explains that there might be two types of massacres. On the one hand, there are those that are part of strategic plans and end up in history books, narrating the plot of the wars of which these massacres were a part. On the other hand, there are the pointless historical events, events which do not belong to any strategic plan and do not have any strategic effects. These events resemble the traumatic events Ankersmit tells us about. They are traumatic in the sense that it is not possible to make them part of a coherent narration about the history of the war they were part of. This leads Corinth to the thought that there are two histories: the logical and chronological history we find in history books, and the unnarrated story of the odd traumatic events:

> He thought, one is the history of the spirit, bloody but spiritual, with a purpose and results: Alexander, Caesar, Napoleon – Battle of Marathon, Battle of Dresden, Bombardement of Berlin, Hamburg. That is time, evolution. But beside it, under it, there is an anti-history in the stillness of death, and at certain intervals history sinks away in it. At such times the anti-history of Mao Dun Tanhu, Attila, Tamerlane, Genghisz Khan, Hitler, prevails. Then there is no more thought, no purpose, no results – only nothingness. There is no lapse of time between the massacres of the Huns and the concentration camps of Hitler. They lie side by side at the bottom of eternity. He thought, and there lies Dresden. Massacre of Aquilea, Massacre of Auschwitz – Massacre of Dresden. We smashed up Dresden because it was Dresden, just as the Jews were slaughtered because they were Jews. No further message. Hecatombs dedicated to nothingness, burning in an eternal, dead space outside history. […]

45 Mulisch, The Stone Bridal Bed (see n. 41), pp. 95–96.

> He thought, I shall withdraw into the hills and write the impenetrable, immovable anti-history book in which the Massacre of Dresden is no longer obscure compared with the Battle of Dresden and the Battle of Marathon, but in which Napoleon and Miltiades are mentioned in a footnote at the bottom of the page; the anti-history of nothing fighting against something, the anti-biography of men who never existed: Hitler, Corinth [...].[46]

In this scene, Corinth contrasts the history of meaningful events with the history of meaningless events. The first type of history is that which centers around development and change, whereas the second centers around eternity, death and silence. These histories represent two perspectives on historiography. The history of the spirit can be considered to be the 'official historiography', which constructs the past as a logical narrative and places the events in a chronological order. The history of death, however, relates to those events that do not fit into the logical order of the historiographical narrative – events that do not fit, for instance, because they are too painful to imagine, or because they did not influence the course of history that followed them. In that sense, Corinth considers Hitler's massacres to be a-historical or non-historical. This is because, first of all, they are scarcely conceivable. Secondly, in post-war Europe these massacres are mostly suppressed from the collective memory, which may lead one to conclude that, consequently, they did not influence post-war European history. The same holds for Corinth's own actions during the war, which are excluded from the postwar historiographic story of the liberation.

Thirdly, Mulisch represents the historical trauma by creating a character who experiences the past as traumatic. The notion of trauma here can be considered to be purely psychological in nature – it refers to the psychological experiences of one human being. At one point, Mulisch compares Corinth to the archeologist Schliemann. This 'heroic warrior' did not find a historical city, but rather a metaphorical accumulation of nine different temporal layers. The same holds true for Corinth, who came to Dresden to understand the one historical moment of 1945, but ended up with a theory in which he declares the historical moment to be part of the anti-history of timelessness. We might conclude from this that Corinth did not succeed in making the traumatic experience part of a logical, temporally structured narrative. Corinth fails to come to terms with his trauma. In spite of his serious attempt to bridge the gap between his present identity in American post-war society and his former identity in wartime, he ends up staring at a note that says: 'prohibited'. The only thing that is left for him is to look across a deserted wasteland:

> He crumbled the cutting and threw it into the fire which was seeping through the stones in eddies. Wiping the blood from his scars with his sleeve, he looked into the flames. The car existed only as a transparent ghost in the blazing glow. A few yards down was a

46 Mulisch, The Stone Bridal Bed (see n. 41), pp. 96–97.

> notice, fallen across the road, PROHIBITED – EVEN FOR PEDESTRIANS.
> He got up again and crept behind an overgrown mound, where he could not see the fire but could look across the deserted wasteland.[47]

We may conclude that Mulisch has constructed his novel in such a way that temporal coherence is frustrated and transformed into spatial coherence. The moment represented by this text is captured metaphorically in other historical and fictional moments of war and massacre. This way, the novel represents the unsolved friction between these two ways of dealing with historical experience. The whole novel revolves around Corinth's failing attempts to come to terms with his past. At the end of the novel, Corinth is looking into an abyss, with his burning car behind him. If anything, it shows that he has not found a way to reconcile the past with the present. His experiences as a war bomber remain traumatic: buried in the past and not integrated into his own life story.

4 Trauma and myth

In the literary works of Harry Mulisch, we can find a fascinating contribution to the debate about traumatic experience. Mulisch never uses the concept of trauma explicitly, but it emerges as the overall structuring principle of his historical novels. We might say that Mulisch uses the aforementioned 'esthetics of trauma' in his early novels in which he wanted to come to terms with the historiography of evil. What he introduces into the discussion is the concept of myth. This links up quite well with Ankersmit's conception of myth as a 'liminal phenomenon' that tells the story of a transgression of a fundamental boundary.[48] Mulisch has represented the historical event of the bombing of Dresden by creating a character that experienced the past as a witness, as a perpetrator and as a victim. The character tries to gain access to his suppressed past, but finds himself facing a boundary he cannot cross.

At the same time, the narrator of the novel has managed to describe the historical moment twice in an indirect, artificially represented way: by narrating the memories of the victims and by using a Homer-like narrator. Not only Corinth gets stuck on the fracture between past and present, but the narrator equally fails to represent the past in a direct way. To represent this historical moment, the narrating historian needs language, but words fail to enable one to bridge historical distance. With this construction, Mulisch creates a literary representation of the theoretical problem of the opposition between official historiography (the 'coherent' and 'reliable' story of canonical history) and

47 MULISCH, The Stone Bridal Bed (see n. 41), p. 160.
48 ANKERSMIT, The sublime dissociation of the past (see n. 23), p. 319.

memory (the individual experiences of the past of someone who has not managed to turn the past into a coherent story). Mulisch thematizes – in the development of the main character and in the construction of the novel – the distance between the experienced historical moment (history as a 'now') and the linguistic representation of the historian (history as a 'then'). In that sense, the novel reflects on the problems of historiography and narrativity.

It becomes clear that Mulisch does not simply believe that the novelist is able to recreate the past as a now while the historian is not. Rather, he does something else: he represents the past as a traumatic experience in Ankersmit's sense of the term. With *The Stone Bridal Bed*, Mulisch has written a mythological text that highlights the traumatic experience of an American war bomber and his inability to live in the 'world of change' as a result of his traumatic experiences in the Second World War. In doing so, Mulisch frames the contrast between the official chronological story of history and the personal stories of the victims, which are anything but logical and chronological. In dramatizing the gap between the historical and the pre-historical, he tries to revive the potential of the old myths by creating contemporary myths in which characters deal with the traumatic events of World War II. The fact that these characters are not able to solve their traumas suggests that, if anything, Mulisch wants to show us, in the words of Cathy Caruth: 'the legacy of incomprehensibility at the heart of the catastrophic experience'.[49]

49 CARUTH, Unclaimed Experience (see n. 27), p. 58.

Wouter Schrover

Reading Literature through Medical Sociology: The Doctor-Patient Relationship in Thomas Rosenboom's *Public Works* and a Poem by Neeltje Maria Min*

1 Introduction

Since medicine is both a science and a profession, it involves many different kinds of knowledge. This is reflected by the organizational structure of present-day faculties of medicine, with departments oriented to different diseases and disorders (such as internal medicine, obstetrics, paediatrics) as well as departments concerned with, for instance, the anthropological, sociological, psychological, and ethical aspects of medicine. Literature, likewise, engages with the range of bodies of knowledge through its ability to represent all these aspects. It can actively evaluate current views and engage in debates, both overtly and more indirectly.[1] Thus, texts can overtly refer to specific ideas, concepts, or theories, as in the acclaimed novel *Publieke werken* (*Public Works*, 1999) by Thomas Rosenboom, which refers to both pharmaceutical and biomedical knowledge.[2] The novel describes the use of contemporary medication and discusses notions of health and illness, but it can also be related to bodies of knowledge that are less explicitly referred to. Medical sociology, for example, can offer fruitful insights into the novel's representation of the doctor-patient relationship, even though this discipline is not specifically mentioned in the text. The reader can infer the book's relation to medical sociology not because it is explicitly mentioned, but through certain congruent elements and a more general, thematic corre-

---

* This article is a product of the PhD-project *The Art of Dying. The Representation of Euthanasia and Assisted Suicide in Literature and Film* (2010–2014), funded by the Netherlands Organisation for Scientific Research (NWO). I would like to thank Ben Peperkamp for reading earlier versions of this article and Sarah Davidesko for proofreading the final text.

1 Ben Peperkamp, 'Wetenschap in de moderne Nederlandse literatuur, van 1850 tot heden', in: *Leonardo voor het publiek: Een geschiedenis van de wetenschaps- en techniekcommunicatie*, Frans J. Meijman, Stephen Snelders and Onno de Wit (eds.), Amsterdam 2007, pp. 243–252.

2 Thomas Rosenboom, *Publieke werken*, Amsterdam 1999.

spondence between text and academic discourse. Of course, the reader has an active role here in arguing the relevance of such a specific body of knowledge.[3]

The doctor-patient relationship is also of significance in other Dutch literary works. In this essay I will, besides *Public Works*, specifically discuss an untitled poem by Neeltje Maria Min from her collection *Een vrouw bezoeken (Visiting a Woman)*, published in 1985.[4] I will first argue the relevance of medical sociology in interpreting these texts and subsequently address the different ways each text expresses ideas of a medical sociological kind. More specifically, I will examine the way poem and novel evaluate the notion of interdependency, such as it is discussed by the Dutch sociologist Abram de Swaan in his seminal 1981 essay 'The Medical Regime' ('Het medisch regiem').[5] By means of these evaluations, both texts, although from distinct genres and published in widely different years, offer a substantial and original reflection on the relationship between doctor and patient.

De Swaan describes individual persons as junctions in an ever-changing network of interdependencies. Whether a person is in a position of relative dependence or relative independence is determined by the power others have over that person and the power that person has over others. The balance of power between self and others continuously shifts during a lifetime. In childhood and old age, individuals are largely dependent on a small number of other people; but in adulthood they are much less dependent on others, while others are mostly dependent on them. In some relationships the balance of power is more or less equal (for example, the relation between friends), while in others the balance is unequal (between a mother and child). In the context of medicine, the latter applies to the doctor-patient relationship. This does not mean the patient is completely powerless, as de Swaan makes clear:

> [T]he patient [is] someone in a lesser – more dependent – position, yet still […] someone who engages in the relationship, for example by selecting and arranging his symptoms; by implicitly or explicitly negotiating diagnosis and therapy; by taking up or ignoring medical instructions; by extracting information or by simply ignoring it; by doctor shopping or by playing health care providers off against each other. This does not falsify the theory of medical dominance, but corrects and confirms the notion of an asymmetrically dependent relationship between physician and patient. The doctor is in

3 For methodological reflection on the issue of which textual properties signal a literary work's engagement with (academic) knowledge, see Mary Kemperink and Leonieke Vermeer, 'Literatuur en wetenschap: Een dynamische en complexe relatie', in: *Nederlandse Letterkunde* 13, no. 1 (2008), pp. 33–66, here pp. 44–45 and 54–55.

4 Neeltje Maria Min, *Een vrouw bezoeken*, Amsterdam 1985.

5 Abram de Swaan, *De mens is de mens een zorg: Opstellen 1971–1981*, Amsterdam 2009, pp. 151–219. For the reception and undiminished relevance of de Swaan's essay, see Annet Mooij, 'Voorwoord', in: *De mens is de mens een zorg: Opstellen 1971–1981*, by Abram de Swaan, Amsterdam 2009.

> a position of power, but relies at the same time on the patients of his practice for maintaining this position, and is therefore required to show a certain degree of amiability towards individual patients.[6]

In other words, as it is possible for the patient to assert himself, it follows that the doctor is not fully independent. De Swaan thus draws attention to the fact – as is done in numerous other medical sociological publications[7] – that the seemingly powerless position of the patient is not that powerless at all.

In discussing the representation of the doctor-patient relationship in Min's poem and Rosenboom's novel and the ensuing implications for the interdependence of doctor and patient, I will use Howard Brody's *The Healer's Power* (1992) as a theoretical framework. Brody proposes a theory of power in the doctor-patient relationship that is based on earlier work by medical sociologists. He distinguishes three components of that power, namely Aesculapian, charismatic, and social power. Aesculapian power comprises of knowledge about the body and diseases, practical skills, and experience in the application of this knowledge and these skills. It is an impersonal kind of power, which means it can be acquired by anyone with the necessary intellectual and social capacities. Charismatic power refers to a doctor's personal qualities, such as courage and kindness, which cannot be learned, as they are personality traits that are independent of his or her disciplinary knowledge and skill. This kind of power concerns the doctor as an individual. Social power is about the capacity of doctors, as members of the medical profession, to determine sound medical knowledge. This also means that doctors can rule who is ill and who is well and

---

6 '[D]e patiënt [is] iemand in een weliswaar mindere – afhankelijkere – positie, maar toch ook [...] iemand die binnen die verhouding actief ingrijpt, bijvoorbeeld door zijn klachten te selecteren, te ordenen, door impliciet of met zoveel woorden over de diagnose en de therapie te onderhandelen, door voorschriften al dan niet op te volgen, door informatie af te dwingen of juist te negeren, door te winkelen of door het medisch personeel onderling uit te spelen. Dat logenstraft de visie van medische dominantie niet, maar corrigeert die en bevestigt de notie van een asymmetrische afhankelijkheidsrelatie tussen arts en patiënt, waarin de machtsbalans uitslaat ten gunste van de dokter die toch tegelijkertijd voor het behoud van zijn positie aangewezen blijft op zijn patiëntenbestand als geheel en daarom ook tegenover afzonderlijke patiënten een zekere mate van voorkomendheid moet tonen.' De Swaan, De mens is de mens een zorg (see n. 5), pp. 155–156. All translations are mine, unless otherwise indicated.

7 E.g. Talcott Parsons, *The Social System*, New York 1951, pp. 428–479; J.M.D. Boot, *Inleiding in de medische sociologie*, 7th ed., Assen 2001, pp. 77–79; Charles L. Bosk, 'The Social Construction of Illness', in: *Encyclopedia of Bioethics*, Stephen G. Post (ed.), New York 2004, pp. 1066–1070, here p. 1067; Deborah Lupton, *Medicine as Culture: Illness, Disease and the Body*, 3rd ed., Los Angeles 2012, pp. 114–120. The doctor-patient relationship is often discussed in a larger context, in which other actors, such as health insurers and patients' associations, exert their influence on the doctor-patient relationship. See, for example, F.J.A. Beumer and Gabrielle Verbeek, 'Beleid in de gezondheidszorg' in: *Introductie in de gezondheidszorg: Structuur en functioneren in de praktijk*, A.M.C. Scherpenisse and Gabrielle Verbeek (eds.), Houten/Diegem 2002, pp. 179–208.

determine whose problems are medical and whose are existential: 'the physician's word on the subject is sufficient to set in motion various social roles and practices (such as the 'sick' role) in a way that no word from a lay person could do.'[8] For example, when a person is diagnosed with a serious illness, he/she is relieved from normal social roles (such as working or caring for others), but at the same time is obliged to participate in his/her treatment.[9]

After a brief introduction of the poem and novel under consideration, I will discuss the representation of Aesculapian, charismatic and social power in these works. In my conclusion I will further reflect on the question of how these works are related to the issue of the doctor-patient relationship in medical sociology.

2 Neeltje Maria Min's untitled poem and Thomas Rosenboom's *Public Works*

Een Vrouw Bezoeken (*Visiting a Woman*), Min's second book of poetry, was published almost twenty years after her notorious debut book of 1966, *For Whom I Love, I Want To Be Named* (*Voor wie ik liefheb wil ik heten).* By studying the poem reproduced below from the viewpoint of medical sociology, I aim to do justice to the richness of Min's work.

My body is crawling with streptococci.
I shake and rear up. Higher the fever rises.
Look: 40.5, 6, 7 and so on.
While I lie rambling I fear trouble

If I don't quickly send for a doctor.
They're going to call him. He comes striding along
And bends over me. I seem to be alive still
But – goddammit, it's too late even so.

A small mirror appears above my mouth.
To my alarm I see it doesn't steam up.
I meant well but I succumbed.

It will badly sting the new doctor
That I am his tenth passing away today.
In this way his little business will just never get off the ground.[10]

---

8 Howard Brody, *The Healer's Power*, New Haven/London 1992, p. 17.

9 Parsons, The Social System (see n. 7), pp. 436–439; Bosk, The Social Construction of Illness (see n. 7), p. 1067; Linda Emanuel, Katherine Bennett and Virginia E. Richardson, 'The Dying Role', in: *Journal of Palliative Medicine* 10, no. 1 (2007), pp. 159–168, here pp. 160–161.

10 Mijn lichaam wemelt van de streptokokken./ Ik schud en steiger. Hoger stijgt de koorts./ Kijk: 40.5, 6, 7 enzovoorts./ Terwijl ik lig te ijlen vrees ik brokken// als ik niet snel de dokter

The poem, an Italian sonnet, uses rhyme (abba cddc ecf fce) and rhythm (iambic pentameters) in a rather conventional way. It is basically a narrative about a person who suffers from a bacterial infection, sends for a doctor, but dies before he arrives.[11] What catches the eye is that the different persons in the poem are anonymous and no real individuals. The speaker of the poem discloses little about him/herself: neither age, nor sex, nor any other characteristics. Nor is the identity of 'they' ('ze') in the sixth line clear, although they are probably some significant others. The doctor is established as a male who has just started practicing, but no further information is provided. Taken together, these elements indicate that the poem can indeed be considered to address the doctor-patient relationship. The volta at the end of the tenth line signals a fundamental change in the balance of power between doctor and patient, as I will show below.

Publieke werken (Public Works) is the third novel of the well-known Dutch author Thomas Rosenboom. It won him the prestigious Libris Literature Prize. Moreover, it reached the tenth position in a public vote on the best book ever in the Dutch language.[12] *Public Works* is a historical novel situated alternately in Amsterdam and – more important in the context of this essay – the village of Hoogeveen at the end of the nineteenth century. The local doctor Amshoff is, by order of the municipality, responsible for the health care of the village poor, who live on the outskirts of the village, in the fields ('het Veld'). The village pharmacist, Anijs, accuses Amshoff of miserable neglect of these poor inhabitants and unwillingness to attend them.[13] Anijs, who is both sympathetic towards the poor and desires to rise in social status (in contrast to the village elite, he does not have an academic degree – pharmacy wasn't taught at university when he was young), increasingly sets himself up as a doctor in the course of the novel's

---

komen laat./ Ze gaan hem bellen. Hij komt aangestevend/en buigt zich over mij. Ik lijk nog levend/ maar godverdomme, het is toch te laat.// Een spiegeltje verschijnt boven mijn mond./ Ik zie geschrokken dat het niet beslaat./ Ik heb het goed bedoeld maar ben bezweken.// Het zal de nieuwe dokter danig steken/dat ik vandaag zijn tiende ben die gaat./ Zo komt zijn zaakje nooit eens van de grond.// Min, Een vrouw bezoeken (see n. 4), p. 25. The English translation is mine.

11 The poem stands in a tradition of verse – whether on headstones, in obituaries or just as poems – in which the subject speaks from the dead. See D.M. Schenkeveld, 'Griekse epigrammen op jong gestorven kinderen', in: *De Literaire Dood*, Elrud Ibsch, Andrea Kunne, and Cristina Pumplun (eds.), Assen 1998, pp. 8–18; Jos Versteegen and Victor Vroomkoning (eds.), *Een zucht als vluchtig eerbetoon: funeraire gedichten uit de moderne Nederlandse poëzie*, Amsterdam/Antwerpen 1995, p. 26; Puck Kooij, *Heden gij, morgen ik: gedenken in proza en poëzie*, Amsterdam 2004, pp. 105–110.Worth pointing out in this poem is the use of 'I' both before and after the transition to death; cf. Ernst van Alphen, 'De grenzen van poëzie, ofwel, Faverey's poëtische dood', in: *Forum der Letteren: Tijdschrift voor Taal- en Letterkunde* 35, no. 4 (1994), pp. 295–300.

12 Pieter Steinz, 'Het beste boek voor mannen en vrouwen', in: *NRC Handelsblad*, 12-03-2007.

13 Rosenboom, Publieke werken (see n. 2), p. 28.

story. I will argue that Anijs ultimately fails as a doctor, but I will also demonstrate how the representation of his actions makes clear in what sense doctors are fundamentally dependent on their patients.

3 Aesculapian power

Min's poem starts with a diagnosis: the speaker's body is teeming with streptococci, a bacterial infection that turns out to be not without danger. The provenance of this diagnosis is not made clear, nor is it specified who is taking the temperature referred to in line three, although it is obvious that the latter, for which no special expertise is needed, does not take place in the presence of a doctor. It appears that patients to some extent can also have Aesculapian power. At the same time, the speaker acknowledges the Aesculapian power of members of the medical profession, by stating that recovery depends on the intervention of a doctor and therefore sending for one. In this sense, it is the doctor who is in the position of power; even though establishing death is the only thing he can do when he arrives.

The pharmacist Anijs in *Public Works* begins diagnosing villagers and providing medication in his apothecary when he becomes convinced that doctor Amshoff is failing the poor of Hoogeveen. There are even rumours in the village that Anijs actually performs medical treatments.[14] Later on, Anijs goes out into the fields for a so-called 'public medication' ('algemene medicatie'), at which occasion he indeed does treat the poor villagers. The table on which he displays medication and medical equipment is metaphorically described as 'a small hospital' ('een klein hospitaal').[15] Not only does Anijs provide medicines without prescription, he also administers treatments, for instance by putting leeches on the temples of patients he diagnoses with vertigo.[16] When Lubber, a mentally retarded villager, unexpectedly traps his thumb in the door during the Public Medication, Anijs wins the admiration of the poor citizens by successfully performing a puncture. By means of this minor surgery and by using medical jargon (hematoma, puncture) to explain his doings, Anijs creates the impression that he possesses a considerable amount of Aesculapian power.[17]

In fact, however, Anijs's power is rather limited. Although the pharmacist is highly confident, some of his actions are in fact bizarre. In the case of a boy with a speech impediment, for example, he cuts the frenulum of the tongue (which

14 ROSENBOOM, Publieke werken (see n. 2), pp. 27–28.
15 ROSENBOOM, Publieke werken (see n. 2), p. 187.
16 ROSENBOOM, Publieke werken (see n. 2), p. 193.
17 ROSENBOOM, Publieke werken (see n. 2), p. 192.

connects the underside of the tongue with the floor of the mouth), thus actually worsening the impediment. The limits of Anijs's knowledge also become apparent when he attends to Johanna, a young woman who is pregnant. During the Public Medication Anijs puts his hand 'with his palm against her stomach, *seemingly* automatic, but it was engaging in a world he didn't know' ('met de binnenzijde tegen haar buik, *schijnbaar* werktuiglijk, maar het was een indalen in een wereld die hij niet kende').[18] When Johanna is about to deliver, however, Anijs has no idea about what should be done and the baby is born dead as a result. The pharmacist has severely exceeded the limits of his Aesculapian power, with fatal consequences. It comes as no surprise that when Amshoff learns about Johanna's delivery, he threatens Anijs with a summoning by the board of medical discipline.

More important than the exact amount of Anijs's Aesculapian power, however, is the fact that the poor citizens of Hoogeveen continue to believe in him – even when the baby is stillborn. They know Anijs is not a doctor, but are impressed with his Aesculapian power, which – different from Amshoff – he moreover uses in their favour. Anijs is conscious of this and plays it as a trump card in a discussion with Amshoff:[19]

> 'Indeed, I just started doing something, exactly as you say – because you haven't done anything over the past years,' Anijs readily admitted, flexible but then bending back to finally cause his assailant to lose balance, as in a judo movement: 'But why don't you ask these people themselves what they prefer, your diagnosis or my medicine?'[20]

Although Anijs tries to hide from Amshoff that he too makes diagnoses, it is implied in this passage that Aesculapian power is not simply an asset one possesses, but rather a quality one is credited with by patients. Patients are not at the mercy of the individual doctor or even of the medical profession, since there is always an element of choice. They can choose between different doctors and they can turn to others who also (seem to) have a considerable amount of Aesculapian power and are eager to put their – probably much smaller and not very well-

18 ROSENBOOM, Publieke werken (see n. 2), p. 197, my italics.

19 Raat convincingly argues that this discussion might not really have taken place, but possibly is a figment of Anijs' imagination – see G.F.H. RAAT, [THOMAS ROSENBOOM, *Publieke werken*, Amsterdam, 1999], *Lexicon van Literaire Werken*, A.G.H. ANBEEK VAN DER MEIJDEN, JAAP GOEDEGEBUURE and BART VERVAECK (eds.), Groningen 2004, pp. 1–14, here p. 11. However, this does not at all reduce the meaningfulness of this discussion and the passage cited.

20 "Inderdaad, ik ben maar wat gaan doen, precies zoals u zegt – omdat u al jaren niets doet,' gaf Anijs grif toe, juist om vanuit die meegaande, dan omgebogen judobeweging zijn aanvaller alsnog uit evenwicht te trekken. 'Maar waarom vraagt u deze mensen niet zelf wat ze verkiezen, uw diagnose of mijn medicijn?", ROSENBOOM, Publieke werken (see n. 2), pp. 194–195.

grounded – knowledge and skill to practice.[21] In this sense, doctors need to comply with patients' expectations and are dependent on them for the exercise of their profession.

4 Charismatic power

Charismatic power is not really addressed in the poem by Min. Only the sixth line gives a slight indication of the doctor's personality. The fact that '[h]e comes striding along' ('[h]ij komt aangestevend') might imply something about the doctor's vigour, about his determination to save the patient. These words follow immediately after: 'They're going to call him' ('Ze gaan hem bellen'). Thus, by means of an ellipsis – in the narratological sense of the word – the amount of time between the two events appears to be very confined. This confirms the impression that the doctor acts energetically. Although this quality is in the interest of the patient, it is to no avail: the patient is dead upon the doctor's arrival.

More can be said about the role of charismatic power in *Public Works*. While Amshoff lacks the qualities required for relating to the village poor, charisma is a distinguishing feature of Anijs. In the following passage doctor and pharmacist are contrasted:

> All in all he [Anijs, WS] showed more compassion with the poor than the [assigned] doctor of the poor, being particularly bent on reassuring them. After all, those who were free from any ailment had nothing to worry about, whereas if anything was wrong with someone, it was actually even more important to reassure him. Deterred by Amshoff's stern, aristocratic behavior, people would more and more turn to him directly with their complaints, without firstly consulting the doctor.[22]

The passage makes clear that charisma is not a source of power that *can* be utilized, but one that – at least to some degree – *needs* to be utilized. The importance of a doctor's attitude towards his or her patients cannot be underestimated. In *Public Works*, the poor citizens of Hoogeveen even give up on Amshoff altogether once Anijs begins to put himself forward as an alternative. Not only is Anijs very friendly towards the villagers, he also shows himself bold and decisive, for example in treating Lubber's thumb. At the same time, however, Anijs's lack of integrity – posing as a real doctor while he is no such thing – can

21 E.g. alternative medicine.

22 '[A]l met al toonde hij [Anijs, WS] zich meer begaan met de armen dan de armdokter, waarbij hij het er vooral op toelegde hun gerust te stellen, immers: wie niets mankeerde, hoefde zich geen zorgen te maken, en had iemand wel iets, dan was het eigenlijk nog belangrijker dat hij gerustgesteld werd. Afgeschrikt door het barse, aristocratische optreden van Amshoff wendden de mensen zich steeds vaker direct met hun klachten tot hem, zonder eerst de dokter te raadplegen.' Rosenboom, Publieke werken (see n. 2), p. 27.

be said to outweigh all his other personal qualities, because he ultimately acts at the expense of his patients. In this way, the character of Anijs demonstrates how charismatic power can be used as well as abused.

5 Social power

As already indicated, the provenance of the streptococci diagnosis is unclear. And because the patient dies before the doctor is able to intervene, the poem draws attention to disease as a physiological process – independent of any medical involvement – rather than to sickness as a social role, which is mostly determined by the social power of the doctor.[23] By way of contrast, this power is expressed in the third stanza, when the doctor certifies the patient's death, which is another task reserved for the medical profession. This is rendered with some irony, as the patient only notices – as appears from the phrase '[t]o my alarm' ('geschrokken') – that he/she is dead when seeing that the little mirror does not steam up!

Just before the Public Medication in *Public Works*, Anijs accidentally finds a doctor's white coat. The pharmacist puts it on. Although the reader is not granted a direct view of Anijs's motivation for doing so, donning the white coat can be considered as a strategy – or alternatively as giving in to a secret desire – to claim social power for himself. In addition to his charismatic power, the coat grants Anijs not only the authority of a doctor, but the related belief and trust in him as well,[24] which appears from the fact that the poor citizens choose to be examined and treated by Anijs. Still, they do not consider Anijs a real doctor yet, as is proven by the way a man called Bennemin incites his son, Klein Pet, to thank Anijs after the Public Medication has ended:

> 'Come on, boy,' he [Bennemin, WS] said gravely, 'say thank you, pharmacist.'
> Again the word was too difficult, the lad stood open-mouthed once more, but now Anijs already cast the coattails aside, kneeling humbly before the boy and saying, helping, *correcting, simplifying:* 'Thank you, doctor…'[25]

---

23 For the distinction in medical sociology between disease and illness/sickness, see Katerina A. Christopoulos, 'The Sick Role in Literature and Society', in: *Journal of the American Medical Association* 285 (2001), p. 93.

24 Jannes van Everdingen, 'De leliewitte jas van apotheker Anijs', in: *Ziektebeelden: Essays over literatuur en geneeskunde*, F. Meulenberg, J. van der Meer and A.K. Oderwald, Utrecht 2002, pp. 183–190, here p. 185. Notice that nineteenth-century doctors actually did not wear a white coat, as van Everdingen also makes clear. Rosenboom thus uses an anachronistic element to strengthen his story.

25 "Vooruit jongen,' sprak hij [Bennemin, WS] schor, 'zeg maar: dank u wel, apotheker.' / Weer was het woord te moeilijk, de knaap stond opnieuw met open mond maar reeds wierp Anijs de jaspanden opzij, reeds knielde hij deemoedig voor de jongen neer en zei hij het hem

Bennemin explicitly refers to Anijs as pharmacist, while this passage suggests that Anijs subsequently tries to make it easier for Klein Pet, while correcting his father in the process. Although Anijs later admits to Amshoff – in the discussion already mentioned – that he is not a real doctor, he continues posing as one in front of the inhabitants of the fields. He gives, for instance, a medicine called theriac to Klein Pet with reference to the doctor's social power: 'Come, you do believe the doctor, don't you?' ('Kom, je gelooft de dokter toch wel?').[26] That Klein Pet really considers Anijs a doctor becomes clear when his father assigns him to go and get the doctor because of Johanna's imminent delivery: Klein Pet does not go for Amshoff, but fetches Anijs instead, who indeed puts on his white doctor's coat and goes out into the fields.

The stillborn baby's father turns out to be Lubber, which has not gone unnoticed by the poor villagers. So they actually welcome the outcome of the delivery and raise their hands in admiration to Anijs. Someone shouts: 'Glory to the doctor' ('Ere zij de dokter').[27] By means of his misappropriated social power Anijs is able – aided by his charisma and the complete medical ignorance of the poor citizens – to pretend his intervention was beneficial. The description in this passage of the doctor's coat, representative of the social power of doctors, with the expression of an 'unblemished blazon' ('blank blazoen'), is meaningful in this respect, as the expression refers to a coat of arms connoting honesty and valour.[28] Through this metaphorical description it is illustrated how Anijs manages to preserve his reputation. Although the pharmacist is no real doctor, he definitively has the stature of one in the mind of the poor. The white coat has an important role in creating this conviction.

On the one hand, Amshoff does not use the social power he has as a member of the medical profession; does noet use it – in Anij's view anyway – to assist the poor of Hoogeveen. Anijs, on the other hand, is not entitled to social power, but claims it nevertheless and applies it as well. This confirms the thought, already brought up in the last two paragraphs, that being a doctor is not so much something one is, but something one does – an activity rather than a position.

---

helpend, *verbeterend, vergemakkelijkend* voor: 'Dank u wel, dokter..."; ROSENBOOM, Publieke werken (see n. 2), p. 201, my italics.

26 ROSENBOOM, Publieke werken (see n. 2), p. 274.

27 ROSENBOOM, Publieke werken (see n. 2), p. 299.

28 ROSENBOOM, Publieke werken (see n. 2), p. 300.

6 A relation of interdependency

In the first ten lines of the untitled poem by Min, the patient is represented as someone who is dependent on the doctor, since he/she needs him to get well again, and also as someone who is very much aware of this dependency. The patient acknowledges the Aesculapian power of the doctor and, because of this, delegates treatment to him. The vertical relationship between doctor and patient is reinforced by its representation in line seven: while the patient is lying down, the doctor towers over him/her and needs to bend over him/her. In this way, the dependency of the patient on the doctor is represented spatially. Reading further, the poem appears to confirm this vertical relationship: 'I seem to be alive still, / but – goddammit, it's too late even so' ('Ik lijk nog levend / maar godverdomme, het is toch te laat'). Apart from the play with two different meanings of the Dutch word 'lijk', denoting both 'seem' and 'corpse', in combination with the word 'levend' (alive), what strikes one most is that the subject seems to pity him/herself, since he/she is no longer alive. This also applies to line ten, which reads: 'To my alarm I see it doesn't steam up' ('Ik zie geschrokken dat het niet beslaat'). However, this impression is removed in the next line (which is why there is a volta at the end of the line ten), in which the speaker states he/she meant well, an apology of sorts which appear to be addressed at the doctor. In the last stanza the speaker, showing empathy with the doctor, explains what he/she actually means: because he/she died, the doctor will have no earnings from the medical encounter. This sheds an ironical light on the medical profession, while turning the relationship of dependency between doctor and patient upside down: according to the speaker, the doctor is motivated by the pursuit of gain rather than sheer altruism. Although the patient is dependent on the doctor for regaining his/her health, the request for treatment can also be considered a favour accorded to the physician. In Min's poem, the doctor-patient relationship is represented as being of a contractual nature, in other words: a relation of interdependency.[29] That is also why the patient, empathic as he/she is, is able to feel sorry for the doctor.

The thought that the doctor is nothing without the patient is also expressed in *Public Works*, albeit in a very different manner. Amshoff and Anijs are each other's mirror image in the novel. While the former is a doctor, the latter acts as one; the representation of Anijs's actions makes clear that in order to be ac-

29 In a different sense, interdependency also occurs between the patient and those who are going to call him (line six), probably the patient's significant others. On the one hand, the patient relies on them, yet on the other hand they need to adapt their life in order to help the sick person, for example by calling the doctor. In other words: they make themselves dependent on him/her. For a more extensive analysis of the interdependency between patient and significant others, see GERHARD NIJHOF, *Ziekenwerk: Een kleine sociologie van alledaags ziekenleven*, Amsterdam 2002, pp. 41–43.

knowledged as a doctor, one needs to convincingly act as one as well. Of course, Anijs does not really serve as an example for Amshoff, because Anijs's Aesculapian and social powers are based on delusions. What the representation of his actions does show, however, is that patients need to have the impression that the doctor uses his/her different kinds of power in favour of them. Fruitful relations between doctor and patients can only be realized if the impressions formed by patients correspond to the actual responsible use of Aesculapian, charismatic and social power.

When the mayor of Hoogeveen hears of Johanna's delivery, he tells Anijs that he should be careful not to raise any 'false expectations' ('valse verwachtingen').[30] Yet raising false expectations is exactly what Anijs has been doing. By donning a doctor's white coat, making diagnoses and even giving treatments and performing small surgeries, Anijs managed to give Hoogeveen's poor citizens the impression that he can dispose of the powers attributed to the medical profession. Bearing this in mind, Johanna's pregnancy and delivery of a stillborn can be interpreted in a metaphorical way. As the expectant mother raises the expectation of new life, Anijs's behaviour also raises certain expectations, which he – although he is able to fool the poor who are living on the outskirts of Hoogeveen – eventually cannot live up to. Still, the character of Anijs highlights the importance of belief and trust in the doctor-patient relationship.[31] Between Amshoff and the poor citizens, such relations are not established, as Amshoff is not capable or willing to tailor his behavior to the requirements of these patients. This lack does not affect his general status as a doctor, however, because he has other patients too (to which he apparently relates in an appropriate manner). Yet, it can safely be said that a good doctor should meet the (legitimate) demands of all patients, and that Amshoff has serious shortcomings in this respect.

7 Conclusion

In the history of medical sociology, it has always been claimed that although the doctor is not fully independent, the patient still is in a state of relative powerlessness.[32] By way of counterpoint, both the poem and the novel discussed here stand out for drawing attention to the doctor's dependency on the patient, even though the two works also acknowledge the dependency of the patient on the figure of the doctor: the poem by showing that the patient cannot cure him/

30 Rosenboom, Publieke werken (see n. 2), p. 330.

31 Cf. Lupton, Medicine as Culture (see n. 7), p. 130.

32 E. g. Parsons, The Social System (see n. 7), pp. 428–479; De Swaan, De mens is de mens een zorg (see n. 5), pp. 155–156; Lupton, Medicine as Culture (see n. 7), p. 115.

herself, the novel by representing Anijs's failure. In the poem, it is the patient who is represented as being empathic towards the doctor instead of the other way round. And in Rosenboom's novel the focus is on the necessity for doctors to meet their patients' expectations, rather than on the relative lack of power of these patients. The two works do not as such generate new insights into medical sociology, but do in fact examine the doctor-patient relationship from an original angle, since the fundamental dependence of the doctor on the patient is the focal point in the representation of this relation in both the poem and the novel. In Min's poem, this is achieved by the use of the characteristics of the Italian sonnet, turning the relation of dependency between doctor and patient upside down after the volta. *Public Works* succeeds in doing so by employing the troubled relation between Amshoff and Anijs as the novel's propelling force, demonstrating the failure of both as well as outlining the demands any doctor has to meet. In brief, the manner in which the doctor-patient relationship is represented testifies to an engagement with medical sociology in these works, thus revealing the potential literary works have to evaluate existing ideas, even when those ideas are not overtly mentioned in the text but are rather inferred by the reader.

Liesbeth Minnaard and Joost Haan

The Shaking Palsy in the Low Countries: Representations of Parkinson's Disease in Dutch and Flemish Prose

1 Discovering Parkinson's Disease

In 1817, the English apothecary surgeon James Parkinson (1755–1824) described six individuals with remarkable symptoms in his study *An Essay on the Shaking Palsy.* All had trembling hands, a shuffling gait, stooped posture and an expressionless face. He examined some of them on several occasions and noticed that there was gradual progression of the symptoms. In his study, Parkinson admits that he is not able to provide a good explanation for the disease and he apologizes for the lack of experimental investigations and anatomical confirmation. Parkinson's clinical observations, however, were very accurate and he deserves merit for the recognition of the stereotypical nature of the disease that later came to carry his name. During the era in which he published his book, symptoms such as stiffness and tremulousness were often attributed to alcoholism or to venereal diseases. As his patients included examples who had been 'leading a life of temperance and sobriety' or 'a life of temperance' Parkinson rejected these possibilities.[1] There is only one cause that he speculates on, and that is a worm infection. The reason for this speculation is that one of his colleagues once had a patient with a tremor who was cured by means of 'a vermifuge' (deworming). However, as Parkinson points out himself, that patient was only 'twelve or thirteen years of age.'[2]

In 1876, the renowned French neurologist Jean-Marie Charcot (1825–1893) introduced the eponym 'Parkinson's disease'. This was, by the way, spectacular as Charcot almost always named diseases after himself or after countrymen such as Gilles de la Tourette and Pierre Marie (id).[3] Opting for a foreigner this time, he could also have chosen the eponym 'Von Oppolzer's disease', after the Austrian

1 James Parkinson, *An Essay on the Shaking Palsy*, London 1817, pp. 10, 14.
2 Parkinson, An Essay on the Shaking Palsy (see n. 1), p. 30.
3 David R. Kumar, Florence Aslinia, Steven H. Yale and Jospeh J. Mazza, 'Jean-Martin Charcot: The Father of Neurology', in: *Clinical Medicine & Research* 9 (2011), pp. 46–49.

scientist who in 1860 performed the first post mortem investigation on a patient with the characteristic symptoms. The question whether political issues might have played a role in favouring an Englishman over an Austrian has not yet been answered. In more recent decades, many new insights have produced a more complete and accurate picture of Parkinson's disease. It was found, for example, that the disease is caused by a combination of genetic and environmental factors, and that structural abnormalities in the so-called 'basal ganglia' (mainly in the substantia nigra – the 'black nucleus') play a crucial role. What occurs is a dysfunction of neurotransmitters and their receptors, especially of dopamine. Impaired memory (even dementia) and mood disturbances (sometimes up to depression) can be part of the clinical picture. Problems with passing water, sexual functions and blood pressure control can also occur. What is known by now and what is disputably the most tragic aspect of Parkinson's disease, is that there is no cure – the only treatment is aimed at easing the symptoms. Parkinson drugs contain dopamine or related compounds and often have severe side-effects. These side-effects include hallucinations and so called 'response-fluctuations' in which the patient's body unpredictably switches between an 'on'- (with an excess of uncontrollable movements) and an 'off'-mode (stiff and immovable).

2 The Fiction of Parkinson's Disease

This article will now attempt to demonstrate that Parkinson's disease has not only inspired doctors and scientists. The various mysterious and intriguing symptoms have also encouraged many novelists to depict protagonists with Parkinson's disease in their work. Examples can be found in the works of William Shakespeare, Charles Dickens, Samuel Beckett, Martin Walser, Rohinton Mistry, John Updike, J.M. Coetzee, François Mauriac, Michael Robotham and Jonathan Franzen, to name some of the more well-known authors. Also the popular book *Awakenings* (1973) by the American neurologist Oliver Sacks features several characters with Parkinson's disease. Strictly spoken this is not a work of fiction, but the narrative is strongly romanticized (Haan and Meulenberg, 2009), and was even adapted into a major feature film (with Robert de Niro as one of the patients and Robin Williams as dr. Sacks).[4]

4 William Shakespeare: *Henri IV, Troilus and Cressida*, Charles Dickens: *David Copperfield* and *Little Dorrit*, Samuel Beckett: *Murphy, Footfalls*, a.o., Martin Walser: *Beyond all Love,* Rohinton Mistry: *Family Matters*, John Updike: *Rabitt Redux,* J.M. Coetzee: *Diary of a Bad Year,* François Mauriac: *Desert of Love,* Michael Robotham: *The Suspect*, Jonathan Franzen: *The Corrections.* Scholarly work that addresses these novels: L. Fogan, 'The neurology in Shakespeare', in: *Archives of Neurology* 46 (1989), pp. 922–924; Joost

Whereas several articles have been published on international (mainly Anglophone) works of fiction that explore the Parkinson theme, this article will focus on literary writing from the so called Low Countries that deals with the same topic.[5] It presents a selection of six novels in which a central character (often the protagonist) suffers from Parkinson's disease.[6] Aside discussing the various ways in which these works depict Parkinson's disease, we also examine the ways in which the disease impacts on the plot of the narrative and the narrative function that Parkinson's disease performs within the larger story. The question that we will address is not only in how far and how Parkinson's disease plays a role in determining the course of events, but also how it triggers reflection on various other dimensions of human existence. We will argue that depictions of Parkinson's disease and its symptoms in these works of fiction often function as metaphors that enable reflection on complicated and often precarious existential issues.

Before we start our analyses it seems useful to have a quick glance into the field of medicine again, in order to point out some associations between this field and that of literature (and literary studies).[7] The use of metaphors is considered

---

HAAN, 'Protagonists with Parkinson's disease', in: *Literary Medicine: Brain diseases and doctors in novels, theater, and film*, Basel 2013; JULIEN BOGOUSSLAVSKY and SEBASTIAN DIEGUEZ (eds.), *Frontiers of Neurology and Neuroscience*, 31 (2013), pp. 178–187; JOOST HAAN and FRANS MEULENBERG, *De trillende tuinman en andere parkinsonbeelden*, Houten 2009; KERRIE L. SCHOFFER and JOHN D. O'SULLIVAN, 'Charles Dickens: The man, medicine, and movement disorders', in: *Journal of Clinical Neuroscience* 13 (2006), pp. 898–901; RAGNAR STIEN, 'Shakespeare on Parkinsonism', in: *Movement Disorders* 20 (2005), pp. 768–769; H. VOSS, 'The representation of movement disorders in fictional literature', in: *Journal of Neurology, Neurosurgery and Psychiatry* 83 (2012), pp. 994–999; OLIVER SACKS, *Awakenings*, Pennsylvania 1973. Cf. Joost HAAN and FRANS MEULENBERG, *De trillende Tuinman*, Houten 2009.

5 This topic has not been the object of literary research yet. The Dutch scientists H. VAN DER BRUGGEN and G. WIDDERSHOVEN refer to the novels *Een grote blauwe cirkel* [A big blue circle] by P. LOECKX and *Ik was een meisje met grote ogen en een strik* [I was a girl with big eyes and a ribbon] by H. VAN DAELE in an article for the journal *Medicine, Health Care and Philosophy* 7 (2004), pp. 289–301. Most of the novels discussed in our article have not been translated into English. JEROEN BROUWERS' *Bezonken rood* (Amsterdam 1981), translated as *Sunken red* (New York 1988) by Adrienne Dixon, is an exception. Translations of citations, unless mentioned otherwise, by JH.

6 Our selection leaves out works of fiction in which minor characters suffer from Parkinson's disease, as is the case in JAN WOLKERS' *Brandende liefde* [Burning love] (Texel 1981) and in the eponymous story from *De meisjes van de suikerwerkfabriek* [The girls from the sugar factory] (Amsterdam 1983) by T. DE LOO.

7 The study of the whole spectrum of associations between medical topics and literary texts is known as 'narrative medicine' (R. CHARON, 'Narrative medicine: Form, function, and ethics', in: *Annals of Internal Medicine* 134 [2001], pp. 83–87.) This spectrum contains patients writing about their illnesses (CHARON, p. 83), doctors writing about patients (CHARON, p. 83), students learning to write patient stories (A. A. KAPTEIN, A.C. LYONS, A.S. PEARSON, S. VAN DER GEEST, J. HAAN, F. MEULENBERG and J.M. SMITH, 'Storying stories', in: *Medical Edu-*

very important within medicine, because 'metaphors are inherently creative and meaning expanding'.[8] Especially since Susan Sontag's *Illness as Metaphor* (1978), the classical work on the subject of medical metaphor, this importance of metaphors in relation to the understanding of disease has been broadly acknowledged.[9] In the contact between doctor and patient, metaphors are often used to transfer meaning and make serious information less threatening.[10] Rosenman argues that 'metaphors are vital in medicine by allowing us to conceptualize the unseen', but simultaneously warrants caution as: 'tired metaphors can blinker our view and can lead us down well trodden, but erroneous paths'.[11] It is here, in 'reanimating' such 'dead' metaphors or at least bringing them up for discussion, that fiction, according to Macneil, can play a distinctive role.[12]

Although we principally subscribe to this assumption and our analyses indeed demonstrate the novels' use of both common and more innovative metaphors, in this article we will go a step further by looking beyond the illness-related significance of (medical) metaphors. We will show how the broad spectrum of intriguing aspects that are embodied by, in this case, Parkinson's disease provides ample opportunities for the exploration of matters as diverse as relationships, memory, psychic and behavioral problems, and perceptions of the

cation Development 2 [2012], pp. 24–26), and so-called 'bibliotherapy', described as the therapeutic effect of books (S.J. Jack and R. Ronan, 'Bibliotherapy', in: *School Psychology International* 29 [2008], pp. 161–182). A special educational situation is formed by group readings and discussions by medical students of diseases depicted in novels, for example on autism (S.R. Wooden, 'Narrative medicine in the Literature Classroom: Ethical Pedagogy and Mark Haddon's *The Curious Incident of the Dog in the Night-Time*', in: *Literature and Medicine* 29 [2011], pp. 274–296).

8 H. Brody, *Stories of Sickness*, Oxford 2003. Examples of medical disciplines where metaphors are used to enhance communication between doctors and patients are: pulmonary disease (A.C. Arroliga, S. Newman, D.L. Longworth and J.K. Stoller, 'Metaphorical medicine: Using metaphors to enhance communication with patients who have pulmonary disease', in: *Annals of Internal Medicine* 137 [2002], pp. 376–380), dementia (H. Zeilig, 'Dementia as a cultural metaphor', in: *The Gerontologist* 54 [2014], pp. 258–67) and pain syndromes (Stephen Loftus, 'Pain and its metaphors: A dialogical approach', in: *The Journal of Medical Humanities* 32 [2011], pp. 213–230); and Arthur W. Frank, 'Metaphors of pain', in: *Literature and Medicine* 29 (2011), pp. 182–196).

9 Susan Sontag, *Illness as Metaphor*, New York 1978. Examples are: S. Rosenman, 'Metaphor in clinical practice', in: *Australian Family Physician* 37 (2008), pp. 865–866; V.S. Periyakoil, 'Using metaphor in medicine', in: *Journal of Palliative Medicine* 11 (2008), pp. 842–844; P.U. Macneil, 'The arts and medicine: A challenging relationship', in: *Medical Humanities* 37 (2011), pp. 85–90. Commonly used metaphors in medicine are those associated with war ('fighting cancer'; Periyakoil, p. 842), sports ('winning or losing' 842) and machines ('body as machine' 843).

10 Metaphors are also used to differentiate between diseases that resemble another. See L. Plug, B. Sharrack and M. Reuber, 'Seizure metaphors differ in patients' accounts of epileptic and psychogenic nonepileptic seizures', in: *Epilepsia* 50 (2009), pp. 994–1000.

11 Rosenman, Metaphor in clinical practice (see n. 9), p. 866.

12 Macneil, The arts and medicine: A challenging relationship (see n. 9), p. 89.

self. As it turns out, representations of Parkinson's disease in the selected works of fiction generally come down to much more than what we technically consider the symptoms of the disease.

3 (Not) Accepting Parkinson's Disease

The first novel that we discuss is *Een grote blauwe cirkel* [A big blue circle] (1994), written by the Flemish author Paula Loeckx. Marcus Holten, one of the main characters in this novel, has Parkinson's disease. An external narrator describes how his hands shake and his handwriting has become illegible – like an 'artistic scrawl' as his secretary puts it.[13] When Marcus raises himself from a chair, he becomes dizzy. He has problems when walking, the speed of his steps is gone and his gait is shuffling and irregular. The novel describes how Marcus has become 'rigid in body and mind', even so much so that his face is said to resemble a mask.[14] Dopamine treatment helps to undo some of the afflictions, but simultaneously this treatment causes severe side effects.

Central in *Een grote blauwe cirkel* is Marcus' struggle with the acceptance of his illness. Denial appears to be the novel's central theme: denial by the Parkinson victim Marcus as well as by Judith, his wife, who considers herself to be a victim of the disease as well. At first, Marcus denies having Parkinson's disease: 'No, he did not have the disease. He had a nervous tick; his thumb and index finger rubbed against each other continuously, but that was all.'[15] His denial even goes as far as refusing to mention the name 'Parkinson.'[16] As the illness progresses, however, it becomes increasingly difficult to deny its reality. Marcus starts to need the help of Judith for dressing and washing, and he begins to visit a psychologist for mood disturbances. The fact that he has become impotent strongly troubles his self-perception as a male: it makes him feel castrated.

More and more, Marcus realizes the inevitability of his disease which prompts him to search for an explanation: he wants to understand why it is him who has fallen victim to this illness. Rather than relieving his mind, however, this search leads him into a web of reproach, guilt and penance. This happens, for instance, when he thinks back of his childhood: 'Standing in the corner, being sent to bed early, no dessert, a tap on the cheek, flick on the pants, terms of abuse, harangues, hits on the bare bottom.'[17] The main cause of this misery, described in his childhood recollections, seems to be his father, although Marcus himself refrains

13 Loeckx, Een grote blauwe cirkel (see for reference n. 4, J. Haan and F. Meulenberg), p. 13.
14 Loeckx, Een grote blauwe cirkel (see n. 13), p. 49.
15 Loeckx, Een grote blauwe cirkel (see n. 13), p. 5.
16 Loeckx, Een grote blauwe cirkel (see n. 13), p. 9.
17 Loeckx, Een grote blauwe cirkel (see n. 13), p. 24.

from downright accusations and forgivingly suggests that probably his father also had his own problems. In his words: 'Maybe father had too much work, too many sorrows, too many children [...]'.[18] Nevertheless, the result of his father's behaviour on Marcus' self-esteem is devastating: 'I have never been good enough as I was, just, myself, a little hesitant boy'.[19]

As already mentioned, it is an external narrator who tells the story of Marcus' downfall. The focus in the twenty-four chapters is, however, divided between Marcus (eleven chapters) and Judith (thirteen chapters). The 'Marcus chapters' deal with his struggle to cope with the disease and to simultaneously keep Judith's support. By use of flashbacks as the one described above, it becomes clear that a major part of Marcus' upbringing consisted of punishment. Now Marcus feels punished again, this time by the disease. Also Judith has problems accepting his illness. She is ashamed of him when he drops his book in church; she cannot accept his impotence and she finds his shuffling gait repulsive. The adulterous relationship that she starts seems an answer to the growing repulsion that she feels towards her husband.

Already in chapter three, the first chapter focalized by Judith, Timothy, her future lover, is introduced. As readers we witness how, after initial hesitation, Judith responds to Timothy's advances. The remaining of the 'Judith chapters' describe how she struggles with a dilemma caused by her split feelings: these oscillate between the wish to remain 'honest' to her diseased husband on the one hand and the desire to continue the relationship with her lover on the other.

At a certain point in the narrative, Judith goes on a trip with Timothy as an escape out of the home situation with Marcus. He, however, finds out about this and from this moment onwards his tremor and also his despair become worse. This downward movement is best illustrated in the scene where Marcus finds himself shouting 'stop, stop shaking!' to his own 'hated hand.'[20] It is in this moment of utmost despair that Marcus decides that only a positive attitude towards his disease can help him. He hopes to get Judith's support in this, but in the course of the novel this hope appears to be in vain: she is no longer on his side, but instead choses for herself and her lover.

Aside denial and acceptance, the loss of control over one's body is another important theme in the novel. In their article 'Being a Parkinson's Patient: Immobile and Unpredictably Whimsical' Van der Bruggen and Widdershoven describe this process as follows: 'To the Parkinson's patient the body is first something one *is*, then something one *has*, and finally something one *no longer*

18 Loeckx, Een grote blauwe cirkel (see n. 13), p. 39.
19 Loeckx, Een grote blauwe cirkel (see n. 13), p. 39.
20 Loeckx, Een grote blauwe cirkel (see n. 13), p. 125.

has – almost in chronological order.'[21] This description applies to Marcus as well. At a certain point, Marcus looks at his body-parts from a distance, his movements are called artificial. The space that his increasingly uncontrollable body occupies progressively becomes smaller, first being limited to the house, then to one room, a wheelchair, his bed. This reduction of Marcus' mobility, and thus of his existence, is symbolized in several scenes that describe how he is unable to stand up from a chair or to rise from his bed. Van der Bruggen and Widdershoven argue that it is especially the contrast between excess (the tremor) and lack of movement (stiffness, also called rigidity), as well as that between being 'immobile and unpredictably whimsical' that appeals to novelists' imagination.[22] It is the disease's contradictory combination of petrifaction and slowing down with a continuous and rapid movement of the hands that seems to offer unique opportunities for addressing conflicts within characters. In fact, it is this contrast that can make the sufferer of Parkinson's disease become a contradiction within him- or herself, as seems to be the case with Marcus.

Een grote blauwe cirkel provides a bitter insight in the problems individuals can have in dealing with a serious disease such as Parkinson's. The novel shows that coming to terms with a situation of illness depends on many factors, that can include marriage problems, education, prejudices, etc. The narrative even seems to suggest that these factors contribute to the disease by increasing its symptoms, or that they are in some way intertwined with the disease itself. The novel, for example, prompts the reader to consider whether Marcus is impotent because of his disease or because of the problems in his marriage, which in their turn can again be a result of his disease. A similar question arises in relation to his depression: is the depression a reaction to his disease, an intrinsic component of the disease, or a result of the problems with his wife? By opening up these various possibilities the novel's depiction of Parkinson's disease offers more than a mere representation of the disease. It appears that within the narrative, the disease not only functions to illustrate fundamental aspects of being human, such as our self-image and our relation to our body, but it also serves as a catalyst that throws doubt on the protagonists' relationship. Parkinson's disease more or less forces Marcus to put his fate completely in Judith's hands. Judith, however, who is only indirectly affected by the disease and still in full control of her self, makes an ambivalent decision about her relationship with Marcus. She tells Timothy that she is going to join Marcus on a six week journey to Holland, but nevertheless promises Timothy to phone him twice a week.[23] As a reader, one's empathy shifts from Marcus to Judith. Marcus is the one with the disease, Par-

21 Van der Bruggen and Widdershoven, Being a Parkinson's patient (see n. 5), p. 292.
22 Van der Bruggen and Widdershoven, Being a Parkinson's patient (see n. 5), p. 290.
23 Loeckx, Een grote blauwe cirkel (see n. 13), p. 136.

kinson's actual victim, but his way of dealing with the situation – his initial denial, then his attempt to master it without prospects, and then a complete surrender in which he puts his fate, and thus all responsibility, in someone else's hands – in the end does not produce much sympathy.

Judith, in her turn, does her best to envision the impact of the disease on her husband, but is simultaneously overwhelmed by the impact of the disease on her own situation. The fact that she chooses to start an affair can be considered disloyal, but she 'defends' herself by pointing out that Marcus himself had many affairs in the time that he was still healthy. It seems that Parkinson's disease in this novel is just one element in a complex human relationship, in which factors such as personal history, ambitions, expectations, and frustration play a role as well. A disease can shift the balance and change the overall situation. That is what this novel most clearly shows. For Judith, it seems, there is an escape, whereas Marcus is caught in the ever-tightening grasp of being a Parkinson patient.

4 Mother, Son and Parkinson

The second work that we will discuss is the short autobiographic novel *Bezonken rood* [*Sunken Red*] by the Dutch author Jeroen Brouwers. In a retrospective narrative, this novel describes in horrible detail the occurrences in the Japanese internment camp Tjideng in 1945. This camp, located on the isle of Java, at that time part of the Dutch East Indies (now Indonesia),[24] was inhabited by women and children under the age of ten. In 1945, Jeroen, the first-person narrator of *Bezonken rood*, was five years old. He lived in one of the huts with his grandmother, mother and sister. Using flashbacks, he describes how the days in the camp were filled with hunger, disease, death and, one of the most shocking elements, the sadism of the Japanese guards. In the eyes of a five year old, however, the routine in the camp looks innocent. Some things even seem funny to him, such as the marching of the Japanese guards and the punitive expeditions in which all women and children had to sit in the burning sun for hours and hop like frogs.

When Jeroen's mother dies, thirty years later, her death prompts the now adult Jeroen to go back to his memories and to reinterpret their mother-son relationship. He admits to himself that he is, in fact afraid, to go to her funeral, out of shame about how he has treated and neglected her. By the end of her life,

24 Indonesia, the current name of the archipelago in South East Asia, dates back to the 18th century, but in the time that the islands were subjected to Dutch colonial rule the name 'Dutch East Indies' was mostly used. After gaining independence in 1949, the name Indonesia was introduced again as the official name of the new nation-state.

his mother suffered from Parkinson's disease: 'her head and hands trembled, her mouth fell open and her tongue hung out.'[25] Jeroen did not visit her during the last years of her life and had never even seen her disease: 'I never saw it, because I did not want to see it.'[26] Now, he takes tranquilizers to avoid anxiety attacks. Thinking back in an effort to understand his present state of mind, he realizes that it was in the camp that he lost the love for his mother.

His anxiety attacks appear directly related to his childhood experiences in the camp. Images from the camp seem to have taken possession of him. He remembers how a guard raped a Dutch woman. How beautiful his little girlfriend Nettie looked after her horrible death. How his grandmother slowly wasted away and died, and how he could not bear the smell of her dying body. The most penetrating image, however, is that of his mother. How she had to stand outside for days and nights in the sun and in the rain as a punishment for small offences. After (or as a result of) this torture, Jeroen does not recognize her as his mother anymore. She has become skinny as a skeleton, she has lost her hair and her breasts have disappeared. To the small boy she does not even look human anymore. Retrospectively, witnessing the repeated torture of his mother turns out to have been a traumatizing experience. Especially one particular instance of violence has been of crucial impact on the later mother-son-relationship. In the scene that describes this violence, the mother is beaten by the guards in front of her son. They kick and hit her everywhere, also between her legs, a spot that to Jeroen, literally and symbolically, the site of his origin:

> It is as if the Japs, with their weapons, mean to beat my mother into the ground right through the asphalt. [The Japanese guard named] Sone personally kicks her between her legs with his boots that jingle as if there are bells on them, and I witness it personally. Beware, Sone. I am that little boy in the crowd and my eyes nearly pop out as I watch. [...] My mother bleeds where I came out of her with a head like a cobblestone. I feel her pain between my own legs, as if I myself had received a bayonet thrust in that place; my mother's wounds will have to be stitched up with a curved needle.[27]

The climax of this dramatic scene is located in the naive disappointment of the little boy Jeroen: 'My mother was the most beautiful mother; at that moment I ceased to love her' after which the narration shifts to the adult Jeroen who adds that 'from that moment I lost my way.'[28] Here the loss of the mother and the loss of orientation in life are brought together. Looking back after so many years makes him realize that this was a formative moment in which he learned that

---

25 Brouwers, Sunken Red (see for reference J. Haan and F. Meulenberg n. 4), p. 14.
26 Brouwers, Sunken Red (see n. 25), p. 14.
27 Brouwers, Sunken Red (see n. 25), pp. 121–122.
28 Brouwers, Sunken Red (see n. 25), p. 122. In the same scene the young boy even concludes: 'now I want a different mother, because this one is broken.'

loving someone makes you vulnerable: you have a lot to lose. It is this experience that makes him develop a distaste for life, and a longing to no longer exist.

There are also feelings of shame which grow on Jeroen in the narrative present, thus constituting a link between past and present, but also between his mother and himself. The major link between mother and son in the present, however, is Parkinson's disease: Jeroen not only suffers from attacks of fear, but he also develops symptoms of Parkinson's disease. Like his mother, he trembles, has a mask-like face, walks with difficulty and becomes increasingly immobile. And this is where fear and fact meet: to a certain extent Jeroen has become (like) his mother.

Like in Loeckx' *Een grote blauwe cirkel*, depictions of Parkinson's disease in Brouwers' *Bezonken rood* touch on existential themes. Here, it is the pathological parallel between mother and son that constitutes an extra trigger in Jeroen's feelings of shame and fear. In this sense, the novel is much more than a 'neutral' pathography, or a biography of himself and his mother. Within the narrative, aspects of the mother's Parkinson's disease work to evoke and direct Jeroen's reaction to his past as well as to his present situation. It is as if he perceives of the present through a mirror that is located in the past. He feels that his own petrifaction in fact already started in the concentration camp when he was a toddler. It was already there and then that he had become rigid, anxious, depressed, and bothered by tremors. Simultaneously, in close interconnection with this petrifaction, the horrible occurrences in the camp effected the loss of love for his mother, a state of emotional deprivation continuing to the present day. In a similar way that Jeroen no longer felt able to love his mother, he has lost the ability to love himself. It is Parkinson's disease, and especially the repetition of this disease within the disturbed family structure, that enlarges the tragic bond between the unloved (or too much loved) mother and her son.

5 Terminal Parkinson's Disease

Our third example, the autobiographical narrative *Uitdorsten* (*Thirsting out*) by the Dutch writer A.F.Th. van der Heijden was first published, together with another autobiographical narrative titled *Asbestemming* (*Ash destination*) in the collection *De Requiems (The Requiems*, 2003).[29] Whereas *Asbestemming* describes the death of first-person narrator Adri's father, *Uitdorsten* focuses on the death of his mother, who suffered from a severe form of Parkinson's disease.

29 In 2007 *Uitdorsten* is reprinted as an independent publication. The full title now is *Uitdorsten. Klein requiem voor mama, mam, ma* [Thirsting out. Small requiem for mummy, mum, ma].

Again, we see the by now familiar description of Parkinson's disease symptoms. The narrator describes how his mother's hands shake, how she looks in frozen bewilderment, and how her movements have turned into a shuffling gait. He regularly does so in a tongue-in-cheek way, for instance when he compares her unwilful and rather awkward hand movements with the waving of the queen. However, despite the fact that her illness heavily restricts her agency, the mother responds to the joke by mumbling a word that ends on '-aus'.[30] In that moment, Adri does not understand his mother. Only later he realizes that this syllable could either have referred to 'Claus' (the husband of the Dutch queen Beatrix, who suffered from Parkinson's disease) or to 'Paus' (pope John Paul, who suffered from the disease as well): 'fellow-sufferers in the battle against Parkinson.'[31] This belated insight points out a scene of misunderstanding that tragically depicts the heavy limitations that Parkinson's disease sets not only to the sufferer's self-control, but also to this person's interaction with others. Simultaneously, however, the particular representation of the situation of misunderstanding that pivots on word-fragments and failed communication also bring about an ironic, even humorous reading-effect.

The narrative describes how the mother, while growing more and more unstable, starts to fall quite regularly. It happens several times that she has been lying on the floor for hours before someone finds her and helps her to get up. It is because of these problems that she desires to move to a safer place, a place where she is better looked after. Finding such a place, however, appears difficult; 'nowhere was room for her'.[32]

At a certain point, the mother is admitted to a home for the elderly in Eindhoven. After a couple of months there, Adri talks to a doctor and discusses his conversation with his mother:

> 'Mama, I want to discuss a couple of things the doctor said to me yesterday evening on the phone...' Whispering, squeaking she says: 'He is lying'. 'Lying... about what?'. After a lot of what I understand: 'Faith... trust... not to be trusted.' 'Why is he not to be trusted?' '...lying...' 'He lies... that you do not want to be helped by 'sleeping', as he mentioned it?' Then she starts, squeaking as an animal, to cry quietly. 'Dead... Not dead...' 'You do not want to die. Of course not. Let's not run ahead of things.'[33]

Despite Adri's attempts at reassurance, his mother remains convinced that they are going to murder her by denying fluids. She is afraid that they want to 'thirst her out'.

30 A. F. Th. van der Heijden, 'Uitdorsten', in: *De Requiems*, Amsterdam 2003 (see for reference J. Haan and F. Meulenberg n. 4), p. 474.
31 Van der Heijden, Uitdorsten (see n. 30), p. 474.
32 Van der Heijden, Uitdorsten (see n. 30), p. 453.
33 Van der Heijden, Uitdorsten (see n. 30), p. 457.

Soon after, a doctor again talks to Adri, his brother and his sister in order to come to a decision about how to proceed and especially also when to stop the treatment of their mother. Adri asks him to make sure that their mother gets sufficient liquids, adequate medication, and tube feeding. Moreover, he requests that if all this turns out ineffective, everything will be done so that she has a soft way of slowly passing away. The doctor agrees, but only after describing the apparent advantages of 'thirsting out'. He explains that the aim of this procedure is definitely 'not to let someone die, but to decrease suffering of someone who is dying already. [In this situation] thirst is not experienced as thirst.'[34] To Adri's surprise, the doctor nevertheless vehemently refuses to call 'thirsting out' a form of euthanasia.

In *Uitdorsten*, we again see that the theme of Parkinson's disease is linked to the discussion of other existential issues, but in a different way than in the novels previously discussed. Here, the focus is not so much on Parkinson's disease itself, but it is used as a stepping-stone for discussing controversial themes such as euthanasia and end-of-life decisions. *Uitdorsten* gives voice to various perspectives on the matter and raises difficult medical and ethical questions about how to deal with such a situation. It is the cynicism of the helpless narrator in combination with the anxious mother that brings about the most poignant affective insights in the matter. For instance, in the scene where the mother starts crying, when she hears that her sons have convinced the doctor to give her more to drink. In this situation, Adri reacts as follows: 'Here she lies crying from gratitude that the hangman has loosened the halter for a while to give her some extra air.'[35]

Some weeks after the conversation with the doctor, very 'late at night', an acquaintance tells him that his mother is very sick.[36] In that particular moment Adri has a very dry throat caused by a hangover (in Dutch: 'nadorst'), and is also slightly trembling because of this. Some minutes later, while he is preparing himself to drive to Eindhoven, the telephone rings. His mother has died. In this moment the parallel between mother and son is striking: as if her symptoms (thirst, trembling) are transposed onto him. The dry throat after his alcohol over-consumption constitutes an acrid link: as if in the moment of the announcement of her death he himself experiences her 'thirsting out'.

The stepping-stone function of Parkinson's disease for the discussion of end-of-life-questions is even more clear in the scene that takes place after the mother's passing away, when the doctor proposes to do an autopsy 'to check

34 Van der Heijden, Uitdorsten (see n. 30), p. 462.
35 Van der Heijden, Uitdorsten (see n. 30), p. 462.
36 Van der Heijden, Uitdorsten (see n. 30), p. 463.

whether she really suffered from Parkinson's disease'.[37] The proposal sounds amazing to Adri and starts off a range of questions in his head. Does this not imply, if it turns out that his mother was indeed not suffering from Parkinson's disease, that she has been taking the wrong medication for many years? And an even more piercing question: does this mean that she could have been saved, if only the right diagnosis had been made? A more reassuring inner voice tells Adri that his mother simply had all the symptoms that are considered typical for Parkinson's disease. 'Just like prince Claus' she shuffled, suffered from bouts of depression, and had a blocked posture. In the case that she had not been suffering from Parkinson's disease, she suffered from a disease that imitated Parkinson's down to the minutest details: 'Now we only need the name of this plagiary disease, and we are where we want to be.'[38]

6 Parkinson in a Soldier

Like in Brouwers' *Bezonken rood*, the colonial past features as a point of reference for the main protagonist in the fourth novel that we discuss: Maria Vonk's *Oude soldaten sterven niet* [Old soldiers never die] (2008). Piet, the first-person narrator in the novel, served as a soldier in the Dutch forces in the former East-Indies, both before and after the Second World War. In this capacity, he participated in the now heavily contested 'police actions', the euphemism used in the late 1940's (and long after) to refer to the colonial war against the Indonesian fighters for independence. In the narrative present, Piet is a sufferer of Parkinson's disease. He lives in a nursing home out of necessity, because he is no longer able to get out of bed himself. He needs help to go to the toilet and wears diapers, a clear indication of his dependence. His disease causes stiffness, trembling hands, and great difficulty with walking. Besides this all, Piet is also very confused. Often he does not understand why he is sitting among these old people and at several occasions he starts crying without a concrete reason. The reader learns about Piet's present situation in the chapters with odd chapter numbers. The even-numbered chapters are dedicated to the past and, through the use of flashbacks, provide a more or less chronological account of Piet's life-story.

The story of Piet's life is not a very happy one. He spent his childhood in Amsterdam, together with his ten siblings and his father. His mother died when he was still very young. The father is described as a very unsympathetic character. He earns some money, but spends it all without thinking of his responsibility for the family. He not only treats his children badly, he even abuses his

37 Van der Heijden, Uitdorsten (see n. 30), p. 471.
38 Van der Heijden, Uitdorsten (see n. 30), p. 471.

oldest daughter by forcing her to have sex with him. Piet remembers how he and the other children could hear her cry, at one occasion Piet even witnesses the abuse. Another sister has tuberculosis and one day suddenly disappears. The reader can only guess what has happened to her, but it is clear that the father does not mind too much, as it means that he has one mouth less to feed.

At a certain point, Piet manages to escape from this precarious home situation by joining the army. Soon afterwards, he is sent to the Dutch colonial territories in South-East-Asia. There he learns to speak Malay and, as he himself in disturbingly euphemistic language announces, 'paints the town red'.[39] After three years of service, he returns to the Netherlands again where he now meets Mien who is soon to become his wife. They get married out of 'necessity': she is pregnant.[40] Mien feels upset about this, but Piet is extremely happy. In 1946, Piet is conscripted to return to the Dutch Indies, this time to participate in the aforementioned 'police actions'.

Whereas in these even-numbered chapters, Piet presents a quiet sober depiction of his life, these occurences return as memories in the odd-numbered chapters that are set in the present. This applies in particular to what happened in what is now Indonesia: these occurrences return as ghosts, as demons from the past. Piet clearly struggles with his past, and his general confusion only seems to increase this effect. As the reader starts to realize, Piet is not only suffering from Parkinson's disease, but it is also Alzheimer's disease that disturbs his memory. The symptoms of the latter importantly impacts on the narrative. Piet's cognitive, Alzheimer-related problems, but also his apparent naivety, make him a very unreliable narrator.

Dutch national history and Piet's personal memories grow more and more intertwined. At times it seems as if he is hallucinating, experiencing the horrors of his military mission in the former colony anew. 'The massacres, the screaming children, the raped and murdered women, the extreme fatigue and especially the loneliness and my longing for her…'[41] It is striking that the content of these hallucinations does not seem to affect Piet's judgment on his presence in the colony when he is in a clearer state of mind. In one suchlike moment for instance, Piet is vaguely aware of the fact that the military actions in the former Dutch colony are not beyond controversy. Despite the traumatic memories that terrorize his mind during hallucinations, he nevertheless defends the actions as necessary interventions at that time in history. This happens, for example, in the scene in which Piet remembers arriving in Rotterdam by boat, after a long period

39 Maria Vonk, *Oude soldaten sterven niet*, Amsterdam/Antwerpen 2008 (see for reference Haan and Meulenberg n. 4), p. 35.

40 Vonk, Oude soldaten sterven niet (see n. 39), p. 83.

41 Vonk, Oude soldaten sterven niet (see n. 39), p. 147.

of service in Indonesia. The crowd in the harbor 'welcomes' him and his fellow-soldiers with aggression, calling them murderers.[42] In the narrative present Piet responds to this memory by postulating: 'But we have killed no one. On the contrary, we have helped the poor residents as much as we could.'[43]

The combination of Parkinson's disease with Alzheimer's disease, a combination that is actually not uncommon, confuses the symptoms of both diseases considerably. In *Oude soldaten sterven niet*, it is Parkinson's disease that predominantly establishes the image of Piet's physical deterioration and of his helplessness. On the contrary, the confusion and loss of memory, features that grow more and more central to the odd-numbered chapters, appear primarily connected to Alzheimer's disease. Together these illnesses contribute to the depiction of a painful and ambivalent process of simultaneous self-discovery and loss of self. Or as Piet phrases it, in a combined moment of self-evaluation and self-denial: 'There are mirrors everywhere. I try not to look in them, because then I see a little old fellow. And I am afraid that the little old fellow could be me.'[44]

7 Parkinson in a Girl

The interference of Parkinson's disease with Alzheimer's disease also plays an important role in Henri Van Daele's short novella *Ik was een meisje met grote ogen en een strik* (*I was a girl with big eyes and a ribbon*, 1991), our fifth case. However, while Vonk's novel focused on the tribulations of a male protagonist, the Flemish writer Van Daele presents his readers with a female protagonist, the eponymous 'girl with big eyes and a ribbon'. As the novella's title already indicates, the first-person narrator is a girl no more; on the contrary, in the present of the narrative, 'Moe' as she is now called, is an old woman, hospitalized and suffering from both motoric disruptions, such as trembling, mumbling and decreased mobility, and confusion. As the narrative form used is that of the monologue, the reader realizes that Moe is as much aware of her disease as she is of her physical and mental deterioration. For instance, when she cynically comments on the path-breaking findings of the name-giver of 'her' disease: 'Parkinson is a chap who took notice of hands. A doctor for the hands. He also studied drooling. And people who fall off stairs. When you describe a disease for the first time, you are allowed to give it your own name. It is a way to become

42 Vonk, Oude soldaten sterven niet (see n. 39), p. 141.
43 Vonk, Oude soldaten sterven niet (see n. 39), p. 142.
44 Vonk, Oude soldaten sterven niet (see n. 39), p. 166.

famous, searching for diseases.'[45] Her cynical comments on the broad range of pills that she has to take because of her diseases can be seen as another proof of her critical awareness of her situation: 'One for songs and stories. One for my hands. One to keep my head upright. One against drooling and one against falling. And then there is the upper-pill, to learn to regulate all other pills.'[46]

As we saw in the previous case of Piet, also Moe's memories get mixed up with hallucinations. This becomes evident, for example, when she starts talking to her husband and her father-in-law who both have been dead for years. Also, her mentioning of improbable situations works to illustrate her confusion: in the one moment she thinks she is on a trip with the cycling champion Eddy Merckx and with the famous Belgian singer Will Ventura; in another she believes that movie star Farah Fawcett is one of her nurses.[47] The reader realizes very well that Moe is not a reliable narrator. This, however, does not mean that one cannot identify with her and her fate. On the contrary, Moe's is a moving story, as it enables the reader to experience her growing dependence and confusion in the process of reading.

It is the particular narrative frame-work within which Moe's monologue is presented that in its turn works to undo this identificatory effect. *Ik was een meisje met grote ogen en een strik* opens with an instruction for reading that emphasizes the fictional character of the text and is signed 'H.v.D.': 'This is not a report, but a story. Readers who think they recognize themselves or a situation that is known to them in what follows, I want to ask to keep the definition of both genres explicitly in mind, irrespective of how much the words that follow will move them.'[48] What follows after this warning, is a listing of the characters in the text, as if we are dealing with the listing of the cast in a theatre play. In this list, Moe is introduced as one of the characters: 'Almost seventy. More than 10 years Parkinson. Housewife. Four children. Widow of Bi-Beer (nickname).' The list not only introduces the characters, among them 'several nurses (overworked)' and 'several patients (who complain about the food…)', but also positions them in relation to each other.[49] About Moe's husband, Bi-Beer, the list for instance informs us that he, despite his death in 1983, is '[s]till very present'.[50] Thus, the list functions to underline the monologue's fictional character.

45 Henri Van Daele, *Ik was een meisje met grote ogen en een strik* (see for reference J. Haan and F. Meulenberg n. 4), p. 16.

46 Van Daele, Ik was een meisje met grote ogen en een strik (see n. 45), p. 42.

47 Van Daele, Ik was een meisje met grote ogen en een strik (see n. 45), p. 24.

48 'Dit is geen reportage, maar een verhaal. Lezers die zichzelf of een toestand die hen bekend is, menen te herkennen in wat volgt, wil ik vragen de definities van beide genres uitdrukkelijk voor ogen te houden, hoezeer de woorden die volgen hen ook aangrijpen', Van Daele, *Ik was een meisje met grote ogen en een strik* (see n. 45), p. 5.

49 Van Daele, Ik was een meisje met grote ogen en een strik (see n. 45), p. 7.

50 Van Daele, Ik was een meisje met grote ogen en een strik (see n. 45), pp. 6–7.

At the very end of Moe's affectively impactful monologue we find another 'neutralizing' intervention. In a kind of postscript a Belgian professor in Neurology 'Prof. Dr. R. Dom Kliniekhoofd Neurologie Universitaire Ziekenhuizen K.U.-Leuven' (Chairman in Neurology of the Academic Hospital in Leuven, Belgium) provides some matter-of-fact background information on the cause, course, symptoms and treatment of Parkinson's disease.[51] This postscript has no direct relation whatsoever with Moe's dramatic monologue and in terms of style the medical text even forms a striking and sobering contrast to the preceding text. As if the writer, by concluding with a presentation of facts, again wants to point out that Moe's story has been fictitious, and warn the reader not to take it at face value. Together with the framing preceding the monologue, the postscript works to create a distance between the reader and Moe's moving story. In a more critical vein, it can even be argued that this framing works to undo the affective impact of the story by turning Moe's monologue into a spectacle. As such, her account transforms into a medical case-report, and she – disputably – ends up as an exemplary 'freak' in a freak-show.

8 Hallucinating Parkinson's Disease

Our last case-study, the short novel *Duivelskermis* (*Devil's carnival*, 2007) by Gerrit Krol, differs from the previous ones in that Krol (who passed away in 2013) himself actually suffered from Parkinson's disease. This means that Krol could draw on the 'inside knowledge' of experience that the other writers lack. Krol has never made a secret of his disease and referred to it in various interviews.[52] However, also in the introduction of *Duivelskermis*, Krol relates about aspects of his disease and how they impact on his daily life. It is on this paratextual level that the by now familiar Parkinson's disease's symptoms are presented to the reader: Krol narrates how he suffers from trembling hands, has problems starting up, feels uncertain when he is walking and has inclinations to fall. Besides, he informs the reader that he experiences very lively hallucinations.

It is the particular narrative form of the introduction that forcefully makes the reader aware of the shifting personalities caused by Parkinson's disease. The opening lines of the piece are written in the third-person singular, as if providing objective information about the various aspects of the disease: the tremor, the walking problems, the growing hesitation. Then, after a few lines, Krol switches

51 Van Daele, Ik was een meisje met grote ogen en een strik (see n. 45), pp. 89–91.
52 D. Serdijn, 'Op zoek naar Maria in Zuid-Limburg', *NRC Handelsblad* 2007; A. Fortuin, 'Het Gedemoniseerde Hoofd. Gerrit Krols nieuwe Roman is een Pijnlijke Nederlaag', *de Volkskrant* 2007.

to a first-person narrative and describes his own hallucinations, and especially the frightening demons that have started to haunt his mind. Then, in the following lines, this first-person narrator directly includes the reader in his reflections, by using a generalized 'you': 'They are in your toilet, walk in your garden. They are passengers on the back seat of your car. And you do not notice.'[53] This strategy has a threatening effect: the use of the generalized 'you' underlines the seeming arbitrariness of who falls victim to the disease, and in doing so causes feelings of discomfort in the reader. The message that this can happen to anyone, and that if so you will not even notice, is clearly very disturbing.

In a next step, Krol emphasizes that the most important feature of the hallucinations that often come with the disease is that the person suffering from them does not recognize them as such. He describes the extreme difficulty to distinguish between reality and hallucination. The climax of this warning message about the mercilessness of Parkinson's disease comes in the last paragraph of the introduction, when he writes: 'Sometimes you are a demon yourself.'[54] This sentence makes clear that not only your perception can be hallucinatory, but also who and what you are, your self-understanding. This seems the ultimate uncertainty: when suffering from Parkinson's disease there is nothing that one can be sure of, not even oneself. It is this chilling insight that also pervades the narrative of *Duivelskermis.*

The protagonist and first-person narrator of *Duivelskermis* is named Albert (rather than Gerrit), a gesture that works to underline the fictional character of the novel and that, after the autobiographical revelations in the introduction, frustrates an all-too-easy autobiographical reading. Albert, however, suffers from very much the same symptoms as described in the introduction. He, too, struggles with stiffness, hesitation, trembling, and extreme slowness, this last being a factor that especially hampers him when trying to make love. Moreover, he suffers from emotional disturbances, on-off phenomena (fluctuating symptoms of the disease) and hallucinations in which demons and devils torture his mind.

At the beginning of the novel, Albert relates how he starts on a journey to Maastricht. There, he hopes to find Maria, an old love of his. His search appears very chaotic, mostly as a result of the fact that his thoughts are constantly dominated by hallucinations. The reader is prompted to accompany Albert on his journey, but soon finds out that this journey is predominantly a struggle with

53 Gerrit Krol, *Duivelskermis*, Amsterdam/Antwerpen 2007 (see for reference J. Haan and F. Meulenberg n. 4), p. 6.
54 Krol, Duivelskermis (see n. 53), p. 7.

his hallucinations.[55] What is real, what is fantasy? It is not only Albert who cannot distinguish between actual experiences and hallucinations, but also the reader struggles to get a grip on what is happening in the narrative. For instance in the sequence in which Albert attends a so-called 'décolleté contest ' (a beauty contest of sorts) together with his friend Josefina. He easily gets aroused, which he explains by pointing out that Parkinson's disease makes him horny.[56] Albert reveals how he is allowed to 'mount' several of the competitors in the contest, information that gives reason to doubt. When Albert mentions that he suspects that the breasts of one of these women are made of 'tropical wood', the reader cannot but strongly question the reliability of Albert's narration.

When Albert finally finds Maria, he assesses that she has been pregnant for four years. She has a boyfriend, so Albert leaves her again. Then, he stays with another friend, Irmgard, who expresses her concern about his health situation: 'She started to bother him on Parkinson again. 'How old are you?' 'Thirty' 'Then you do not have Parkinson, father.''[57] Albert stays in bed with Irmgard for two days. During this time, she takes his dopamine drugs away from him, which surprisingly causes Albert's condition to slightly improve. 'I see no demons anymore. Irmgard could have been a demon, but for that she is too beautiful.'[58] This assessment, however, soon turns out premature. A first hint – one that the reader tends to take as a joke – is the following conversation between Albert and Irmgard: ''Do I not have something devilish?', she asked when we were standing in the garden. 'Yes, now that you mention it. You have the outset of horns'.'[59] In the final chapter, titled 'The end', this 'joke' acquires a new dimension. This happens when at a certain point Irmgard teases Albert and challenges him by saying: 'Come get me, if you can.'[60] Albert accepts this challenge and runs after her, at least that is the reality that the narrative presents us with. He stumbles and falls in a hole, which turns out to be a grave, ready and waiting for him. Irmgard stands at the edge of the grave, as if she is the devil tempting him in her trap. According to the novel's final words, she is 'glad with her new acquisition'.[61]

Clearly, this narrative is far from straightforward. Facts are distorted, images are deformed, several realities exist aside each other. This positions the novel within the realm of postmodernism. Ontological doubt, a central theme within postmodernist fiction according to literary theorist Brian McHale (1987), plays

55 KROL, Duivelskermis (see n. 53), p. 6.
56 The word that is used in the Dutch text is 'krols', and – coincidentally? – happens to call the writer's surname to mind.
57 KROL, Duivelskermis (see n. 53), p. 72.
58 KROL, Duivelskermis (see n. 53), p. 76.
59 KROL, Duivelskermis (see n. 53), p. 84.
60 KROL, Duivelskermis (see n. 53), p. 93.
61 KROL, Duivelskermis (see n. 53), p. 93.

an important role in *Duivelskermis*.[62] Albert, and with him the readers, wonder about questions such as: Who are we? Where are we? What is time? What distinguishes *Duivelskermis* from several other postmodern novels, however, is the fact that here these doubts have a concrete cause. It is Parkinson's disease as well as the medication that aims to diminish its impact, that are cause to Albert's disturbed state of mind. It is as if the narrative warns us that, when you are caught by Parkinson's disease, soon enough there is no trace of reality left. The novel also teaches us a lesson about the perception of time, a theme in the novel that is directly connected to Parkinson's disease as well. Many patients with Parkinson's disease suffer from a distorted awareness of time. They are slow and cannot follow the speed of their surroundings. This also applies to Albert, for instance when he thinks that he is thirty years old and that his former lover has been pregnant for four years. Or, when he realizes that his experience of time is not the same anymore: 'my watch now ran backwards much more often'.[63] It is the simultaneous awareness and unawareness of this distorted state of mind that lends the novel its confronting quality.

9 Conclusion

As our analyses of the novels by Loeckx, Brouwers, Van der Heijden, Vonk, Van Daele and Krol have shown, the basic depictions of Parkinson's disease in these works resemble each other quite a bit. Virtually all novels provide the reader with a realistic representation of the disease's elementary symptoms, such as trembling, rigidity, slowness, and an increasing immobility. Besides, all novels address the growing helplessness and dependency on others that strongly affects the patients' lives, and the confusion and feelings of uncertainty that more and more determine their daily existence. In most international novels, which include descriptions of Parkinson's disease, the separate clinical aspects are used as metaphors.[64] The same seems true for the novels that we have discussed here. For example, trembling is often associated with fear, as is clearly illustrated in *Bezonken rood*. The stooped posture often connotes humility and depression as we (again) see in *Bezonken rood*, but also in *Een grote blauwe cirkel* and *Uitdorsten*. Hallucinations symbolize the growing distance between the patient and 'reality', as in *Duivelskermis*, *Oude soldaten sterven niet* and *Ik was een meisje met een grote strik*. In this sense, we agree with Van Der Bruggen and

62 Brian McHale, 'From Modernist to Postmodernist Fiction: Change of Dominant', in: *Postmodernist Fiction*, New York/London 1987, pp. 3–25.
63 Krol, Duivelskermis (see n. 53), p. 64.
64 Haan, Protagonists with Parkinson's disease (see n. 4).

Widdershoven that fictional texts on Parkinson's disease can give insight in the altered corporality, realization of a change in the passing of time, altered notion of space, and sense of loss of identity.[65]

Although there are many similarities in the descriptions of the disease, the main emphases that the novels put on the disease differ. *Een grote blauwe cirkel*, for example, focuses on how a lack of acceptance of the disease puts social relations under pressure. In *Bezonken rood* the symptoms of the disease are 'mirrored' from mother to son, but in the son they come to function as an expression of guilt. End-of-life decisions are central in *Uitdorsten*, whereas hallucinations form the core of *Duivelskermis.* Finally, *Oude soldaten sterven niet* and *Ik was een meisje met een grote strik* emphasize the common co-occurrence of Parkinson's disease with Alzheimer-like cognitive deterioration.

Strikingly, each novel except for *Een grote blauwe cirkel*, features a first-person narrator who presents the process of deterioration from a subjective perspective and a position of personal involvement. In three of the discussed novels (the ones by Vonk, Krol, Van Daele), this narrator suffers from Parkinson's disease him- or herself. In two others (the ones by Brouwers and Van der Heijden), the Parkinson's disease patient is the mother of the (male) first-person narrator. The novels by Krol, Brouwers and Van der Heijden seem to contain autobiographical elements (Krol suffered from Parkinson's disease; the name of the narrator of *Bezonken rood* is Jeroen, the same as that of the writer; the narrator of *Uitdorsten* is Adri, which is the first name of A.F.Th van der Heijden). These texts can be seen as examples of so-called autofiction, which is a genre between autobiography and fiction in which author, protagonist and narrator are the same. Marie Darrieussecq defines autofiction as 'a fiction of strictly real events and facts' and associates the genre with 'shaking notions of reality', a phrasing that strikingly applies to our examples in both a figurative and literal sense.[66] The apparent popularity of autofiction in the representation of Parkinson's disease might well have to do with the way in which the autobio-

65 Of course, when confronted with a 'real' patient with Parkinson's disease, a doctor will do his utmost best to empathetically realize the impact of the disease on the patient. Nevertheless, a medical 'representation' will for many reasons in most instances mainly focus on functional disturbances such as walking impairment, problems with speech or with swallowing and loss of balance. For example, the most used clinical scale of impairment in Parkinson's disease, the so-called 'Hoehn& Yahr scale', categorizes affected patients in 7 stages based on motor symptoms, balance problems, dependency on caregivers and 'confinement to bed or wheelchair unless unaided' (Margaret M. Hoehn and Melvin D. Yahr, 'Parkinsonism: Onset, progression and mortality', in: *Neurology* 17 (1967), pp. 427–442). A fictional representation can be supplementary to such an 'objective' measurement by also describing how it 'feels' to have this disease.

66 Marie Darrieussecq, 'Fiction in the first person, or immoral writing', in: *L'Esprit Créateur* 50 (2010), pp. 70–82.

graphical dimension of this fiction increases the emotional appeal of the narratives. The idea that there is an, albeit fictional, truth in the depicted experiences helps to stir empathy on the part of the reader.

As we already stated in the introduction the 'basic' symptoms of Parkinson's disease often intertwine with or trigger the carving out of other, existential issues. It may not come as a surprise that the physical and mental loss of control of the Parkinson's patient coincides with existential doubts concerning a more general loss of self. Also, the fact that this loosing grip on one's life can have a strong impact on the patient's relationship to the surrounding world – to close relatives, other persons, objects, language and space – is a central theme in the novels discussed. A question that several of the novels pose, however, is whether it is solely Parkinson's disease that puts pressure on the relational self, or whether the disease rather functions to reveal relational structures that were already problematical beforehand?

The narratives that tell the Parkinson's experience from within seem to have the most direct affective effect, prompting the reader to join as it were in what is a highly disturbing experience. In the biographically inspired narratives by Brouwers and Van der Heijden, the Parkinson's disease of the mothers functions both as a fearful mirror, that forces the narrators to reflect on their own identities, and, related to this, as an instigation to rethink and reassess the mother-son relationships. Again existential issues such as love, care, and responsibility are central to the narratives that present Parkinson's disease as the initial source of discomfort.

All in all, the novels offer adequate and important insights in what, especially from a lay perspective, is still a mysterious and in many ways intimidating illness. At the same time, however, these novels move beyond being solely pathological narratives by deploying the 'shaking palsy' to address existential issues that concern – and bother – us all.

Stephan Besser

Mixing Repertoires: Cerebral Subjects in Contemporary Dutch Neurological Fiction

1 Introduction

First scene: The fictitious writer makes a note in his diary: 'I am my brain [*Ik ben mijn hersenen*]. It is fourteen centimetres wide, roughly seventeen centimetres long and about nine centimetres high. It weighs close to one and a half kilograms and contains billions of nerve cells that ceaselessly form new connections with one another at an incredible speed. Every day on average a hundred thousand of them perish.'[1] We know that the writer has first-hand personal experience with the death of neurons and the alleged convergence of brain and self: after a near-fatal accident, he suffers from a severe form of aphasia, a condition he tries to improve by keeping a diary to order his thinking and rehearse his linguistic skills, with limited success.

Second scene: The animal rights activist is upset with her lover who cannot seem to get an erection, in spite of extended stimulation. She taunts him with a reproachful syllogism: '[Y]our dick is controlled by your brain, and your brain is who you are [*je hersenen dat ben je zelf*]. So whose fault is it?' The vitriolic comment soon turns into an argument between the two lovers about the detrimental influence of international terrorism on the man's sexual performance and the woman's not-so-secret crush on Osama Bin Laden. Osama, she argues, is at least a 'strong' man: 'Otherwise he wouldn't be able to serve an entire harem'.[2]

Ik ben mijn hersenen/Je hersenen dat ben je zelf: these two invocations of the identity of brain and self stem from two recent Dutch-language novels, Bart Koubaa's *Het gebied van Nevski* (*Nevki's Area*; 2007) and Charlotte Mutsaers's *Koetsier Herfst* (*Coachman Autumn*; 2008), both published years before brain

1 Bart Koubaa, *Het gebied van Nevski*, Amsterdam 2007, p. 123 (all translations of Dutch texts by SB).
2 Charlotte Mutsaers, *Koetsier Herfst*, Amsterdam 2008, pp. 285, 286.

researcher Dick Swaab's popular science book with a quite similar title – *Wij zijn ons brein* (2011) – became a bestseller in the Netherlands. According to the deterministic view of identity Swaab presents in his book, there is not much leeway for the modification of the specific genetic and neural setup that defines who we are: an individual's character traits, health dispositions, and sexuality are essentially predetermined and fixed by the allegedly hardwired structures in her brain.[3] To be sure, neither Koubaa's nor Mutsaers's novels simply embrace such a brain-based and deterministic conception of personhood. Instead, *Het gebied van Nevski* constantly oscillates between a serious, knowledgeable engagement with neuroscientific theories and the parodic exaggeration and playful subversion of their alleged philosophical implications; the remark 'I am my brain', for instance, is swiftly followed by the somewhat puzzling and relativizing addition 'I am my arm.'[4] Similarly, Mutsaers's female protagonist's witty syllogism can be read precisely as a critical comment on the great explanatory power currently granted to the 'brain' in everyday life situations of every kind without much consideration of the plausibility of such claims.

At the same time, the two novels are certainly not indifferent towards or simply dismissive of what has been called the 'brain hype'[5] in contemporary western societies. Like numerous other literary works of the last ten to 15 years in the Netherlands and elsewhere they show a remarkable fascination with – and aesthetic and discursive investment in – the findings of neuroscience and what has been called the 'ideology of brainhood',[6] i.e. the conviction that human beings *are*, rather than simply *have*, a brain. In this article, I will explore the ways in which three recent Dutch novels – Robbert Welagen's *Porta Romana* (2011), Jeroen van Rooij's *De eerste hond in de ruimte* (*The First Dog in Space*; 2010), and Yves Petry's *De maagd Marino* (*The Virgin Marino*; 2010) – engage with this notion of brainhood. While these novels are not focused on the specificities of neuroscientific knowledge in a way that for instance Koubaa's *Het gebied van Nevski* is, they do show how important and influential neurological conceptions of personhood have become in Dutch fictions in recent years. I will show that

3 Dick Swaab, *Wij zijn ons brein: van baarmoeder tot alzheimer*, Amsterdam 2010.

4 Koubaa, Het gebied (see n. 1), p. 124. For an extended analysis of Koubaa's novel see Stephan Besser, 'From the Neuron to the World and Back: The Poetics of the Neuromolecular Gaze in Bart Koubaa's 'Het gebied van Nevski' and James Cameron's 'Avatar'', in: *Journal of Dutch Literature* 4, no. 2 (2013), pp. 43–67.

5 Margriet van der Heijden, 'De hersenhype', *NRC Weekblad* 29-1-2011, pp. 19–23.

6 Fernando Vidal, 'Brainhood, Anthropological Figure of Modernity', in: *History of the Human Sciences* 22, no. 1 (2009), pp. 5–36, here p. 6. Recent Dutch literary texts that deal with neuroscientific knowledge and the phenomenon of brainhood include Thomas Oosterhoff, *Dans zonder vloer*, Amsterdam 2003; Joke J. Hermsen, *Blindgangers*, Utrecht, Amsterdam and Antwerpen 2012; Daan Heerma van Voss, *De vergeting*, Amsterdam 2013 and Hanna Bervoets, *Efter*, Amsterdam/Antwerpen 2014.

these engagements with the notion of brainhood neither lead to a reductionist conception of personhood nor to the reinforcement of a strict boundary between the normal and the pathological in neurological terms, as some literary critics have argued for the case of recent Anglo-American 'neuronovels'. By displacing the notion of brainhood and engrafting it in various new contexts and constellations, they rather push and extend the boundaries of what a neural perspective on subjectivity and mental disorders can mean. I will argue that the ways in which they do that are significant for the more general patterns of diffraction and dissemination of brainhood in contemporary neuroculture.

2 Literature and Neuroculture

My following analyses are based on an understanding of 'neuroculture' as the interdiscursive circulation of neuroscientific knowledge and the fascination with the brain as the source and substrate of human conduct and subjectivity. This definition is based on Suzanne Anker and Giovanni Frazzetto's description of neuroculture as the 'incorporation of neuroscience knowledge into our life, culture and intellectual discourses',[7] although it should be emphasized that neuroscience itself is a cultural endeavour as well; the production of scientific brain facts is thus thoroughly influenced by its social and cultural contexts.[8]

In a number of seminal publications, historians of science, Fernando Vidal and Francisco Ortega have described the 'neurocultural universe' as an expanding network of practices, technologies, and discourses that presently shows a certain tendency to claim cultural hegemony in western societies. Like other critics of present-day 'neuromania'[9] they point to the remarkable fact that the adjective '*neuro*' has recently gained almost 'magical qualities' in the most diverse social contexts and spheres of life.[10] A striking example of this trend is the emergence new social and academic fields, such as neuroeconomics, neuroeducation, or neuroaesthetics, which redefine the epistemology and practice of various disciplines from a neurological and brain-centered perspective.[11] Be-

7 Giovanni Frazzetto and Suzanne Anker, 'Neuroculture', in: *Nature Reviews Neuroscience* 10 (2009), pp. 815–821, here p. 819.

8 Suparna Choudhury and Jan Slaby (eds.), *Critical Neuroscience: A Handbook of the Social and Cultural Contexts of Neuroscience*, Chichester 2012.

9 Paolo Legrenzi and Carlo Umiltà, *Neuromania: On the Limits of Brain Science*, Oxford 2011.

10 Fernando Vidal and Francisco Ortega, 'Approaching the Neurocultural Spectrum: An Introduction', in: Francisco Ortega and Fernando Vidal (eds.), *Neurocultures: Glimpses into an Expanding Universe*, Frankfurt/M. 2011, pp. 7–27, here pp. 9, 14.

11 Legrenzi and Umiltà, *Neuromania*, pp. 41–102. For a critique of the expensive and hegemonic tendencies of contemporary neuro-discourses also see Jan Slaby, 'Perspektiven

yond such more or less institutionalized contexts the cultural dissemination of the 'brain' is also apparent in popular and literary culture, for instance in a number of recent art-house and mainstream films like *Avatar* (2009), *Pacific Rim* (2013), and *The Fountain* (2006), as well as in computer games, artworks, a recent wave of 'neuronovels',[12] and a new sub-genre of autobiographical disease narratives that have been termed 'brain memoirs'[13]. In addition, the critical and affirmative reflection on the 'neuro revolution'[14] by artists and theorists such as Catherine Malabou, Warren Neidich, or Patricia Pisters has become part of the interdisciplinary feedback loops of contemporary neuroculture as well.[15] I will, therefore, situate my analysis of the reworkings of brainhood in the novels by Welagen, van Rooij, and Petry in this broader, interdiscursive context instead of merely looking at the relationship between literature and (neuro)science.

One of the areas in which the impact of the 'neuro' currently makes itself felt is the vast realm of the conceptions and practices of the self, i. e. the various ways in which people conceive of themselves as subjects and fashion their identities in relation to culturally specific possibilities and constraints.[16] According to Ortega and Vidal, contemporary neuroscience has a powerful offer to make in this context, namely the notion of the 'cerebral subject', an anthropological figure they see as providing the confusing landscape of contemporary neuroculture with a 'certain unity'.[17] Drawing upon sociologist Alain Ehrenberg's notion of the *sujet cerebral*,[18] Vidal defines the cerebral subject as a brain-based conception of the self, according to which 'the human being is specified by the

---

einer kritischen Philosophie der Neurowissenschaften', in: *Deutsche Zeitschrift für Philosophie* 53, no. 3 (2011), pp. 375–390, and, from a psychological perspective, JAN DERKSEN, *Bevrijd de psychologie uit de greep van de hersenmythe*, Amsterdam 2012.

12 Some recent examples from the Anglo-American context are E.L. DOCTOROW, *Andrew's Brain*, New York 2014; RICHARD POWERS, *The Echo Maker*, London 2007; IAN MCEWAN, *Saturday*, New York 2005, and JONATHAN LETHEM, *Motherless Brooklyn*, New York, 1999.

13 JASON TOUGAW, 'Brain Memoirs, Neuroscience, and the Self: A Review Article', in: *Literature and Medicine* 30, no. 1 (2012), pp. 171–192. Prominent examples of this genre are SIRI HUSTVEDT, *The Shaking Woman, or a History of My Nerves*, New York 2009 and SUSANNA CAHALAN, *Brain on Fire: My Month of Madness*, New York 2012.

14 ZACK LYNCH and B. LAURSEN, *The Neuro Revolution: How Brain Science is Changing Our World*, New York 2009.

15 See for instance CATHERINE MALABOU, *What Should We Do with Our Brain?*, transl. by SEBASTIAN RAND, New York 2008; ARNE DE BOEVER and WARREN NEIDICH (eds.), *The Psychopathologies of Cognitive Capitalism: Part One*, Berlin 2013; PATRICIA PISTERS, 'Het neurobeeld: confrontatie met de waanzin', in: *Parmentier* 21, no. 1 (2012), pp. 31–38.

16 See for instance NIKOLAS ROSE and JOELLE M. ABI-RACHED, *Neuro: The New Brain Sciences and the Management of the Mind*, Princeton/Oxford 2013; VICTORIA PITTS-TAYLOR, 'The Plastic Brain: Neoliberalism and the Neuronal Self', in: *Health* 14, no. 6 (2010), pp. 635–652; FRANCISCO ORTEGA, 'Towards a Genealogy of Neuroascesis', in: ORTEGA and VIDAL (eds.), Neurocultures (see n. 10), pp. 31–48.

17 VIDAL and ORTEGA, Approaching the Neurocultural Spectrum (see n. 10), p. 16.

18 ALAIN EHRENBERG, 'Le Sujet cérébral', in: *Esprit* (November 2004), pp. 130–155.

property of 'brainhood', i. e. the property or quality of *being*, rather than simply *having*, a brain.' In this view, an individual is therefore in every regard sufficiently characterized by the specific properties of her *brain*, whereas other organs, the body as a whole, or the social, cultural, or natural surroundings of a person only matter in relation to the neural matter in one's head: show me your brain and I tell you who you are. Following Ehrenberg, Vidal argues that the dominance of this reductionist conception of subjectivity can be used to explain the 'emphasis on interiority at the expense of social bonds and contexts' in western and westernized societies and the individualism characteristic of these societies.[19] Importantly, Ortega and Vidal nevertheless stress that brainhood is *not* the only way to fashion identities and that it always coexists and mixes with other ontologies: '[I]ndividuals are generally not one kind of subject alone.'[20] People might be fascinated by neurobiological explanations of behavior and personality types ('the brain of the introvert, adolescent, schizophrenic' etc.), follow nutritional advice to enhance their 'brain fitness'[21] or be convinced by the neuro-determinism of Dick Swaab's bestseller and nevertheless *also* hold religious beliefs, see a psychiatrist, and conceive of their own personality and behaviour in terms of psychological theories that may not be compatible at all with a neuromaterialist reduction of mind to brain. Even in a time in which notions of the 'synaptic self'[22] and 'neuronal man'[23] abound, people can and do make use of 'multiple and often inconsistent and contradictory repertoires for describing and managing personhood and selfhood, which are activated and deployed in different contexts, and in different departments of life',[24] as sociologists of science Nikolas Rose and Joelle M. Abi-Rached point out.

Such a flexible and hybrid mix of different forms of personhood, however, does not necessarily go without saying. Mixing repertoires is neither obvious nor without dispute in reality or in literary texts, especially when it comes to the genre that has traditionally been identified with the representation of subjectivity: the novel. In his influential article 'The Rise of the Neuronovel', published in 2009, literary critic Marco Roth states that we currently witness a transformation of the novel of consciousness or psychological novel into a new form of novelistic writing, namely 'the *neurological novel*, wherein the mind becomes the brain'. For Roth, this transformation reflects a larger 'cultural sea change' from Freudianism and poststructuralist theory to scientific essential-

19 Vidal, Brainhood (see n. 6), pp. 6, 7.

20 Vidal and Ortega, Approaching the Neurocultural Spectrum (see n. 10), p. 17.

21 Ortega, Neuroascesis (see n. 16), p. 32.

22 Joseph LeDoux, *Synaptic Self: How Our Brains Become Who We Are*, London/New York 2002.

23 Jean-Pierre Changeux, *Neuronal Man: The Biology of Mind*, New York/Oxford 1985.

24 Rose and Abi-Rached, Neuro (see n. 16), p. 221.

ism, the medicalization of difference, and a 'new reductionism of mind to brain' that explains 'the proximate causes of mental function in terms of neurochemistry, and ultimate causes in terms of evolution and heredity'. Discussing Ian McEwan's 2005 novel *Saturday* as a prime example of this trend, Roth points to two characteristics of the recent wave of neurological fictions that are both closely related to the much broader critique of neuro-reductionism. From a discursive and ideological perspective, *Saturday* seems highly dubious to Roth because of the novel's 'stark biological determinism' and the strict distinction between 'mental normals' – the neurosurgeon Henry Perowne, his barrister wife, and his artist children – and the 'subnormal' character Baxter, 'a violent thug suffering from the incurable, genetic brain-wasting disease Huntington's chorea'. From a poetological and aesthetic perspective, Roth fears that neurological explanations of human conduct might lead to an impoverishment of the metaphorical abundance characteristic of the older novel of consciousness. If neurological conditions such as Huntington's disease in *Saturday* or Capgras delusion in Richard Powers's *The Echo Maker* are nothing but contingent biological phenomena, how can they say anything about the social, cultural, and political environments in which they appear? The 'aesthetic sensation' a reader gets from a hard-boiled neuronovel may thus not be 'the pleasure of finding the general in the particular, but a frustration born of the defeat of the metaphoric impulse'.[25]

While this certainly is an ominous development in Roth's view, all scholars of recent neurological fiction, including Ortega and Vidal, have not shared his critical assessment. In a recent review article on the topic they argue that the neuronovel is neither a new phenomenon, as Roth suggests, nor in principle equivalent with neuroreductionism or 'cerebral solipsism'.[26] To make their point that neuronovels generally convey *ambivalence* about the claim 'that the nature of personhood is essentially cerebral or brain-based'[27] they discuss a number of analyses of Richard Powers's *The Echo Maker* that show the novel's commitment

25 Marco Roth, 'The Rise of the Neuronovel', in: *n+1*, no. 8 (2009), pp. 139–151, here pp. 139, 140, 144, 149.

26 Francisco Ortega and Fernando Vidal, 'Brains in Literature/Literature in the Brain', in: *Poetics Today* 34, no. 3 (2013), pp. 327–360, here p. 343. Ortega and Vidal cite the role of phrenology in Victorian literature as an example of the long history of neurological fiction in western literature (pp. 333–334). Another example are representations of the brain as biological sources of human conduct in naturalist fiction, for instance in Marcellus Emants' novel *Een nagelaten bekentenis* [*A Posthumous Confession*] (1894). For the long literary and cultural history of 'brainomania' see also George Rousseau, 'Brainomania': Brain, Mind and Soul in the Long Eighteenth Century', in: *British Journal for Eighteenth-Century Studies* 30, no. 2 (2007), pp. 161–191 and Anne Stiles, *Popular Fiction and Brain Science in the Late Nineteenth Century*, Cambridge 2012.

27 Ortega and Vidal, Brains in Literature (see n. 26), p. 332.

to the so-called '4EA approach' in cognitive neuroscience and theories of consciousness. This acronym refers to a wide range of approaches that study the mind as an embodied, embedded, enacted, extended, and affective phenomenon and therefore reject any form of cerebral solipsism.[28] Drawing on Gary Johnson's remarks about the potential of neuroscientific knowledge 'to refresh and redeem the field of literature',[29] they state that for many writers of contemporary neuronovels the new scientific approaches to the brain mainly function as a reservoir for new fictional devices and narrative tools, for instance in the attempt to find creative responses 'to the exhaustion of the traditional consciousness novel'.[30] Similarly, Valeria Gennero has argued that the notion of the cerebral subject 'opens the way to new forms of formal experimentation'[31] in the same way that the literary experiments of high modernism did in relation to Freudian conceptions of the psyche.

While the novels by Welagen, van Rooij, and Petry indeed provide intriguing examples of the kind of formal experiments Johnson and Gennero track, I will nevertheless argue that the aesthetic and discursive dimensions of literary texts cannot be disentangled as easily as some of the formulations by Ortega and Vidal can seem to suggest.[32] As we will see, it is very well possible that a literary work that explicitly criticizes, ridicules, and deconstructs certain forms of neuroscience or notions of brainhood *at the same time* also represents a huge *investment* in that very same knowledge, for instance by giving it a special role in the text's symbolic economy, valuing the specific intellectual flavour of certain tropes over others, or simply representing this knowledge as relevant, interesting, or even glamorous. Such complex investments, I will argue, cannot be

28 John Protevi, *Political Affect: Connecting the Social and the Somatic*, Minneapolis 2009, p. 4. Important representatives of this host of approaches are Antonio Damasio with his research on the corporeal dimensions of emotion and cognition, Andy Clark's investigations of the ways in which human cognition is inherently related to its natural and technological environments and Francisco Varela, Evan Thompson and Eleanor Rosch with their research on the embodied and enactive mind (*The Embodied Mind: Cognitive Science and Human Experience*, Cambridge MA 1991).

29 Gary Johnson, 'Consciousness as Content: Neuronarratives and the Redemption of Fiction', in: *Mosaic* 41, no. 1 (2008), pp. 169–184, here p. 340.

30 Ortega and Vidal, Brains in Literature (see n. 26) p. 340, 342.

31 Valeria Gennero, 'Larger Than Our Biologies: Identity and Consciousness in Contemporary Fiction', in: Francisco Ortega and Fernando Vidal (eds.), Neurocultures (see n. 10), pp. 311–327, here p. 311. The implications of neurological knowledge for an author's 'formal and rhetorical choices', rather than just on the level of plot, have also been emphasized by Stephen J. Burn, 'Mapping the Syndrome Novel', in: Tim Lustig and James Peacock (eds.), *Diseases and Disorders in Contemporary Fiction: The Syndrome Syndrome*, New York 2013, pp. 35–52, here p. 36.

32 In their very insightful article, Ortega and Vidal state for instance that for many writers of neuronovels the notion of brainhood is 'mainly a literary tool' and the brain 'mainly a trope'. Ortega and Vidal, Brains in Literature (see n. 26), pp. 330, 348.

reduced to the question in how far a literary work 'endorses' or 'subverts' the notion of the cerebral subject. Nevertheless, it will be relevant to study how these investments affect the distinction between the normal and the pathological that Marco Roth talks about. If the workings of the 'normal healthy brain'[33] can best be studied in pathological cases, as neuroscientist Vilayanur S. Ramachandran claims, then how can literary fiction make use of this insight, and with what results for the notion of cerebral normalcy itself?

3 *Porta Romana:* A Tale of Two Traumas

Robbert Welagen's short novel *Porta Romana* tells the story of a severe case of cerebral trauma. The narrative centers on Emilio Lastrucci, a 52 year-old inconspicuous businessman, who becomes the victim of a violent robbery. During a diner appointment with a mysterious woman, Emilio is lured into a trap, overpowered by four men, and forced to transfer all of his savings to the assailants. He can only escape the situation by throwing himself through a window, landing on a balcony two floors below. The fall causes a cranial fracture and substantial damage to Emilio's long-term memory, 'the part of the brain where autobiographic events are being stored, the episodic memory',[34] as his doctors explain to him. As a result, Emilio loses almost every recollection of his life before the incident and, hence, any connection to his former identity. In an attempt to regain his memory he travels to Florence, the city of his childhood and youth, and talks to old friends and family members. However, none of the places and people from his past seems able to bring back Emilio's recollection of his life before the traumatic event.

For readers interested in the literary pathology of the cerebral subject, *Porta Romana* offers an intriguing narrative combination of two different forms of trauma. One of them can tentatively be described as 'Freudian', in the twofold sense that it links the loss of memory to repression, i. e. a form of forgetting that is unconsciously motivated, and that it explains the impact of the traumatic event through its relation to a previous conflict in the psycho-sexual biography of the subject.[35] The other, strikingly different form of trauma, can be described as neurological and caused by a cerebral lesion *devoid* of any relation to a

33 Vilayanur S. Ramachandran, *The Tell-Tale Brain: Unlocking the Mystery of Human Nature*, London 2011, p. x.

34 Robbert Welagen, *Porta Romana*, Amsterdam 2011, p. 25.

35 For an overview of the Freudian conception of trauma see Ruth Leys, *Trauma: A Genealogy*, Chicago and London 2000, pp. 18–41 and Jean Laplanche and Jean-Bertrand Pontalis, *The Language of Psycho-Analysis*, transl. by Donald Nicholson-Smith, London 1988, pp. 465–469.

hermeneutics of the subject. There is, in other words, no deeper psychic meaning to be discovered in the traumatic event: the wound is the wound and nothing else, even though it can change the personality of the patient beyond recognition. Such a form of trauma has recently been theorized by French philosopher Catherine Malabou in terms of what she calls 'cerebrality', i. e. the exclusive 'causal value' of physical damage inflicted upon brain function and their capacity to determine the 'course of psychic life'. Importantly, this concept of the 'cerebral event' does 'not allow an interpretation of the lesion or the trauma that aligns it with a 'previous conflict''.[36] Although Malabou does not use the term herself, this view can be seen as the acknowledgment of the dark, destructive side of the cerebral subject: if we essentially *are* our brains, as Malabou assumes, then we are our cerebral lesions as well, without any safety net provided by the continuities of the psyche and its libidinal economy. According to Malabou, this 'is the great metaphysical teaching of neurobiology today: not to consider brain damage as an isolated possibility, rare things that happen in hospitals, but to consider them as a constant possibility'.[37] Being a cerebral subject means the possibility of becoming somebody else at every moment.

In *Porta Romana*, this tension between psyche and cerebral subject is of central importance for the meaning-making of the narrative itself. It already comes to the fore at the very beginning of the novel, in a metaphor of memory employed in the description of Emilio's arrival in the city centre of Florence. Inexplicably fascinated by the light yellow colour of a house's wall at dusk, Emilio attempts to trigger an act of memory:

> Looking at the yellow spot was the only thing Emilio did, hoping that something might happen. A connection in his brain, an association, an image. But nothing happened. That was because of the gaps that had been burned into the thin tracing paper [*het dunne kalkpapier*] of his memory. Somewhere there, behind his eyes.[38]

As a metaphor of memory, the term 'tracing paper' here is vaguely reminiscent of Sigmund Freud's famous comparison of the mental apparatus and the mnemic system with a *Wunderblock*, a mystic writing pad that is able to record 'permanent traces' (*Dauerspuren*)[39] even if they are erased on the 're-writeable' surface of perception. The spatial logic here is one of surface and depth: memory

---

36 Catherine Malabou, *The New Wounded: From Neurosis to Brain Damage*, New York 2012, pp. 2, 8.

37 Noëlle Vahanian, 'A Conversation with Catherine Malabou', in: *Journal for Cultural and Religious Theory* 9, no. 1 (2008), p. 9.

38 Welagen, Porta Romana (see n. 34), pp. 12–13.

39 Sigmund Freud, *Notiz über den 'Wunderblock', Studienausgabe*, Alexander Mitscherlich, Angela Richards and James Strachney (eds.), vol. 3, Frankfurt/M. 1975, pp. 363–369, here p. 365. Cf. Douwe Draaisma, *Metaphors of Memory: A History of Ideas about the Mind*, Cambridge 2000, pp. 7–9, 20–23.

appears as a form of drawing or writing that leaves meaningful inscriptions in the deeper layers of the psyche even beyond the conscious recollection of the subject. The therapeutic process then might aim at dissolving the blockages that make certain memories inaccessible. To be sure, *Porta Romana* does not present a coherent psychoanalytic theory of memory and trauma in any way. Nevertheless, the novel constantly alludes to the trope of the search for a hidden meaning in lost memories and supports these allusions by various references to texts and artworks that evoke associations with psychoanalysis, such as Alfred Hitchcock's film *Vertigo*, the dreamlike cityscapes in the paintings of Giorgio di Chirico, and Marcel Proust's *In Search of Lost Time.*

Besides this notion of a text or traces of memory, the metaphor of the 'tracing paper' also supports a quite different, neurobiological conception of memory in which the paper does not figure as a medium of writing but as a tissue or membrane damaged by physical force. In this reading of the metaphor, the emphasis is not on the imaginary topology of surface and depth implied in the transparency of the 'paper' – something is calked through – but on the lateral connections *within* this tissue, namely the neural networks 'within his brain' that are physically disrupted and seem to represent the biological correlates of memory in the above quote ('an association, an image'). Similar to neurobiological theories of trauma, the 'gaps' in the paper then signify a 'literal imprint of an external trauma' that does *not* have a semantic dimension, but is simply a wound or a hole without any meaning.[40]

At certain moments during his wanderings in Florence it seems that the repression or unconscious evasion of potentially disturbing memories might indeed partly cause the stubborn persistence of Emilio's amnesia. In a dream, for instance, a younger version of himself urges him to 'stay out of my city', i.e. the Florence of his childhood. Later on in the novel, Emilio accidentally meets his former girlfriend Giulia who first is surprised that he doesn't seem to recognize her and assumes that he might have 'repressed' the memory of their unpleasant break-up almost thirty years ago.[41] This assumption recalls the psychoanalytic conception of trauma, according to which, as historian of psychology Ruth Leys points out, the external trauma derives its 'force and efficacity entirely from internal psychical processes' understood to be fundamentally shaped 'by earlier psychosexual desires, fantasies, and conflicts'.[42] As a matter of fact, the encounter with Giulia does seem to bring some memories of Emilio's former self from the 'depth' to the 'surface' of his consciousness. The only impression,

40 Cf. Ruth Ley's critical assessment of neurobiological theories of trauma proposed by physician Bessel van der Kolk and others in: Leys, Trauma (see n. 35), pp. 239, 249.
41 Welagen, Porta Romana (see n. 34), pp. 55, 126.
42 Leys, Trauma (see n. 35), p. 21.

however, that Emilio gets from these elusive 'fragments' [*flarden*] of memory is that his previous life might have been just as lonely, empty, and devoid of meaning as his post-traumatic existence.[43]

On the whole, the novel thus constantly postpones and defers the promise of the revelation of a hidden meaning that the narrative logic of repression and psychic trauma hold up. In a literary and novelistic modality, this systematic evacuation of meaning from trauma quite closely resembles the general line of argument in Catherine Malabou's aforementioned study on *The New Wounded*, in which she sets out to theorize 'the kind of injuries or wounds or brain damage that psychoanalysis never took into account'.[44] These 'new wounds' include neurodegenerative disorders (Alzheimer's or Parkinson's disease), as well as the cerebral damage caused by various forms of sexual and political violence, natural disasters, and Post-Traumatic Stress Disorder: every form of trauma that effects the 'neuronal organization' of the victim's brains. Malabou emphasizes that these traumatized cerebral subjects can experience a 'radical rupture' in their psyche that literally makes them '*someone* else'. Drawing on research into post-traumatic personality disorders, she argues that the 'cool', detached, and almost zombie-like psyches of the victims are the result of the disruption of 'cerebral auto-affection' and thus of the 'link between emotion and cognition'.[45]

Although Welagen's quiet, introspective, and elegiac novel couldn't be further away from Malabou's global panorama of meaningless political violence, natural disasters, and degenerative brain diseases, her theory of trauma is a valuable tool for detecting a deep sensibility for the sinister sides of the cerebral subject in *Porta Romana*. While critics have mostly read Welagen's novel as an atmospherically orientated literary exercise in mild nostalgia and sepia-toned melancholy,[46] this approach makes it possible to see Emilio's constant sense of isolation and irreality, his lack of emotions, and feeling of being placed under a 'bell jar'[47] as symptoms of a cerebral trauma that cannot be cured because it doesn't have a story and because there is no continuous psyche to return to: a self after the loss of self and a 'wound with no hermeneutic future'.[48]

This is not to say that Welagen ultimately 'opts' for a cerebral conception of subjectivity in which the brain *is* the mind or neurological notions of memory

43 Welagen, Porta Romana (see n. 34), p. 128.
44 Vahanian, A Conversation with Catherine Malabou (see n. 37), p. 8.
45 Malabou, The New Wounded (see n. 36), pp. 11, 48, 47.
46 Arjen Fortuijn, 'Het gevaar schuilt in iedereen', in: *NRC* 03-06-2011; Arie Storm, 'Revisor-proza met een twist', in: *Het Parool* 08-06-2011; Joost de Vries, 'Negen kopjes koffie', in: *De Groene Amsterdammer* 30-06-2011; Dirk Leyman, 'Elegant kabbelende roman van Robbert Welagen', in: *De Morgen* 20-07-2011.
47 Welagen, Porta Romana (see n. 34), pp. 22, 72, 88.
48 Malabou, The New Wounded (see n. 36), p. 8.

and trauma replace psychological ones. *Porta Romana* shows that, as Ortega and Vidal point out, the cerebral subject can coexist and blend with other conceptions of personhood and create new aesthetic and narrative possibilities through this interaction. In this regard, the novel is quite similar to other products of contemporary neuroculture, such as the US-American TV series *The Sopranos* (1999–2007), *Six Feet Under* (2001–2005), or *Dexter* (2006–2013), which all in their own ways mix the representation of brainhood with other forms of subjectivity. In the specific case of Welagen's novel, this qualified investment in the cerebral subject and the 'neurologization of memory'[49] facilitates a subtle teasing of the 'readerly meaning impulse'[50] and ultimate withdrawal of the pleasures of explanation and narrative closure.

4 *De eerste hond in de ruimte:* The Neurology of Techno-Capitalism

A severe case of brain damage also plays an important role in Jeroen van Rooij's debut novel *De eerste hond in de ruimte* (2010). The book is dedicated to the British musicologist and musician Clive Wearing, who is probably one of the most famous patients in history of neurology. In 1985, Wearing contracted an infection with the Herpes simplex virus that attacked his central nervous system and severely damaged his hippocampus. Since that time, Wearing suffers from an extreme form of anterograde and retrograde amnesia, meaning that his brain is unable to store any new memories. Since his short-term memory span now only lasts 7 to 30 seconds, Wearing is constantly under the impression of just having awoken or having regained consciousness after a period of absent-mindedness. The diary he began to keep for therapeutic reasons is filled with crossed-out notes, such as the following:

> 2:10 pm: this time properly awake… 2:14 pm: this time finally awake. … 2:35 pm: this time completely awake […] At 9:40 pm I awoke for the first time, despite my previous claims.[51]

De eerste hond in de ruimte features an anonymous character, mostly referred to as 'a middle-aged man', who suffers from exactly the same form of extreme amnesia and who constantly fills a diary with brief and subsequently crossed-out descriptions of his first real awakening to consciousness. In the narrative and symbolic order of the novel this ghostly human being arguably represents more

49 Ortega and Vidal, Brains in Literature (see n. 26), pp. 346–349.
50 Roth, The Rise of the Neuronovel (see n. 25), p. 149.
51 Cf. Oliver Sacks, *Musicophilia: Tales of Music and the Brain.* Revised and extended edition, Basingstoke/London 2011, p. 203.

than just an unfortunate case of memory loss: besides pointing to his lack of identity, the namelessness of the 'middle-aged man' also invites an allegorical interpretation of his disorder in relation to a broader condition of a disturbed sense of temporality and memory that appears as a pathological characteristic of the technologically and economically advanced society that the novel depicts. Here, we thus deal with a neurological condition that does *not*, as Marco Roth suggests, defy any metaphorical interpretation as a more general sign of the times.

De eerste hond in de ruimte is structured as a rhythmic orchestration of about 20 'voices', i. e. the thoughts, actions, and experiences of various characters that appear in different typefaces and that are comprised of snippets varying from a few sentences up to several pages in length. Together they constitute a present-day *Sinfonie der Großstadt* (Walter Ruttmann, 1927) in the form of a textual exploration of daily life in a big European city – probably Berlin – to the soundtrack of post-millennial techno music. The increasingly interacting storylines revolve round the attempt of a mysterious, seemingly extramundane character called 'the daymaker' to find a way to prevent an impending shortage of days on Earth. Through the daymaker's musings it becomes clear that the manufacture of a day is an extremely labour-intensive and time-consuming task that the humans in the city do not seem to value much anymore. Having heard of the 'middle-aged man', the daymaker sets out to find this person for whom even *one* day would be more than enough for all eternity and to somehow devise a solution for the larger problem from his condition. During this mission, the daymaker encounters a group of young ravers, also referred to as 'the beautiful ones', who spend their days and nights in the flourishing techno-scene of the city, organizing parties, popping pills, and, above all, enjoying the sublime experience of becoming one supra-individual techno-body of ecstatic dancers. The symbolic opposition between day and night here is clear: whereas the daymaker equates the experience of a carefully crafted 'day' with the sensory experience of natural 'colours, the nuances of the seasons, the subtle smells that arise from freshly baked bread', the members of the techno avant-garde enjoy a nocturnal lifestyle full of flashlights, digital music and the chemical enhancement of their feelings. Their communal experiences are routed through technology: 'Our smiles are luminous and the light they radiate is amplified and passed on through the laser beams above our heads.'[52]

Paradoxically, it is precisely this restless, highly mediated lifestyle whose manifestations closely correspond to the depiction of Clive Wearing's amnesia in the novel. Empty repetitions of the same, a loss of memory, and temporal disorientation: these are the symptoms the ravers Jonas, Micha, Ellen, and Lisel

52 Jeroen van Rooij, *De eerste hond in de ruimte*, Amsterdam 2010, pp. 38, 50, 56; 33; 36.

experience after a period of extensive partying as well. Jonas, for instance, notices that he is not able to distinguish between the different days (and nights) of the week anymore; his memory of distinct events begins to disappear. Ellen, in turn, is unable to watch films on DVD for more than 30 minutes: not quite as short as the attention span of Clive Wearing, but certainly a hint that the day-maker's intended *solution* looks a lot like the *problem* the techno-lifestyle generates.[53] It is thus for good reasons that critic Joost de Vries notes that 'the entire city is some kind of Clive Wearing, a city that gets up again every day and has forgotten everything'.[54] Hence, it is not too far-fetched to argue that the individual neuropathology of amnesia here closely corresponds to the social pathology of an advanced media and techno culture that operates according to the principles of high capitalism. It becomes clear, for instance, that the techno-lifestyle of the young ravers significantly contributes to a constant extension of the zone of labour and consumption from daytime into the night. This chrono-economic development is illustrated by the example of a continuously overtired snack bar owner who is forced to serve 'the beautiful ones' until the morning hours in order to find a temporal niche in the fierce competition with other fast-food stores.[55] In the novel's frantic story world, the 24-hour party people thus figure as an avant-garde of the 24/7 service economy.[56]

Significantly, film scholar Patricia Pisters describes a quite similar configuration of temporal disorientation, neurological imagery, media culture, and capitalism in her analysis of what she terms the 'neuro-image' in contemporary cinema. Drawing on Deleuze and Guattari's notion of schizoanalysis, Pisters argues that we currently witness the emergence of a new cinematic imagination in which the spectators literally enter the 'brain-world' of the characters – think of films such as *Inception* (2010), *Being John Malkovich* (1999), and *Eternal Sunshine of the Spotless Mind* (2004) – and in which the pathological and the critical aspects of the protagonists' altered mental states cannot be separated. An emblematic character in this regard is the delirious and paranoid lawyer Arthur Eden in Tony Gilroy's film *Michael Clayton* (2007). In a pivotal scene in the film, Eden experiences a moment of critical clarity about his involvement in the amoral business activities of his law firm when he walks across Times Square at night and is paralyzed by the vortical stream of flashing lights and digital-screen

53 Van Rooij, De eerste hond in de ruimte (see n. 52), p. 52.

54 Joost de Vries, 'De beat beukt', in: *De Groene Amsterdammer* 16-06-2010.

55 Van Rooij, De eerste hond in de ruimte (see n. 52), p. 37.

56 Van Rooij's description of this lifestyle shows striking similarities with Jonathan Crary's analysis of the chrono-economics of contemporary capitalism, including its neurological consequences, in: Jonathan Crary, *24/7: Late Capitalism and the Ends of Sleep*, London/New York, 2013.

images.[57] Similarly, the ravers in *De eerste hond in de ruimte* feel 'beaten senseless by the stream of images' and 'permanent flood of nonsense' that reaches them via media screens.[58] Eden's altered state of mind is attributed to a chemical imbalance in his brain but at the same time also reflects the insanity of the capitalist system around him.[59]

Given the novel's neurological sensibilities, it seems very fitting that this ambivalence of pathology and critique in *De eerste hond in de ruimte* is expressed by a subspecies or variation of the cerebral subject, namely the so-called 'neurochemical self'. Sociologist of science Nikolas Rose has introduced this term in order to characterize a host of pharmaceutical technologies and views of the self established on a brain-based, post-psychoanalytic conception of personhood. According to Rose, it seems that individuals in 'psychopharmacological societies' are beginning 'to recode their moods and their ills in terms of the functioning of their brain chemicals, and to act upon themselves in the light of this belief.'[60] Prominent literary examples of this tendency can be found in the character Gary Lambert in Jonathan Franzen's *The Corrections*, a 'hero of neuro-reductionism',[61] who interprets his mental states in terms of brain chemistry: 'Various chemicals that floodgates had been holding back all afternoon burst loose and flooded Gary's neural pathways. A cascade of reactions initiated by Factor 6 relaxed his tear valves and sent a wave of nausea down his vagus'.[62] Henry Perowne in McEwan's *Saturday* also constantly interprets the modulation of his consciousness and feelings as results of events at the neurochemical level.[63] Similarly, the young adults in van Rooij's novel experience and manage their selves in neurochemical terms (although there are hints that some of them might have old-fashioned psychological problems as well).[64] As experienced users of MDMA/ecstasy pills and modulators of their mental states, the ultimate goal of the ravers is to transport their identities into a state of 'flux' in which the boundaries between individual bodies and minds disappear. This deterritorialization of subjectivity during the raves is described by Jonas as a 'sort of

57 Patricia Pisters, *The Neuro-Image: A Deleuzian Film-Philosophy of Digital Screen Culture*, Stanford 2012, pp. 1–4.
58 Van Rooij, De eerste hond in de ruimte (see n. 52), pp. 64, 66.
59 Pisters, Het neurobeeld (see n. 15), pp. 31–38.
60 Nikolas Rose, 'Neurochemical Selves', in: *Society* 41, no. 1 (2003): pp. 46–59, here pp. 46, 59.
61 Gennero, Larger Than Our Biologies (see n. 31), p. 312.
62 Jonathan Franzen, *The Corrections*, New York 2001, p. 156.
63 'An habitual observer of his own moods, he wonders about his sustained, distorting euphoria. Perhaps down at the molecular level there's been a chemical accident while he slept – something like a spilled tray of drinks, prompting dopamine-like receptors to initiate a kindly cascade of intracellular events'. Ian McEwan, *Saturday*, New York 2005, p. 5.
64 Cf. van Rooij, De eerste hond in de ruimte (see n. 52), p. 57.

collective love, a rhythmic love, a love of being one [...]. This is what I believe in, even if it is a chemical form of love.'[65]

Unlike the neural 'solipsism' of the cerebral self, this desire for connectedness emphasizes the interaction with others on a somatic, neurochemical, and technological basis; the ravers literally want to move 'out of their heads'. The novel pathologises this techno-delirium (by likening it to a neurological condition) but also embraces its beauty, utopian promise, and aesthetic possibilities. In one of the self-reflective moments of the narrative, Jonas describes a DJ set of techno musician Koze as a magical polyphony of voices, not unlike the novel itself:

> The voices, the voices, the voices, black voices and white voices, men and women, clear and distorted, soulful and mechanical, voices you understand and voices that just make noises, Koze has them all. Differences still exist, but everything is complete and fits, falls into place and yet keeps its own sound, its own colour.[66]

Given the novel's profound interest in the materiality of thinking and feeling it is probably no coincidence that the euphoria and pathology of altered states in *De eerste hond in de ruimte* form a network of neurological references and allusions that includes the eerie case of Clive Wearing, the prisoner of his brain, as well.

5 *De maagd Marino:* Spiritual Materialism

The biological materiality of thinking and feeling is also an issue of great concern in Yves Petry's 2010 novel *De maagd Marino*, a challenging and unsettling literary exploration of the relations of mind and matter, fiction and science, and brain and spirit [*geest*]. Although this persistent concern with the cerebral matter of thought and personhood might not immediately be visible at the surface of the novel, it is a constant and determining presence in its complex symbolic order and curious narrative form. It manifests itself, among other things, in a number of seemingly casual remarks on the workings of the brain. The narrator, for instance, claims that reading numerous works of world literature has made his brain 'complex and obstinate'. He muses about the pernicious influence of religious thought on the plasticity of neural networks – false religiosity might make a brain 'brittle' – or suspects that the brains of the inhabitants of big cities are in the process of becoming 'increasingly smaller'

65 Van Rooij, De eerste hond in de ruimte (see n. 52), p. 32.
66 Van Rooij, De eerste hond in de ruimte (see n. 52), p. 171. Hans Demeyer has described the novel as a 'technotrack' and pointed to the utopian dimension of the raves. Cf. Hans Demeyer, "I Want You in My Arms': Utopie en nostalgie bij John Maus en Jeroen van Rooij', in: *Dietsche Warande & Belfort* no. 2 (2013), pp. 244–253.

since modern city life is detrimental to mental independence. All of this brain talk, however, should not be taken too seriously since the same narrator, a literary scholar, repeatedly mocks what he regards as the pedantic reductionism of many neuroscientists and explicitly makes fun of the 'pious tone' these scientists assume when they talk about the brain as 'the most complex piece of matter in the entire universe'. But then again, this very narrator *himself* turns out to be nothing but a materialized spirit in someone else's skull, or, to be precise: 'an electromagnetic oscillation in the lobes of the brain' of the man who killed him.[67]

Such a twisted and substantial investment in the 'brain' can seem a little odd for a novel inspired by a real-life case of consensual murder that rather invites associations with psychiatric disorders and mental illness. This real-life event is the case of the so-called 'Rotenburg Cannibal', Armin Meiwes, who in 2001 met with his voluntary victim Bernd Jürgen Brandes in order to eat his severed penis; Meiwes later killed Brandes and ate parts of his body. In *De maagd Marino*, the victim is the narrator Bruno Klaus, a literature professor at a Belgian university, and the perpetrator is the 37 year-old computer technician Marino Mund. The novel starts after Klaus has already been killed and Marino awaits his trial in prison. Bruno still exists as a mental presence in Marino's head, and dictates to him the story of their relationship that forms the narrative of the novel.

In the conflict between brain, spirit, and psyche as figures of personhood that the novel plays out, the psyche is the weakest element. Remarkably, the account of their relationship that the defendant writes down for Bruno refrains from any psychosexual explanation of Marino's inclinations towards cannibalism. There are some brief allusions to Marino as 'little Oedipus', the 'dominant role' of his mother in his life, and the strange coincidence between his first homosexual experience and the death of his father. Such possible psychological explanations, however, are thoroughly discredited by the description of the trial in which the psychiatric report on Marino is exposed as an empty form of courtroom folklore. Marino is pressured to come up with a convincing story because the jury wants 'a visible and comprehensible soul [*geest*], a coherent object in an universe governed by psychological gravity and time'. In a rather Foucauldian twist the urge for a psycho-sexual explanation thus appears as a strategy of disciplinary power to humanize delinquency and give the defence lawyers something to work with. Even one of the psychiatrists himself does not seem to believe in his profession: 'I do not take psychology that serious. Nobody takes it that seriously anymore.'[68]

While the psyche thus appears as a rather unconvincing conception of sub-

67 Yves Petry, *De maagd Marino*, Amsterdam 2011, pp. 222, 62, 199, 91.
68 Petry, De maagd Marino (see n. 67), pp. 34, 21, 160, 144.

jectivity and medium of storytelling, the spirit [*geest*] and the brain form an unlikely alliance as figures of personhood and human identity. In bringing them together, Petry manages to combine two diametrically opposed positions in the recent Dutch public debate on issues of subjectivity and consciousness, namely the brainhood ideology of scientists like Dick Swaab and a spiritualist position represented by, among others, cardiologist Piet van Lommel in his 2007 popular science book *Eindeloos bewustzijn* [*Endless Consciousness*]. In this publication van Lommel questions the 'biological basis' of consciousness and tries to make plausible that consciousness is *not* a product of the brain but present *outside* of human beings and animals as well. Citing the principles of quantum mechanics and accounts of near-death experiences of patients worldwide, van Lommel argues that the brain is merely a sort of receiver terminal for the 'non-local' wave functions that form consciousness as a supra-individual phenomenon: 'Our brain can be compared to a television set that receives information from electromagnetic fields and decodes them into images and sounds and with a TV camera that encodes images and sounds in electromagnetic waves'. Not surprisingly, Dick Swaab has criticized van Lommel's attempt to move beyond a 'purely materialistic'[69] point of view in consciousness research as a form of 'spiritual' and 'anti-scientific' obscurantism, arguing that the various paranormal states of mind van Lommel discusses in support of his theory can very well be explained in terms of brain physiology.[70]

In *De maagd Marino*, Petry paradoxically combines a cerebral and a spiritual view of consciousness and subjectivity in his very own brand of spiritual materialism. Whereas Bruno Klaus' outlook on human life can be roughly identified with a humanist perspective (i. e. '*geest*', as in *geesteswetenschappen* or humanities), Marino's mother stands for spiritual experiences in a religious sense (she is a devotee of a Christian sect called *Spiritus Semper*) and Marino, the computer technician, for a scientific and materialist view of human existence. These various perspectives are constantly mixed up, in a figurative as well as in a literal sense. The desired cannibalistic act, for instance, can be seen as a 'perverse Eucharist'[71] that stands in a long religious and literary tradition of the mystical union between body and spirit. Marino Mund's experience of his position in the world, in turn, is described as a mystical experience as well: lying in his garden on a sunny Pentecost afternoon, Marino experiences a moving cosmic harmony between the frantic activity of the molecules of his body and the slow rhythms of

69 Pim Van Lommel, *Eindeloos bewustzijn: een wetenschappelijke visie op de bijna-dood ervaring*, Kampen 2008, pp. 16, 24, 25.

70 Swaab, Brein (see n. 3), pp. 361–368, here p. 367.

71 Johan Goud, 'Spirituality and Eroticism: Corpus Mysticum in Contemporary Dutch Literature', in: *Present-Day Spiritualities: Contrasts and Overlaps*, Elisabeth Hense, Frans Jaspers and Peter Nissen (eds.), Leiden 2014, pp. 141–162, here pp. 148–149.

the celestial bodies in the universe. Significantly, this experience then is described in terms of brainhood:

> Who knows, maybe he owed this special feeling simply to some minor epileptic attacks in his temporal lobes. [...] Every mental state is a brain state, our most sober thoughts no less than our mystical flashes.

The strange position in which the deceased narrator finds himself – as an 'electromagnetic oscillation' in Marino's brain – adds yet another twist to the complex entanglement of brain and spirit in the novel. In a curious similarity to van Lommel's wave function theory of consciousness, the talk about 'electromagnetic waves' here facilitates the notion that 'death is not the end' and that the spirit can move on to a new home; remarkably, Bruno Klaus himself also mentions that all empirical evidence provided by neuroscience will not withhold him from conceiving of himself as 'an independent spirit floating above his body'.[72] At the same time, the biological and molecular materiality of this spirit seems crucially important for the novel as well, in particular in light of the assertion that 'every mental state is a brain state' and nothing else. *De maagd Marino* thus produces a strange hybrid of neurology and spiritualism that forms the narrator of the text: a cerebral subject without a body and without a brain.[73]

6 Concluding Remarks

The three novels under scrutiny are not exclusively focused on the cerebral subject or employ it as their sole anthropological figure – and it would be difficult to find *any* literary text that does this. Nevertheless, in all three works by Welagen, van Rooij, and Petry the notion of brainhood – the idea that human beings essentially *are* their brains – is 'consubstantial to the narrative'[74] in the sense that it influences and shapes the poetics and narrative form of the texts. In *Porta Romana*, the protagonist's cerebral lesion frustrates the search for a hidden meaning of the trauma and the expectation of narrative closure; in *De eerste hond in de ruimte*, a neurological syndrome turns into an ambivalent allegory of social pathology and critique; in *De maagd Marino*, the curious figure of a cerebral subject without a brain determines the narrative perspective of the novel as a whole. Reading them as elements of contemporary neuroculture thus

72 Petry, De maagd Marino (see n. 67), pp. 77, 222.

73 Anthropologist Nicolas Langnitz has recently described similar forms of 'mystic materialism' in current reconfigurations of psychedelic culture and brain research in Nicolas Langnitz, *Neuropsychedelia: The Revival of Hallucinogen Research since the Decade of the Brain*, Berkeley, Los Angeles and London, 2013, pp. 204–242.

74 Ortega and Vidal, Brain in Literature (see n. 26), p. 328.

not only makes it possible to detect unexpected connections between these texts but to see how brainhood, here, indeed functions as a stimulant for 'new forms of formal experimentation'[75] and stylistic innovation reminiscent of the earlier liaison of the genre of the novel with the fields of psychology and psychoanalysis.

But what does this mean for the alleged discursive hegemony of the cerebral subject in contemporary neuroculture and the role of literature in its dissemination? As pointed out in the beginning, I do not believe it is possible or convincing to distinguish between the aesthetic and the discursive dimension of literary texts: both are part of an *investment* in specific forms of knowledge – and a divestment from others – that makes these knowledges valuable, relevant, and interesting even if they are ridiculed or contradicted. The more general conclusion to be drawn from my readings is therefore not that the neurological fictions by Welagen, van Rooij, and Petry subvert rather than support the figure of the cerebral subject; instead, I suggest seeing them as examples of a general pattern in the cultural circulation of brainhood that Ortega and Vidal mention as well. Rather than leading to a general neuro-reductionism, as Marco Roth seems to fear, the dissemination of the cerebral subject necessarily leads to its dissolution, contamination and mixing with other conceptions of personhood. In the novels under scrutiny we therefore see a blending of cerebral subjects with neurochemical selves, psychological accounts of subjectivity, and spiritual and religious notions of personhood.

At the same time, the investments in the cerebral subject in these three novels prove to dissolve rather than to reinforce a strict boundary between the normal and the pathological in neurological terms. In *De eerste hond in de ruimte*, one of the ravers raises the question of whether the 'normal' perception of reality is any more reliable or authentic than one influenced by chemical stimulants,[76] while in *Porta Romana*, the question remains undecided whether the protagonist's recurrent bouts of paranoia are merely a fabrication of his brain or not. Finally, in *De maagd Marino*, there seems to be no essential difference between mental states caused by epilepsy and 'normal' brain functions, and no reliable possibility to distinguish between them. The fascination with the brain as a medium of storytelling does not have to, but can thus result in an ontological insecurity about what the pathological even is.

75 GENNERO, Larger Than Our Biologies (see n. 31), p. 311.

76 Micha argues that since it is so easy to enter an 'artificial world' by taking pills 'the real world may not be that solid' itself after all. VAN ROOIJ, De eerste hond in de ruimte (see n. 52), p. 71. This notion is supported by the fact that in the storyworld of the novel even 'normal' reality seems to be a fabrication by the daymakers.

List of Illustrations

Cover illustration

Olga van Marion, Lovesickness on Stage: Besotted Patients in 17th-Century Medical Handbooks and Plays

Helmer Helmers, Illness as Metaphor: The Sick Body Politic and Its Cures

Notes on the Contributors

Sander Bax (1977) is Assistant Professor in Literary Studies, Cultural History and Didactics of Dutch Language and Literature at the Department of Culture Studies of Tilburg University. In 2013 he published 'The Nobel Prize and the European Dream. Harry Mulisch's European authorship from a national and an international perspective' in *Journal of Dutch Literature* and in 2015 he published his Dutch monograph on Harry Mulisch, entitled *De Mulisch Mythe* (The Mulisch Myth, 2015).

Stephan Besser (1971) is Assistant Professor of Modern Dutch Literature at the University of Amsterdam and program director of the Netherlands Research School for Literary Studies (OSL). His research focuses on the poetics of knowledge of contemporary neuroculture and the relations of literature, culture and science in general. He is the author of *Pathographie der Tropen: Literatur, Medizin und Kolonialismus around 1900* (2013) on the medical constructions of the tropics in German colonial culture.

Gerard Bouwmeester (1983) is a PhD candidate and research policy advisor at the Faculty of Humanities at the University of Utrecht. His current research interests include the production and reception of medieval miscellaneous manuscripts, especially those containing vernacular short verse narratives. His forthcoming dissertation discusses the (medieval and modern) reception of texts written by the Middle Dutch itinerant storyteller Augustijnken; earlier case studies were published by *Queeste* and the *Journal of the Early Book Society.*

Jaap Grave (1964) was Lecturer for Dutch Literature in Leipzig and Berlin and for Dutch Studies in Nagasaki. Now he teaches Modern Dutch Literature at the Westfälische Wilhelms-Universität in Münster. His research focuses on Dutch Literature in a European context, in particular Multatuli, Transfer, Postcolonialism, and on the History of (International) Dutch Studies.

Joost Haan (1956) works as a neurologist at Leiden University Medical Center and the Alrijne Hospital Leiderdorp. He received his medical degree in 1982, his speciality certificate in Neurology in 1988 and his PhD on 'Hereditary amyloidosis' in 1990. His research is on the genetics of headache and stroke. He (co-) authored many peer-reviewed publications and several books, mainly on clinical genetics. He also published several books on Neurology and Literature, eg. *Migraine als Muze* (2009) and *De Trillende Tuinman en andere Parkinsonbeelden* (2009). His current (PhD) research focuses on *Diagnosis and Literature.*

Helmer Helmers (1977) is Lecturer in Early Modern Dutch Literature and NWO Veni Research Fellow at the University of Amsterdam. He has published widely on Anglo-Dutch cultural and literary exchange in the seventeenth century. His monograph *The Royalist Republic* (2015) discusses Dutch publicity on the English Civil Wars and regicide. He is currently working on a project on the development of Dutch news culture during the Thirty Years' War.

Rick Honings (1984) is Assistant Professor in Dutch Studies at Leiden University. He is specialized in nineteenth-century Dutch literature. In 2011 he published his PhD dissertation *Geleerdheids zetel, Hollands roem! Het literaire leven in Leiden 1760–1860.* With Peter van Zonneveld he published a biography of the Dutch poet Willem Bilderdijk: *De gefnuikte arend* (2013). Currently he is working on his NWO Veni-project *The Poet as Pop Star. Literary Celebrity in the Netherlands 1780–1900.*

Steven Honings (1990) received his medical degree in 2015. During his medical training he did internships on several psychiatric wards and conducted research on the link between personality traits and the risk of Alzheimer's Disease. Currently he is working at Maastricht University on his PhD-thesis on the association between psychotic experiences, suicide and aggression. In 2016 he will start his residency in psychiatry at the Maastricht University Medical Center.

Mary Kemperink (1951) is Full Professor of Modern Dutch Literature at the University of Groningen. She is specialized in the literature and the culture of the fin de siècle of the nineteenth century. Her research focuses more in particular on the mutual relationship between literature and science, see a number of articles and her last book from 2011: *Gedeelde kennis. Literatuur en wetenschap in Nederland van Darwin tot Einstein (1860–1920).* Currently she works on a book on homosexuality.

Frans-Willem Korsten (1959) holds the chair 'Literature and Society' at the Erasmus School of History, Culture and Communication and is Associate Professor in the department of Film and Literary Studies at Leiden University. He published *Lessen in Literatuur* (3rd imprint 2009), *Sovereignty as Inviolability* (2009) and co-edited *Joost van den Vondel. Dutch Playwright in the Golden Age* (2012). In recent years he published on the relation between capitalism and art, and literature and law.

Arnold Lubbers (1981) was post-doc researcher at the University of Amsterdam. In 2014 he defended his PhD dissertation on Dutch book clubs in the early nineteenth century. He had various contributions on that topic published, such as in the forthcoming *Plotting the Reading Experience* and *Texts-Forms-Readings in Europe.* In 2014 he received the James Ollé Award from the Library and Information History Group. He is currently working as policy officer at the Humanities Division of the Netherlands Organisation for Scientific Research (NWO).

Olga van Marion (1961) is Lecturer in Early Modern Dutch Literature at Leiden University, where she has recently finished her NWO Veni Research Project on the creative conceptions and representations of 'the medieval' in early modern plays. She has published widely on intertextual relationships between mythology (Ovid), lifes of saints and literature, on female authorship and underground literature. Her current research focusses on the literary heritage of Leiden and the circulation of theatre in Europe.

Liesbeth Minnaard (1974) is Assistant Professor in Literary Studies at Leiden University. Her research focuses on interculturality in literature and on cultural effects of migration, particularly in Germany and the Netherlands. She is the author of *New Germans, New Dutch. Literary Interventions* (2008) and co-editor of *Literature, Language and Multiculturalism in Scandinavia and the Low Countries* (2013, with Wolfgang Behschnitt and Sarah De Mul) and of *Challenging the Myth of Monolingualism* (2014, with Till Dembeck).

Bettina Noak (1968) is scientific assistant at the Free University of Berlin. She has published mainly on history of Dutch literature of early modern times and on Dutch-German knowledge transfer. At present she is working on a DFG-research project on the topic 'medical case histories in Dutch literature of the seventeenth century'. Recent publications are: Bettina Noak (ed.), *Wissenstransfer und Auctoritas in der frühneuzeitlichen niederländischsprachigen Literatur,* Göttingen 2014 and B. Noak, 'Samen und Worte – sprachliche und natürliche Zeugung bei Johan van Beverwijck und Jacob Cats', in: Lydia Bauer/Antje Wittstock (eds.), *Text-Körper. Anfänge – Spuren – Überschreitungen,* Berlin 2014, 35–57.

Wouter Schrover (1985) teaches modern Dutch literature at VU University Amsterdam, where he recently defended his PhD-thesis on the representation of euthanasia and assisted suicide in contemporary narrative fiction (2015). His main research interests are in literature and medicine, thanatology, and the theory of fictionality. Recent publications include a book chapter in *Death in Literature* (2014) and an article about the fiction/non-fiction distinction in *Tijdschrift voor Nederlandse Taal- en Letterkunde* (2014, 3).

Ronny Spaans (1976) studied Dutch and German language and literature and Comparative Literature at the University of Oslo. He obtained his PhD in 2015 on the thesis *Godenbloed te koop. Exotica, extase en verboden kennis in de poëzie van Joannes Six van Chandelier (1620–1695).* He has received a scholarship from the Norwegian Non-fiction Writers And Translators Association and is currently working on a book about the cultural history of drugs. He has published articles on both Dutch and Norwegian writers.

Mark G. van Vledder (1984) obtained his medical doctor (MD) degree in 2009 from the Erasmus University in Rotterdam. Several years of clinical and experimental research at the Johns Hopkins Hospital (Baltimore, US) and the Erasmus Medical Center (Rotterdam) resulted in his thesis '*Liver Surgery; Imaging and Image Guided therapies*', for which he received his PhD in 2012. He is currently working as a surgical trainee in the IJsselland Hospital (Capelle a/d IJssel).

Hans de Waardt (1952) is Assistant Professor in early modern, viz. cultural history at VU University in Amsterdam. Two recent publications are 'Justus Velsius Haganus: An Erudite but Rambling Prophet', in: Jesse Sponholz and Gary K. Waite (ed.), *Exile and Religious Identity, 1500–1800* (2014, pp. 97–109) and 'Witchcraft and Wealth: the Case of the Netherlands', in: Brian. P. Levack (ed.), *The Oxford Handbook of Witchcraft in Early Modern Europe and Colonial America* (2013, pp. 232–248).